# Transforming Food Environments

# Transforming Food Environments

Edited by

Charlotte E.L. Evans
School of Food Science and Nutrition
University of Leeds
Leeds, United Kingdom

CRC Press
Taylor & Francis Group
Boca Raton London New York

CRC Press is an imprint of the
Taylor & Francis Group, an **informa** business

First edition published 2022
by CRC Press
6000 Broken Sound Parkway NW, Suite 300, Boca Raton, FL 33487-2742

and by CRC Press
2 Park Square, Milton Park, Abingdon, Oxon, OX14 4RN



CRC Press is an imprint of Taylor & Francis Group, LLC



*Library of Congress Cataloging-in-Publication Data*
Names: Evans, C. E. L. (Charlotte E. L.), editor.
Title: Transforming food environments / edited by Charlotte E.L. Evans.
Description: First edition. | London ; Boca Raton : CRC Press, 2022. |
Includes bibliographical references and index.
Identifiers: LCCN 2021044468 (print) | LCCN 2021044469 (ebook) |
ISBN 9780367489663 (hardback) | ISBN 9780367488604 (paperback) |
ISBN 9781003043720 (ebook)
Subjects: LCSH: Nutrition—Social aspects. | Diet. | Food supply. | Food
habits. | Food industry and trade. | Nutrition policy.
Classification: LCC TX357 .T65 2022 (print) | LCC TX357 (ebook) | DDC
641.3—dc23/eng/20211128
LC record available at https://lccn.loc.gov/2021044468
LC ebook record available at https://lccn.loc.gov/2021044469

ISBN: 9780367489663 (hbk)
ISBN: 9780367488604 (pbk)
ISBN: 9781003043720 (ebk)

DOI: 10.1201/9781003043720

Typeset in Times
by codeMantra

*To Zachary and Imogen, for your continual love and inspiration.*

# Contents

# Preface

I have always had an interest in food environments, whether it is the choice of foods served up in schools and hospitals, portion sizes of energy-dense foods or the cost of fruits and vegetables compared with more processed foods. We are well aware that we could eat a healthier diet; however, most of us think that we as individuals are responsible for improving our diets and the food environments around us don't play much of a role. I have never believed this to be the case, and now we have enough evidence to show how important food environments are when it comes to the foods and drinks we choose to eat. When I started out as a dietitian and nutritionist in 1990, I had never heard of the words 'food environment'. In health settings, changing what people eat was almost entirely aimed at changing individual motivation. I spent many hours as a dietitian and research dietitian in clinics supporting people to lose weight before a planned operation or with the aim of reducing blood pressure and cholesterol. It was a frustrating time as I was rarely successful at helping individuals change their diet substantially for prolonged periods of time. The view at that time was that the food environment could not be changed and we just had to live with it. Food environments were guided by market forces, and policy makers wouldn't mess with that. I felt we were often facing a losing battle as it was unfair to expect people to be able to resist large portions of easily accessible, cheap unhealthy food.

No one seemed to be interested in taking responsibility for this shared food environment although more action through environmental approaches was being taken to reduce tobacco use in the 1990s. I took a break to have my two children, which gave me plenty of time and opportunities to reflect on food offered in nurseries and schools. This included the need for age-appropriate portions of nutrient-dense foods in restaurants and cafes rather than food labelled as 'children's food' – almost universally fried foods and completely lacking in vegetables. It wasn't necessarily the same everywhere. Whilst visiting a café in Switzerland with my children aged 4 and 7 years I was surprised that when I ordered two milk shakes, they both got different and age-appropriate sized drinks – both smaller than an adult portion! This was the moment when I realised that the food environment is created by strong cultural beliefs, social norms and expectations but felt strongly that it was possible to change it if there was sufficient public support for change. In 2006 I had the opportunity to work with Professor Janet Cade at the University of Leeds on a project to improve children's packed lunches (lunches prepared at home and taken to school). This was the start of a determined effort to focus my research on food environments and environmental cues around us rather than on individual motivation, to improve the quality of our diets and ultimately our health.

Initially, it was tough to find like-minded individuals. The *Foresight report* published in 2007 with a complex road map of causal factors for obesity included the term 'physical activity environment' on the map but not the term 'food environment'. Instead the food environment consisted of a disparate group of causal factors that were not grouped together. Biological and psychological factors were given more prominence both in the *Foresight report* and government reports looking into research on behaviour change. Not only were there few policies in this area, but also there was less grant funding available to research this important aspect of public health nutrition. Public health bodies were primarily interested in weight management rather than prevention; almost certainly due to financial constraints. The food environment was not thought important as it was obvious that it was possible to choose healthy food because some people managed it successfully, so it must be the fault of individuals if they chose poorly. At a behaviour change conference, I asked a speaker "whose responsibility was it to improve the shared food environment?" but they clearly didn't understand my question. Continued discussion in the media has made it easier to have an opinion on this subject although it has always been more palatable to focus on children so that the rights of adults to freely choose are not challenged. The childhood obesity strategy was published, and although watered down by the new conservative government that came into power in 2010, it was a step forward and covered many aspects of food that aimed to reduce availability and accessibility of energy-dense food. In the UK, the Responsibility Deal was set up in 2011 where food companies were encouraged to reduce salt and trans-fats in a wide range of foods. Attitudes were starting to change, but it was still a difficult time to carry out research in this area. A grant I submitted to the National Institute of Health Research to improve the fast food environment was out of remit if it solely focussed on the environmental outcomes such as portion size or trans-fat content of meals and didn't include diet or health data collected on individuals. Undeterred, I worked on a budget with a fantastic team of PhD students evaluating and reviewing programmes in schools and communities to increase the consumption of fruits and vegetables and reduce sugary drinks as well as researching the fast food environment around schools.

Finally the food environment is now getting the attention it deserves. Interest in a range of food environments has grown enormously and is regularly discussed in the media. We are all stakeholders in our shared food environments and therefore we all have a legitimate view on this topic. Reformulation was the start and now thanks to Public Health England in the UK, this has moved on to reducing portion sizes and free sugars as described in the sugar and calorie reduction reports; and taxing sugary drinks. There is now a renewed focus on the out-of-home sector where portion sizes tend to be larger. The situation has also improved in terms of funding research in this area which has led to exciting discoveries of what works and what doesn't. Conferences on behaviour change are now balanced between researchers reporting on studies aimed at individuals and those taking an environmental approach.

There is still plenty to do. I recently visited a local café and chose a modestly sized doughnut (just right for a snack) only to be told it was a dog treat! In supermarkets, you can still see packets of sweets hanging like Christmas decorations every few feet along aisles selling rice and pasta. Moving forward, it is important that we hear many voices and views on how we could and should improve food environments. The most difficult issues to deal with are the inequalities in diet in the UK and in many other countries. Despite widespread recognition that the food we eat is important, healthy and sustainable foods continue to be less accessible to many parts of the population, especially those living in disadvantaged areas. Therefore, evaluation of all policies is an essential element of changing the food environment. If an action is more successful in households situated in wealthier areas, it is further widening inequalities and cannot be deemed successful. The key aim of reducing inequality is considered in every chapter in this book. Sustainability issues have also come to the fore and improvements in food environments must be kind to the planet as well as equitable.

At the heart of this book is a celebration of easily accessible, great tasting and nutritious food. Eating well should be easy for everyone, not a daily struggle, which is why I felt it important to bring these topics together in this book. This subject crosses many disciplines such as psychology, geography and economics, and I hope it will appeal to students and researchers in many different areas. The first part focusses on different types of environments such as schools and community centres, while the second part looks at different techniques that have been proven to have an impact on food choice. An important aspect of work into the food environment is evaluation, and we have included descriptions of many different ways that we can measure whether changes have been successful. It is my hope that this book will start conversations and give people the confidence to speak up when something isn't right. Do you want to be asked if you want a massive bar of chocolate when you are buying a newspaper or clothing? I hope you enjoy reading this book whether you are a student or researcher dipping into specific chapters, a lecturer thinking about including something on the food environment in your course, a policy maker trying to find out what works or just interested in this topic.

# Acknowledgements

Editing this book has been an incredible journey (and a learning curve!) and couldn't have happened without the help and support of many people along the way. Firstly, I want to thank Randy Brehm at Taylor & Francis. In July 2019 when I pitched my ideas to her and she said it was a really exciting project, I realised for the first time that this book could become a reality rather than just a plan inside my head. I want to thank Randy for helping me to get my ideas to the proposal stage and for the continual positive feedback. I would like to thank Julia Tanner from Taylor & Francis who patiently supported me through the process to submission as I edited my first book.

I want to thank all the authors (55 of you!) who consistently contributed high-quality chapters which has resulted in this book being such an interesting and informative read. It was wonderful working with all of you; some as colleagues at the University of Leeds, some of you who I have met at conferences and some of you who I haven't met in person but hope to do so in the future. Thank you also to all my colleagues at the University of Leeds, both those who contributed to chapters and also those who encouraged me from the side-lines, particularly Bernadette Moore and Janet Cade (who was also an author). Thank you to those who submitted photos, particularly. Steve Leather, who is credited with the picture on the cover of our son at age nine when I started my research into school food environments in 2006.

I also want to thank all my family and friends who supported me over the process and repeatedly listened to my ideas and progress; particularly my sister Susie Evans who read early drafts of the preface and table of contents and answered 'yes' when I asked her whether she thought it would be an interesting book to read; and Anke Taenzer who regularly asked how the book was progressing and always had soothing and encouraging words.

I want to further thank my long-suffering husband, Steve, who has tolerated me talking about wanting to write a book on the food environment for several years before actually submitting the proposal, as well as for his encouragement and unwavering belief in me. I am also eternally grateful for his skills in editing photos and figures throughout the book and listening to me reflecting on different chapters. He has admirably summarised the whole book in six pithy words – 'a bit of everything will help'!

# Editor

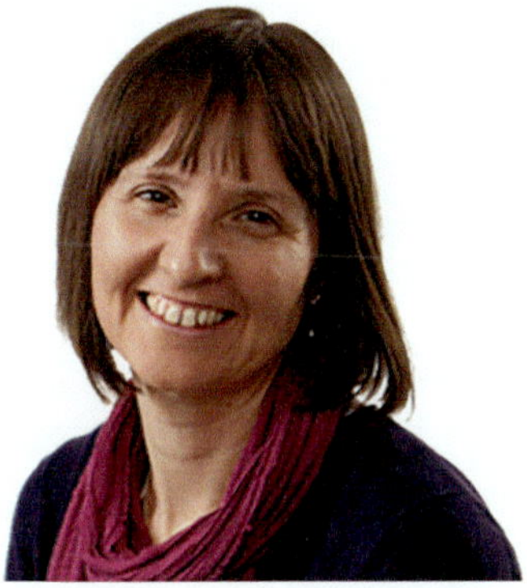

**Charlotte E.L. Evans** is an Associate Professor in Nutritional Epidemiology and Public Health Nutrition at the University of Leeds, UK, with more than 20 years of experience in researching dietary behaviour and food environments. She is dedicated to improving the quality of children's and adolescents' diets, particularly for those on the poorest diets. Her research focusses on making the healthier choice, the easier choice, with experience spanning a range of food environments including schools, hospitals, fast food and nutrition in the media. Another key area of her research is the evaluation of programmes and policies to improve diet quality such as increasing fruit and vegetable consumption and decreasing free sugars. She has more than 100 publications including papers, book chapters, a special issue on adolescent diet as well as conference abstracts. She has also presented her work internationally and has regularly featured on television and the radio communicating hers and others work on diet behaviour. In 2016, she was awarded the prestigious Elsie Widdowson Medal for contributions to Public Health Nutrition by the UK Nutrition Society.

# Contributors

**Katie Adolphus**
School of Psychology
University of Leeds
Leeds, United Kingdom

**Margaret A. Allman-Farinelli**
School of Life and Environmental Sciences
University of Sydney
Sydney, Australia

**Carolyn I. Auma**
School of Food Science and Nutrition
University of Leeds
Leeds, United Kingdom

**Nastasia Belc**
National Institute of Research & Development for Food Bioresources
IBA Bucharest
Bucharest, Romania

**Yael Benn**
Department of Psychology
Manchester Metropolitan University
Manchester, United Kingdom

**Emma J. Boyland**
Department of Psychology
University of Liverpool
Liverpool, United Kingdom

**Maria J. Bryant**
Department of Health Sciences and the Hull York Medical School
University of York
York, United Kingdom

**Janet E. Cade**
School of Food Science and Nutrition
University of Leeds
Leeds, United Kingdom

**Simon Capewell**
Department of Public Health, Policy and Systems
University of Liverpool
Liverpool, United Kingdom

**M. Susan Caswell**
School of Public Health and Health Systems
University of Waterloo
Ontario, Canada

**Christine L. Cleghorn**
Burden of Disease Epidemiology, Equity and Cost-Effectiveness Programme (BODE3)
University of Otago
Wellington, New Zealand

**Chloe Clifford Astbury**
Global Food Systems and Policy Research, School of Global Health
York University
Toronto, Canada

**David M. Dejoy**
College of Public Health
University of Georgia
Athens, GA

**Denisa E. Duţă**
National R&D Institute for Food Bioresources (IBA)
Bucharest, Romania

**Louise Dye**
School of Psychology
University of Leeds
Leeds, United Kingdom

**Cassandra H. Ellis**
Science and Programmes Director
Nutrition Society
London, United Kingdom

**Hannah Ensaff**
School of Food Science and Nutrition
University of Leeds
Leeds, United Kingdom

**Alison Fildes**
School of Psychology
University of Leeds
Leeds, United Kingdom

**Katherine Flynn**
Department of Food Sciences & Technology
ISEKI-Food Association
Vienna, Austria

**Grace Gardner**
Human Nutrition Research Centre
Population Health Sciences Institute
Newcastle University
Newcastle Upon Tyne, United Kingdom

**Marion M. Hetherington**
School of Psychology
University of Leeds
Leeds, United Kingdom

**Teodora-Alexandra Iordache (Manasia)**
National R&D Institute for Food Bioresources (IBA)
Bucharest, Romania

**Alice R. Kininmonth**
School of Psychology
University of Leeds
Leeds, United Kingdom

**Mariko Koide**
United Nations Relief and Works Agency for Palestine Refugees in the Near East
Amman, Jordan

**Naoki Kondo**
Department of Social Epidemiology and Global Health
Kyoto University
Kyoto, Japan

**Vivica I. Kraak**
Department of Human Nutrition, Foods and Exercise
Virginia Polytechnic Institute and State University
Blacksburg, VA

**Clare L. Lawton**
School of Psychology
University of Leeds
Leeds, United Kingdom

**Suzy L. Liddell**
The Trussell Trust
London, United Kingdom

**Ffion Lloyd-Williams**
Department of Public Health, Policy and Systems
University of Liverpool
Liverpool, United Kingdom

**Adam Martin**
School of Medicine
University of Leeds
Leeds, United Kingdom

**Rachel E. McCardel**
College of Public Health
University of Georgia
Athens, GA

**Atsushi Miyawaki**
Faculty & Graduate School of Medicine
The University of Tokyo
Tokyo, Japan

**Anja Mizdrak**
Department of Public Health
University of Otago
Wellington, New Zealand

**Pablo Monsivais**
Department of Nutrition and Exercise Physiology
Washington State University
Spokane, WA

**Sally G. Moore**
School of Food Science and Nutrition
University of Leeds
Leeds, United Kingdom

**Eleonora Morganti**
School of Food Science and Nutrition & Institute for Transport Studies
University of Leeds
Leeds, United Kingdom

**Patti-Jean Naylor**
School of Exercise Science, Physical and Health Education
University of Victoria
Victoria, Canada

**Dana L. Olstad**
Cumming School of Medicine
University of Calgary
Calgary, Canada

**Heather M. Padilla**
College of Public Health
University of Georgia
Athens, GA

**Emma Patterson**
Department of Global Public Health
Karolinska Institutet
Stockholm, Sweden

**Tarra L. Penney**
Global Food Systems and Policy Research, School of Global Health
York University
Toronto, Canada

**Carmen Piernas**
Nuffield Department of Primary Care Health Sciences
University of Oxford
Oxford, United Kingdom

**Madeleine S. Power**
Health Sciences
University of York
York, United Kingdom

**Christian J. Reynolds**
Centre for Food Policy
City, University of London
London, United Kingdom

**Holly L. Rippin**
School of Food science and Nutrition
University of Leeds
Leeds, United Kingdom

**Enid C. Roemer**
Institute for Health and Productivity Studies
Johns Hopkins Bloomberg School of Public Health
Baltimore, MD

**Catherine Rycroft**
School of Food Science and Nutrition
University of Leeds
Leeds, United Kingdom

**Suzanne Spence**
Human Nutrition Research Centre
Population Health Sciences Institute
Newcastle University
Newcastle Upon Tyne, United Kingdom

**Emma Strachan**
Food and Nutrition in Leeds
Leeds City Council
Leeds, United Kingdom

**Ayyoub K. Taher**
Food and Nutrition Program
Environment & Life Sciences Research Centre
Kuwait Institute for Scientific Research
Safat, Kuwait

**Emma Tomalin**
School of Philosophy, Religion and History of Science
University of Leeds
Leeds, United Kingdom

**Elisa J. Vargas-Garcia**
School of Food Science and Nutrition
Department of Health Sciences
Universidad Iberoamericana León
León, Mexico

**Christina Vogel**
MRC Lifecourse Epidemiology Unit
University of Southampton
Southampton, United Kingdom

**Jayne V. Woodside**
School of Medicine, Dentistry and Biomedical Sciences
Queen's University
Belfast, Northern Ireland

**Dorota Zarnowiecki**
College of Nursing and Health Sciences
Flinders University
Adelaide, Australia

# 1 Introduction to the Food Environment

*Charlotte E.L. Evans*
University of Leeds

**CONTENTS**



## 1.1 INTRODUCTION

A definition of healthy food environments:

> Environments in which the foods, beverages and meals that contribute to a population diet meeting national dietary guidelines are widely available, affordably priced and widely promoted.
>
> *(Swinburn et al., 2013).*

Take a moment to look around your immediate environment. What food is easily available to you? Are you more likely to grab whatever is easiest and closest to you or are you willing to walk further, pay more or wait longer for something else you really want to eat? These questions highlight some of the important factors in the food environment. Most people make food-related decisions based on habits and don't expect to spend much time and effort (referred to as agency) on choosing what to eat. We are therefore influenced by what we see and experience, whether it is an advert for a certain food, the availability or the cost of certain foods or cultural beliefs. The main aim of this book is to provide you with substantial evidence that improving our food environment is crucial to our health and well-being.

Although first documented in the 1980s, it is only in the last 10 years that wider interest in the food environment has spread amongst nutritional scientists,

DOI: 10.1201/9781003043720-1

public health policy makers and stakeholders involved in manufacturing, selling and providing food. This chapter provides information on diet and health and the role of the food environment as well as how to make the most of this book.

## 1.2 RELATIONSHIPS BETWEEN DIET AND HEALTH

Evidence from across the globe provides strong and consistent evidence that poor diet leads to higher rates of morbidity and premature death from non-communicable diseases (NCDs) such as cardiovascular disease and some cancers (World health Organization [WHO], 2014). This is true in low-, middle and high-income countries (Lachat et al., 2013). In a large global review of the burden of many diseases, low intakes of fruits, vegetables and wholegrain and high intakes of salt, sugars and fats were identified as the most important factors for good health in the world along with tobacco and alcohol (Lim et al., 2012). It has been estimated that up to 40% of premature NCD deaths could be avoided with a high-quality diet; and poor diet generates more deaths and Disability Adjusted Life Years (DALYs) than tobacco (≈19%), alcohol (≈9%) and physical inactivity (≈2%) combined (Steel et al., 2018).

Obesity is a risk factor for cardiovascular disease as well as some cancers (Riaz et al., 2018) and rates continue to increase in many countries. Overweight and obesity affect 59% of adults in the European region (WHO, 2020) and over 67% of adult males and 60% of adult females in the UK. Furthermore, childhood obesity increases risk of obesity (Ward et al., 2017) and high blood pressure (Umer et al., 2017) in adulthood, and thus reducing childhood obesity has become a major focus of government policy in many countries. In England, obesity now affects over 10% of children starting school (4–5 year olds), and over 20% by the end of primary school (10–11 year olds) (NHS Digital, 2020) and rates are higher for children in poorer households. The recent COVID-19 pandemic highlighted that obesity increased hospital and death rates in people infected with severe respiratory disease (Bornstein et al., 2020), further highlighting the importance of improving health.

An additional diet-related health outcome of particular concern in children includes severe dental decay which reflects high and frequent intakes of dietary sugars and is a common cause of hospital admissions in young children in the UK, particularly children living in low-income households (Public Health England (PHE), 2019). There are high costs associated with these different burdens of disease as a result of consuming poor-quality diets, which add to the costs of our already overburdened health systems and which could be avoided.

The World Health Organization (WHO) defines healthy diets as diets based on nutrient-rich foods, including vegetables, fruits, whole grains, pulses (beans), nuts and seeds, with limited intake of energy-dense foods high in fats (particularly trans and saturated fats), free sugars and salt (WHO, 2014). These foods are also known as discretionary or non-core foods. Many countries have recommendations in place, for example in the UK there is *The Eatwell Guide* (PHE, 2016) shown in Figure 1.1 and in the US the American Heart Association (AHA) has diet and lifestyle recommendations (American Heart Association (AHA), 2017).

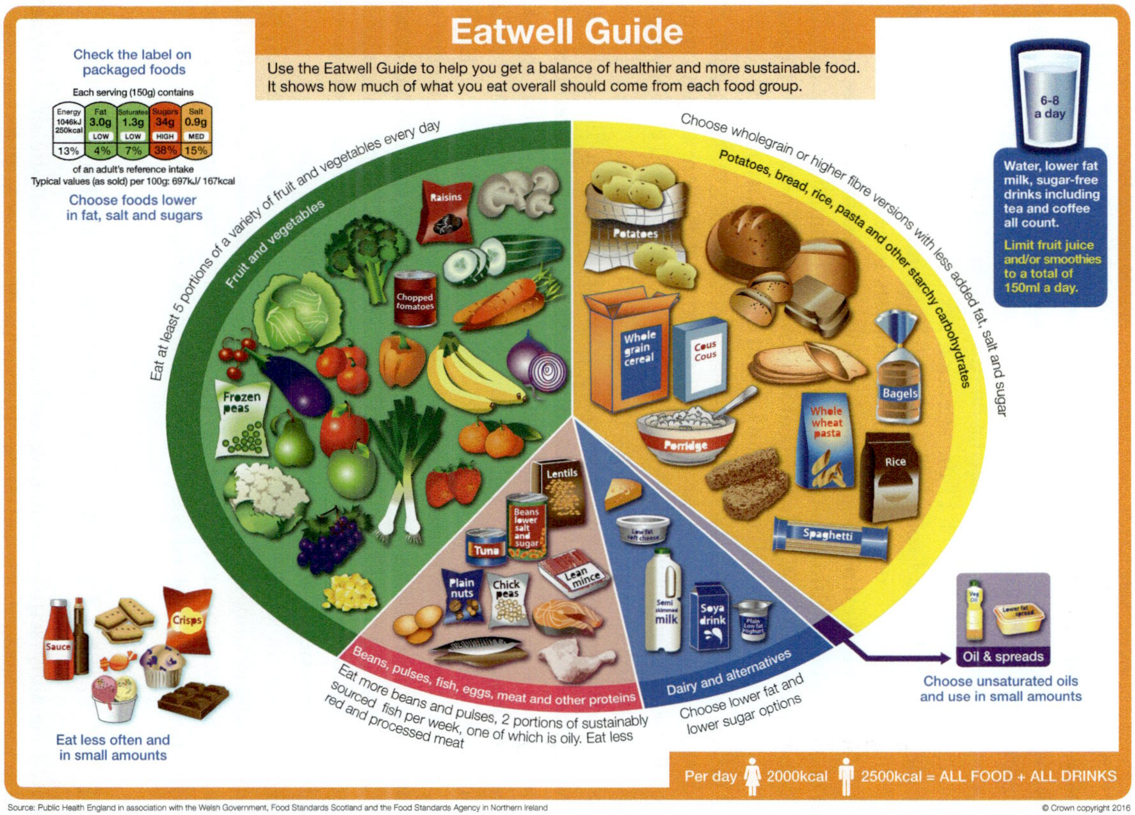


**FIGURE 1.1** *The Eatwell Guide* is sourced from Public Health England in association with the Welsh government, Food Standards Scotland and the Food Standards Agency in Northern Ireland. It is reprinted under the open government licence under crown copyright. (Available from https://www.gov.uk/government/publications/the-eatwell-guide.)

## 1.3 CHANGING DIETARY BEHAVIOUR

Although we might know that eating fruits and vegetables are good for us, that doesn't mean that we eat enough of them; highlighting more than education is needed. Many populations in the world do not currently consume a healthy diet despite the consistent advice and promotion from WHO and other health organisations. In Europe, average intakes of fruits and vegetables in 22 of the 28 EU Member States are currently below the daily 400 g, recommended by WHO (EPHA, 2016) while the average consumption of meat and dairy products remains above recommended levels (EHN, 2017). Although the 5-a-day recommendation to eat five portions of fruit and vegetables per day was introduced in the UK in 2003, nearly 20 years later only about a quarter of the UK population meets the recommendation (Castiglione, 2019).

For the last few decades, much of the attention has been on individuals improving their diets which has had some success, mainly in managing existing obesity or type 2 diabetes but less so in prevention. Economists believe that most of us are time inconsistent, in that even though we plan to consume less in the future or make healthier choices, when the time comes we choose not to (Institute for Fiscal Studies, 2010). On a global scale, huge technological improvements, economic development and globalisation have taken place. In many countries, particularly more recently in low- and middle-income countries, the traditional diet of staple grains, legumes and fruits and vegetables has changed to a dietary pattern that is more reliant on processed foods, foods from outside the home, animal products, refined carbohydrates, edible oils and sugar-sweetened beverages (Popkin, 2015).

There are additional issues related to equity with inequalities in diet and health increasing in many high-income countries. In the UK, intake of fruits and vegetables is only half of the national average in lower-income communities. There are stark inequalities in obesity. In Europe, 20% of adults with a lower education level are obese compared with 12% of those with a higher education (OECD, 2019). In English children, rates of obesity are twice as high for children living in the most deprived areas than in the most affluent areas (PHE, 2020). Worse still, this gap has consistently widened since 2006 in England. The exposure to unhealthy food environments by young people is of particular concern as their health will be disproportionately affected if they experience poor diet over a longer period of their lives.

Despite poor diet choices being potentially avoidable, there are many barriers preventing us making healthy food choices. Different approaches need to be taken and improving the food environment is one method of tackling this complex issue. How research in this area has evolved is described in the next section.

## 1.4 DEVELOPMENT OF FOOD ENVIRONMENT RESEARCH

The WHO's 'healthy settings' initiative embraced a more holistic or ecosystem approach to health promotion based on the 'Health for all' report in 1980, and defined a 'setting' as the place or social context in which people engage in daily activities in which environmental, organisational, and personal factors interact to affect health and well-being (WHO 2021). This holistic or ecosystem approach to health promotion increased in popularity after the 'move towards a new public health' outlined in the Ottawa Charter of 1986, following the first International Conference on Health Promotion (Anonymous, 1986). It stated that 'Health is created and lived by people within the settings of their everyday life; where they learn, work, play, and love'. As Porter wrote in 2007, 'Ottawa steered health promotion away from dominant health education models of individual behaviour change towards a 'socio-ecological' version of health promotion that addresses structural determinants of health' (Porter, 2007). However, due to the polarisation of views on health promotion with systems-based views on the one side and education on the other (Green, 1988), this more holistic ethos has taken time to become universally embedded in public health systems in many countries, particularly where food choice is concerned.

In the UK, a large mapping exercise was carried out to look at the different domains that have an impact on obesity, including diet and physical activity. It quickly became evident that food was influenced by a huge number of interlocking factors (Foresight, 2007). Some of the main domains in the *Foresight Report* included the physical environment, food consumption and individual psychology but, interestingly, not the food environment. Further progress on defining the food environment as a key policy area was made in 2008 when Story et al. (2008) visually represented the key factors that impact on food choice including individual and social networks and physical and macro environments depicted in Figure 1.2. The latter two levels are the main topics covered in this book. Physical environments include places such as school, work and retail environments and macro environments include national policies such as taxes on sugary drinks and reformulation by the food industry.

Swinburn et al. (2013) further refined more precisely what we mean by the food environment. Their socio-ecological (rather than individual) approach gave further credence to the importance of food environments on health which can be defined as 'The collective physical, economic, policy and sociocultural surroundings, opportunities and conditions that influence people's food and beverage choices and nutritional status' (Swinburn et al., 2013). The authors identify food access as key and this has five dimensions: availability, proximity, affordability, acceptability and accommodation (Swinburn et al., 2013). Their framework was adapted from the original by Story and includes four levels (see Figure 1.3) (Kraak et al., 2014).

Interventions at the different levels can include a range of approaches such as provision of information or changing the price. An attempt to rank the intensity of different approaches and interventions was carried out by the Nuffield Council on Bioethics (2007). This ladder of interventions (Figure 1.4) starts at the lowest rung with monitoring the situation and increases in intervention strength to a total ban. It considers the strength of the scientific evidence available on dietary components and health and justification for action that takes into account the acceptability or popularity of public health policies. The rungs of the ladder form the basis of methods covered in this book.

## 1.5 LAYOUT OF THE BOOK

This book is separated into two main parts. The first part includes 11 chapters and covers different places that we regularly inhabit where food is sold or served. It also includes the media environment and how nutritional information is presented to us in

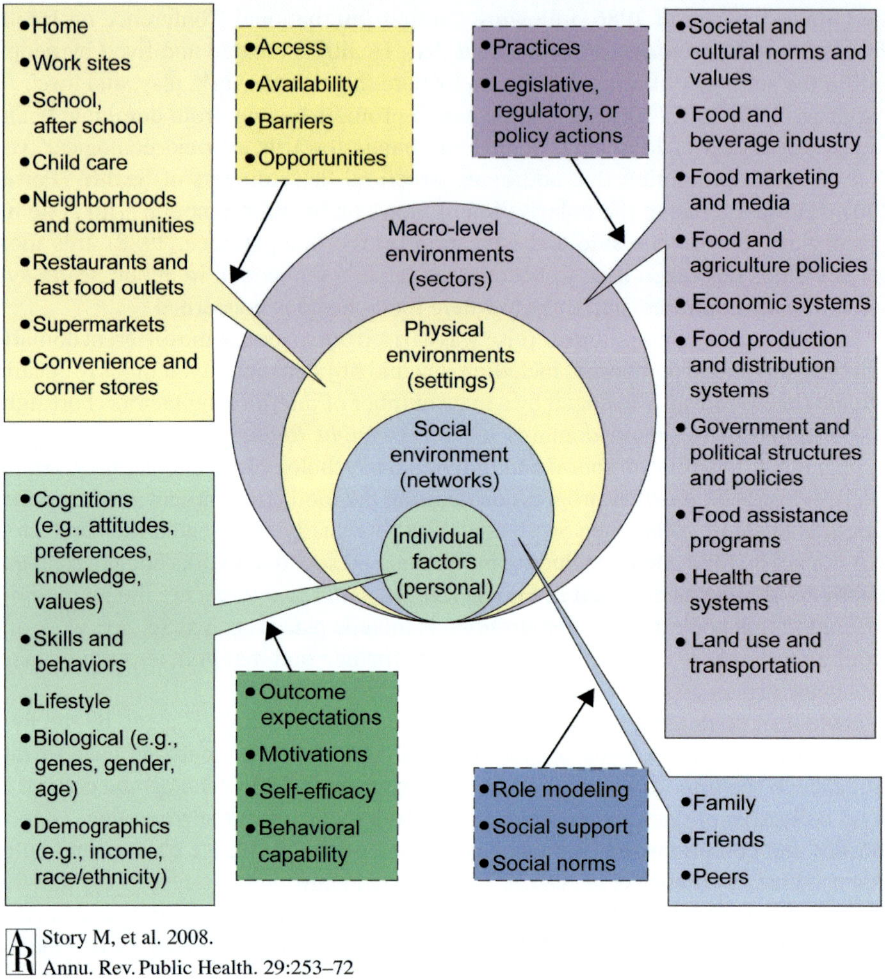


**FIGURE 1.2** Ecological framework for influencers of eating behaviour. (Reproduced with permission from Story et al. 2008. Creating healthy food and eating environments: policy and environmental approaches. *Annu Rev Public Health*, 29, 253–272. https://www.annualreviews.org/doi/abs/10.1146/annurev.publhealth.29.020907.090926.)

newspapers as well as in social media. The second part of this book includes information on different types of actions that can be employed to improve food environments. It is based on the ladder of interventions (see Figure 1.4) and describes a variety of approaches such as labelling and marketing, portion sizes, nudging and price.

### 1.5.1 Places

The majority of food-related spending decisions are made in supermarkets. Most of this food is taken home to consume; therefore, the home and food retail environments are key aspects of this section. However, there are other important places where

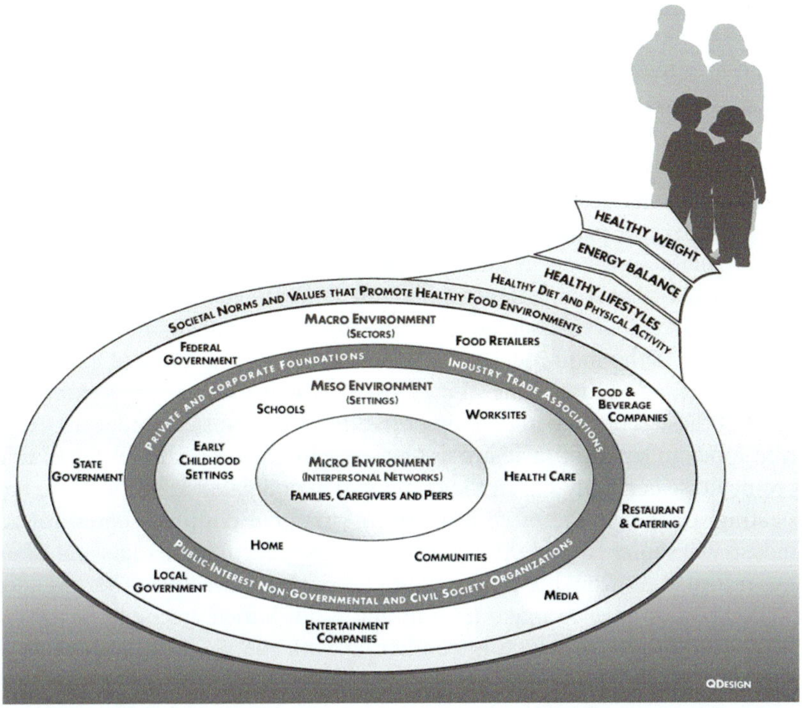


**FIGURE 1.3** Socio-ecological model of the food environment. (Reproduced with permission from Kraak et al. 2014. An accountability framework to promote healthy food environments. *Public Health Nutrition*, 17(11), 2467–2483. Available from doi:10.1017/S1368980014000093.)

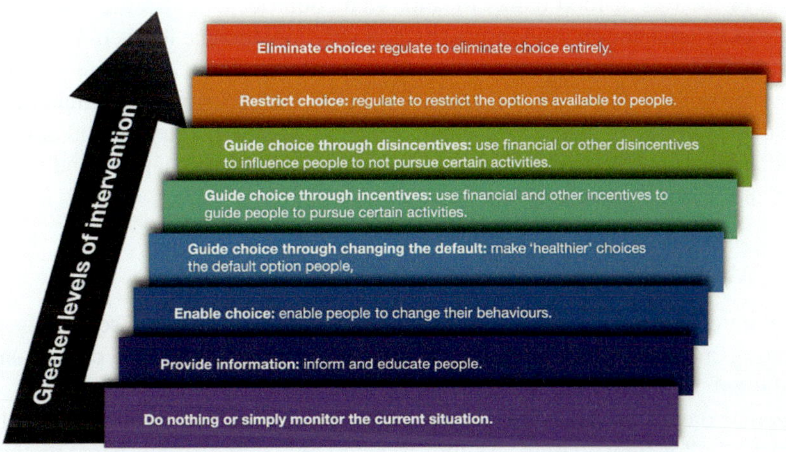


**FIGURE 1.4** Ladder of interventions by the Nuffield Council on Bioethics 2007. (Reproduced under licence CC BY 4.0 from Walls (2015). Available from https://blogs.biomedcentral.com/bmcseriesblog/2015/04/10/solving-obesity-crisis-knowledge-nudge-nanny/.)

we regularly consume meals including schools and work places. Much attention has been focussed on improving food served at schools and ensuring that children eat well while at school. The fact that virtually all children attend school means that this is one of the simplest ways to reach the vast majority of children. Furthermore, improving the food environment and restricting food choice for children has been less controversial than in adults. Community and religious spaces as well as out-of-home restaurants and cafes are also covered.

One of the largest players having an impact on what we eat is the food industry. Food manufacturers are a little behind the scenes and we don't connect with them directly but what companies manufacture determines the choice of food sold in food outlets. There are two chapters covering this topic as there are competing arguments. The role of the food industry is to provide us with a range of safe, palatable and affordable foods and bearing in mind that 80% of foods are processed in some way, most of these foods are not coming directly from farms or producers. However, preferred foods in terms of taste are not necessarily the optimal diet for us to eat in terms of health – certainly not in the combination and balance of foods we are currently eating. Chapter 6 therefore provides information on the essential role of the food industry in supporting healthy choices such as reducing trans-fats and Chapter 7 provides information from the public health nutrition perspective. There is a tension as food companies need to make a profit and foods which are more processed are generally more profitable which is conflicting with the need to promote healthier diets high in less processed foods such as fruits, vegetables and wholegrain products.

An important issue raised throughout this book is equity, and in this context equal access to affordable, healthy and palatable food. Inequalities in diet and health are considered in every chapter. Implemented policies can potentially make the situation worse if they are more successful for those on healthier diets. The situation is particularly difficult for those living with food insecurity in the UK and in many other countries where food insecurity is a daily anxiety for many households. This is discussed in terms of the rise of food banks in some rich countries and also the situation more globally in the chapter on food insecurity and very low-income food environments.

Finally, there are some places that influence our behaviour that are perhaps not usually considered to be places at all. These include nutrition information in the news such as in newspapers or on social media as well as marketing and advertising of food. These virtual environments are also covered in two chapters and bring this section of the book to a close.

### 1.5.2 Methods

Food is an enjoyable part of all of our lives. We therefore need strong reasons for advocating moderation of consumption (either through frequency, portion size or formulation) of foods people love to eat. If the evidence base for beneficial effects of a particular dietary behaviour is weak and/or unpopular, the first step of the ladder is to just monitor the situation. As the evidence builds and strengthens, methods of intervening may also increase, starting with providing information to help people make food-based decisions. This book includes chapters on providing information but particularly providing information at a point when food choices are made such as food package labelling; also categorised as enabling choice. Public health nutritionists are not the only stakeholders developing and designing information related to food; it is also provided by food manufacturers and this type of information is covered in the food marketing chapter. There are also chapters that encompass guiding choice, covered in the chapter on nudging. Nudging includes ways to make the healthier choice the easiest choice such as changing default options or the way foods are presented. Optimising portion sizes provide another way to guide healthy choices; by increasing the availability of smaller portions of energy-dense foods and drinks, the new smaller medium size is considered the new normal. Later in this section is a discussion about the impact of increasing and decreasing price through taxes and subsidies. There are now many countries that have a tax or levy on sugary drinks but do we also need to subsidise the cost of fruit and vegetables to encourage purchasing and consumption?

Over the next two decades there will undoubtedly be more attention paid to the sustainability of our food systems and we discuss what sustainable diets look like with less meat and dairy and more plant-based foods. Novel methods for evaluating the improvements in food environments are discussed, such as interrupted time series analysis originally used by economists but now becoming a popular analysis method for nutritionists. How we can create better food environments as part of a larger system is becoming increasingly important and the systems chapter identifies ways that policy makers can tackle multiple challenges related to equity, sustainability and health at the same time. We finish with a chapter where we focus on future research needed in this area.

## 1.6 CONCLUSIONS

Public health nutritionists and policy makers increasingly agree that a healthy food environment is an important component of improving food choice and in turn healthy populations. Although definitions vary of exactly what is included in food environments, particularly when it is considered within a broader food system with agricultural factors, it is generally agreed that it includes a holistic approach with support at the family, community and national level. Progress has been made in the last decade; however, more action is needed before we can consider our food environment to be healthy. This book brings together the existing evidence base related to a wide range of different environments including physical spaces as well as nutrition-related information and offers solutions that can be used to further improve our access, affordability and equity to healthy food.

## ACKNOWLEDGEMENTS

Thank you to Simon Capewell, Nastasia Belc and Emma Tomalin for their useful references. Thank you to Amelia Lake for reading earlier versions of the manuscript and providing valuable feedback.

## REFERENCES

American Heart Association. 2017. Diet and Lifestyle Recommendations. Available from: https://www.heart.org/en/healthy-living/healthy-eating/eat-smart/nutrition-basics/aha-diet-and-lifestyle-recommendations.

Anonymous 1986. Ottawa charter for health promotion. *Can J Public Health,* 77, 425–430.

Bornstein, S. R., Rubino, F., Khunti, K., Mingrone, G., Hopkins, D., Birkenfeld, A. L., Boehm, B., Amiel, S., Holt, R. I., Skyler, J. S., Devries, J. H., Renard, E., Eckel, R. H., Zimmet, P., Alberti, K. G., Vidal, J., Geloneze, B., Chan, J. C., Ji, L. & Ludwig, B. 2020. Practical recommendations for the management of diabetes in patients with COVID-19. *Lancet Diabetes Endocrinol*, 8, 546–550.

Castiglione, C., & Mazzocchi, M. 2019. Ten years of five-a-day policy in the UK: Nutritional outcomes and environmental effects. *Ecol Econ*, 157, 185–194.

EHN. 2017. Transforming European Food and Drink Policies for Cardiovascular Health. Available from: https://ehnheart.org/publications-and-papers/publications/1093:transforming-european-food-and-drinks-policies-for-cardiovascular-health.html.

EPHA. 2016. Report 1: "A CAP for Healthy Living". Available from: https://epha.org/report-a-cap-for-healthy-living/.

Foresight. 2007. *Trends and Drivers of Obesity* [Online]. Available from: http://www.foresight.gov.uk/OurWork/ActiveProjects/Obesity/KeyInfo/Index.asp.

Green, L. W. & Raeburn, J.M. 1988. Health promotion. What is it? What will it become? *Health Promotion*, 3, 151–159.

Institute for Fiscal Studies 2010. *Dimensions of Tax Design: The Mirrlees Review,* Oxford, Oxford University Press.

Kraak, V. I., Swinburn, B., Lawrence, M. & Harrison, P. 2014. An accountability framework to promote healthy food environments. *Public Health Nutr*, 17, 2467–83.

Lachat, C., Otchere, S., Roberfroid, D., Abdulai, A., Seret, F. M., Milesevic, J., Xuereb, G., Candeias, V. & Kolsteren, P. 2013. Diet and physical activity for the prevention of non-communicable diseases in low- and middle-income countries: A systematic policy review. *PLoS Med*, 10, e1001465.

Lim, S. S., Vos, T., Flaxman, A. D., Danaei, G., Shibuya, K., Adair-Rohani, H., Amann, M., Anderson, H. R., Andrews, K. G., Aryee, M., Atkinson, C., Bacchus, L. J., Bahalim, A. N., Balakrishnan, K., Balmes, J., Barker-Collo, S., Baxter, A., Bell, M. L., Blore, J. D., Blyth, F., Bonner, C., Borges, G., Bourne, R., Boussinesq, M., Brauer, M., Brooks, P., Bruce, N. G., Brunekreef, B., Bryan-Hancock, C., Bucello, C., Buchbinder, R., Bull, F., Burnett, R. T., Byers, T. E., Calabria, B., Carapetis, J., Carnahan, E., Chafe, Z., Charlson, F., Chen, H., Chen, J. S., Cheng, A. T.-A., Child, J. C., Cohen, A., Colson, K. E., Cowie, B. C., Darby, S., Darling, S., Davis, A., Degenhardt, L., Dentener, F., Des Jarlais, D. C., Devries, K., Dherani, M., Ding, E. L., Dorsey, E. R., Driscoll, T., Edmond, K., Ali, S. E., Engell, R. E., Erwin, P. J., Fahimi, S., Falder, G., Farzadfar, F., Ferrari, A., Finucane, M. M., Flaxman, S., Fowkes, F. G. R., Freedman, G., Freeman, M. K., Gakidou, E., Ghosh, S., Giovannucci, E., Gmel, G., Graham, K., Grainger, R., Grant, B., Gunnell, D., Gutierrez, H. R., Hall, W., Hoek, H. W., Hogan, A., Hosgood, H. D., Hoy, D., Hu, H., Hubbell, B. J., Hutchings, S. J., Ibeanusi, S. E., Jacklyn, G. L., Jasrasaria, R., Jonas, J. B., Kan, H., Kanis, J. A., Kassebaum, N., Kawakami, N., Khang, Y.-H., Khatibzadeh, S., Khoo, J.-P., KOK, C., Laden, F., et al. 2012. A comparative risk assessment of burden of disease and injury attributable to 67 risk factors and risk factor clusters in 21 regions: A systematic analysis for the Global Burden of Disease Study 2010. *The Lancet*, 380, 2224–2260.

NHS Digital. 2020. National Child Measurement Programme, England 2019/20 School Year. Available from: https://digital.nhs.uk/data-and-information/publications/statistical/national-child-measurement-programme/2019-20-school-year.

Nuffield Council on Bioethics. 2007. *The Intervention Ladder* [Online]. Available from: http://nuffieldbioethics.org/report/public-health-2/policy-process-practice/.

OECD. 2019. *Health at a Glance 2019*, Paris, OECD Publishing.

Popkin, B. M. 2015. Nutrition transition and the global diabetes epidemic. *Curr Diab Rep*, 15, 64.

Porter, C. 2007. Ottawa to Bangkok: Changing health promotion discourse. *Health Promot Int*, 22, 72–79.

Public Health England 2016. The Eatwell Guide. Available from: https://www.gov.uk/government/publications/the-eatwell-guide.

Public Health England. 2019. Child Oral Health: Applying All Our Health. Available from: https://www.gov.uk/government/publications/child-oral-health-applying-all-our-health.

Public Health England. 2020. Statistics on Obesity, Physical Activity and Diet, England - 2020 [NS]. Available from: https://digital.nhs.uk/data-and-information/publications/statistical/statistics-on-obesity-physical-activity-and-diet/england-2020.

Riaz, H., Khan, M. S., Siddiqi, T. J., Usman, M. S., Shah, N., Goyal, A., Khan, S. S., Mookadam, F., Krasuski, R. A. & Ahmed, H. 2018. Association between obesity and cardiovascular outcomes: A systematic review and meta-analysis of Mendelian randomization studies. *JAMA Netw Open*, 1, e183788.

Steel, N., Ford, J. A., Newton, J. N., Davis, A. C. J., Vos, T., Naghavi, M., Glenn, S., Hughes, A., Dalton, A. M., Stockton, D., Humphreys, C., Dallat, M., Schmidt, J., FLOWERS, J., Fox, S., Abubakar, I., Aldridge, R. W., Baker, A., Brayne, C., Brugha, T., Capewell, S., Car, J., Cooper, C., Ezzati, M., Fitzpatrick, J., Greaves, F., Hay, R., Hay, S., Kee, F., Larson, H. J., Lyons, R. A., Majeed, A., McKee, M., Rawaf, S., Rutter, H., Saxena, S., Sheikh, A., Smeeth, L., Viner, R. M., Vollset, S. E., Williams, H. C., Wolfe, C., Woolf, A. & Murray, C. J. L. 2018. Changes in health in the countries of the UK and 150 English local authority areas 1990–2016: A systematic analysis for the Global Burden of Disease Study 2016. *Lancet*, 392, 1647–1661.

Story, M., Kaphingst, K. M., Robinson-O'Brien, R. & Glanz, K. 2008. Creating healthy food and eating environments: Policy and environmental approaches. *Annu Rev Public Health*, 29, 253–72.

Swinburn, B., Sacks, G., Vandevijvere, S., Kumanyika, S., Lobstein, T., Neal, B., Barquera, S., Friel, S., Hawkes, C., Kelly, B., L'Abbe, M., Lee, A., Ma, J., Macmullan, J., Mohan, S., Monteiro, C., Rayner, M., Sanders, D., Snowdon, W., Walker, C. & Informas 2013. INFORMAS (International Network for Food and Obesity/Non-Communicable Diseases Research, Monitoring and Action Support): Overview and key principles. *Obes Rev*, 14 Suppl 1, 1–12.

Umer, A., Kelley, G. A., Cottrell, L. E., Giacobbi, P., Jr, Innes, K. E. & Lilly, C. L. 2017. Childhood obesity and adult cardiovascular disease risk factors: A systematic review with meta-analysis. *BMC Public Health*, 17, 683.

Walls, H. 2015. Solving the Obesity Crisis: Knowledge, Nudge or Nanny? Available from: https://blogs.biomedcentral.com/bmcseriesblog/2015/04/10/solving-obesity-crisis-knowledge-nudge-nanny/.

Ward, Z. J., Long, M. W., Resch, S. C., Giles, C. M., Cradock, A. L. & Gortmaker, S. L. 2017. Simulation of growth trajectories of childhood obesity into adulthood. *N Engl J Med*, 377, 2145–2153.

World Health Organization. 2014. Global Action Plan for the Prevention and Control of NCDs 2013–2020. Available from: https://www.who.int/publications/i/item/9789241506236.

World Health Organization. 2020. European Health Information Gateway: Overweight. Available from: https://gateway.euro.who.int/en/indicators/h2020_6-overweight/.

World Health Organization. 2021. Health Promotion: Healthy Settings. Available from: https://www.who.int/teams/health-promotion/enhanced-wellbeing/healthy-settings.

# 2 The Home Food Environment

*Alice R. Kininmonth and Alison Fildes*
University of Leeds

## CONTENTS



## 2.1 INTRODUCTION TO THE HOME FOOD ENVIRONMENT

As research into the aetiology of obesity has evolved beyond individual-level determinants to explore environmental influences, the home food environment has become a point of focus. In younger children in particular, the home setting is considered crucial for shaping diets, eating behaviours, and ultimately weight status. Children spend a significant amount of their early life at home and much of their food intake (around 70% for children aged 2–11) is consumed through meals and snacks eaten at home (Chai and Nepper, 2015). Unlike adolescents and adults, young children are entirely dependent on caregivers for their food and experience fewer social and cultural interactions beyond the family. The home is also where children first learn eating-related behaviours, by observing and mirroring those around them (Savage et al., 2007). These dietary behaviours developed during childhood have been shown to track into early adulthood (Bjelland et al., 2013), thereby enduring long after children gain autonomy and leave this environment. Consequently, this chapter reflects the majority of research in this area to date, by focussing on the home food environment as it relates to children (<12 years). It is important to recognise that the home environment does not exist in isolation, rather it is influenced by a range of societal, cultural, political, and economic factors. These aspects and how they relate to childhood diet are depicted in Figure 2.1.

DOI: 10.1201/9781003043720-2 

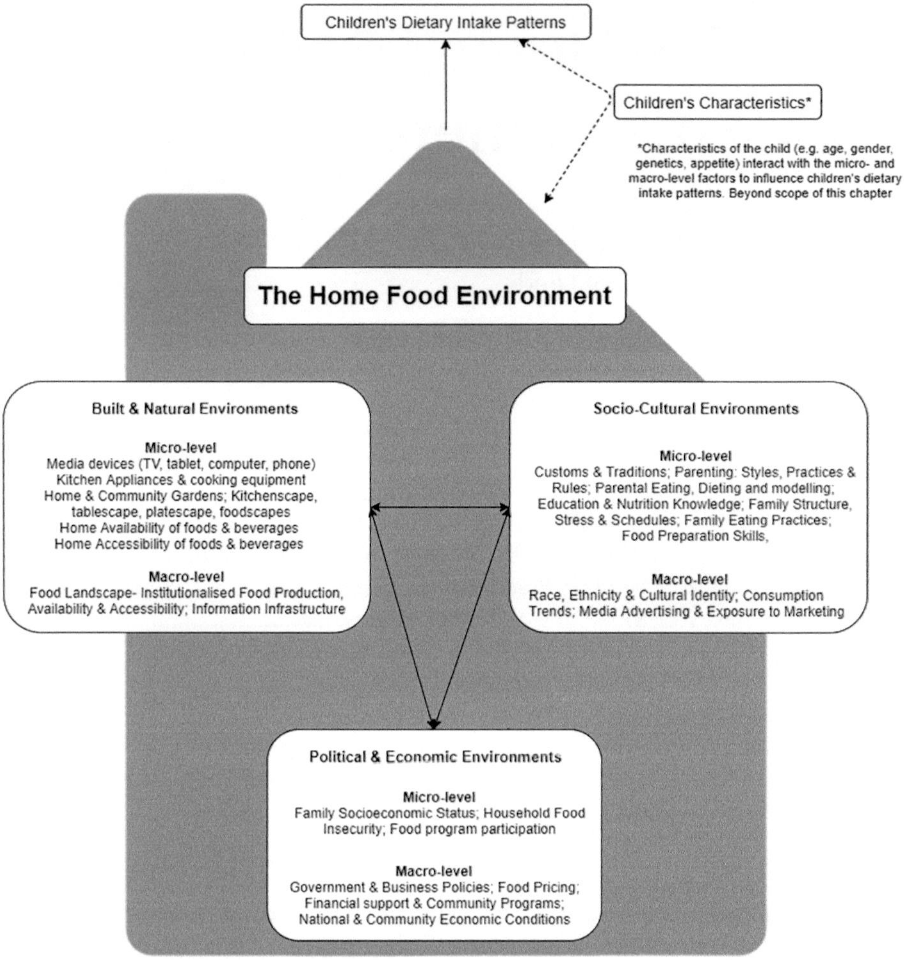


**FIGURE 2.1** Model of the home food environment related to children's dietary intake. The model comprises micro-level (defined as proximal to child's home) and macro-level (exist at community level but have potential to influence a child's home) factors. (Reprinted with permission from Rosenkranz and Dzewaltowski, "Model of the home food environment pertaining to childhood obesity," *Nutrition Reviews* 66, no 3 (2008): 123–140.)

### 2.1.1 Defining the Home Food Environment

The home food environment is multifaceted and complex. Despite the wealth of research in this area, there is little consensus about how to define and measure it. Figure 2.2 provides an overview of key aspects examined to date. Caregivers are fundamental in shaping both the physical and social aspects of the home food environment deemed important for children's health and development. In terms of the physical food environment,

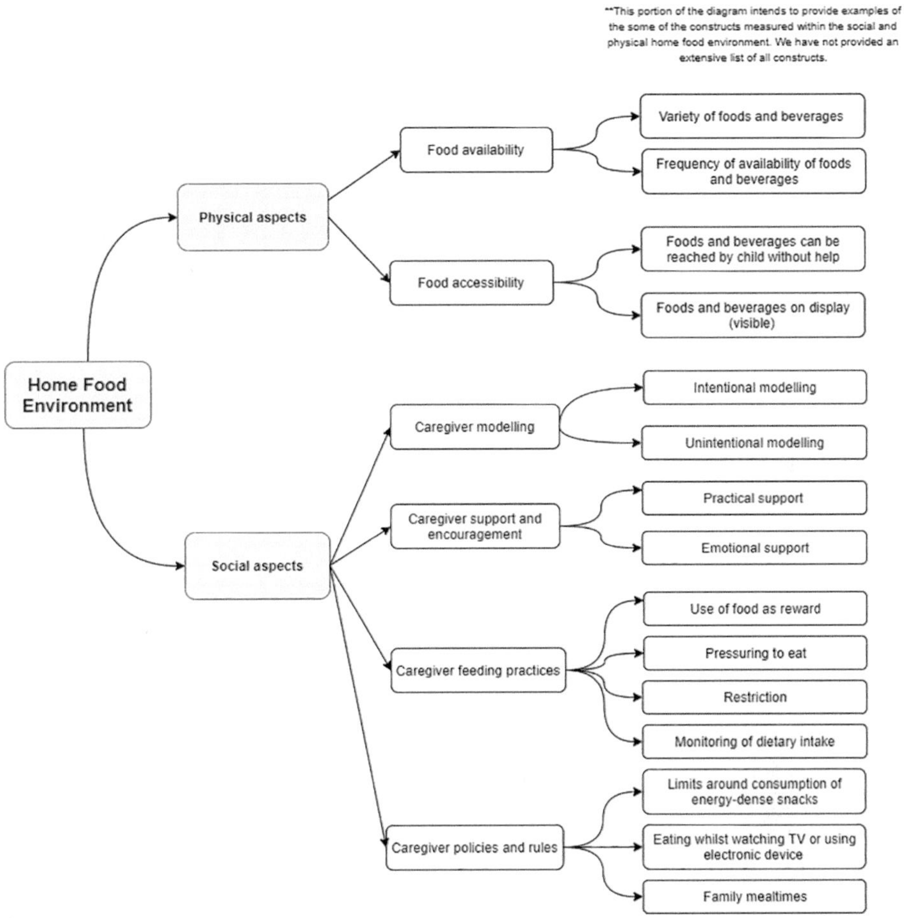


**FIGURE 2.2** Overview of the key aspects within the home food environment split into physical and social aspects, with the final boxes intended to provide some examples (e.g. types of caregiver policies and rules). We have not provided all types captured within each aspect, simply examples.

caregivers act as nutritional gatekeepers for the household, largely controlling (a) the types of foods and beverages available, (b) the quantity of foods and beverages present, and (c) the types and quantities of foods and beverages offered at mealtimes (Savage, 2008). From a social perspective, caregivers act as role models of eating practices and food intake, while also setting rules and structures around food within the home.

### 2.1.2 Measuring the Home Food Environment

Measures of the home food environment can be divided into those that endeavour to capture either physical or social aspects, or both (see Table 2.1). Physical aspects

**TABLE 2.1**
**Methods Commonly Used to Assess the Home Food Environment, Based on Physical and Social Aspects**

| What Is Measured? | Type of Measure | Advantages | Disadvantages | Examples of Validated Tools |
|---|---|---|---|---|
| **Physical factors: availability and accessibility of foods and beverages in the home** | Parent-report inventories or checklist | Relatively low cost and easy to administer on large scale and at multiple time points | Open inventories are time-consuming to complete – high participant burden may result in reduced response rate or incomplete data<br>Potential for self-report biases e.g. social desirability | HOME Inventory Describing Eating & Activity (Boles et al., 2019) |
| | Parent-report questionnaires | Relatively low cost and easy to administer on large scale and at multiple time points | Potential for self-report biases e.g. social desirability | Comprehensive Home Environment Survey (Pinard et al., 2014) |
| | Parent-report telephone interview | Opportunity for interviewer to prompt, probe, or seek clarification to gain information<br>Able to conduct at multiple time points | Labour-intensive and costly to administer<br>Potential for self-report biases e.g. social desirability | Home Environment Interview (Schrempft et al., 2015) |
| | In-home observation | Objective measure, information gained via direct observation by researcher.<br>Social desirability bias reduced (but not eliminated) | Very labour-intensive and costly to administer<br>High participant burden, invasive, and time-consuming to conduct | Observation method (Terry and Beck, 1985) |

*(Continued)*

**TABLE 2.1 (*Continued*)**
**Methods Commonly Used to Assess the Home Food Environment, Based on Physical and Social Aspects**

| What Is Measured? | Type of Measure | Advantages | Disadvantages | Examples of Validated Tools |
|---|---|---|---|---|
| **Social aspects: caregiver feeding practices, caregiver modelling and support, caregiver rules and policies** | Parent-report questionnaires | Relatively low cost and easy to administer on large scale<br>Range of standardized, validated, psychometric measures available | Potential for self-report biases e.g. social desirability | Household Food Rules Scale (Bailey-Davis et al., 2017), Comprehensive Feeding Practices Questionnaire (CFPQ; Musher-Eizenman and Holub, 2007) |
| | Parent-report telephone interview | Relatively low cost and easy to administer on large scale | Labour-intensive and costly to administer<br>Potential for self-report biases e.g. social desirability | Home Environment Interview (Schrempft et al., 2015) |
| | Behavioural observation of parent–child interactions during mealtime | Objective measure, information gained via direct observation by researcher | Labour-intensive and costly – requires specialised equipment and trained researcher to code behaviour<br>Some designs have limited ecological validity<br>High participant burden, invasive, and time-consuming to conduct<br>Potential for unnatural behaviours and social desirability bias resulting from observation | Family Mealtime Coding Scale (Blissett et al., 2016) |

within the home food environment include the **availability**[1] and **accessibility**[2] of foods and beverages. Availability is commonly measured by assessing the frequency with which foods and beverages are present in the home (i.e. "How often do you have fruit in the home?") and the amount or variety of these (i.e. "What types of fresh fruits do you have in the home?") (Schrempft et al., 2015). Accessibility is assessed in terms of the physical location or visibility of foods and beverages in the home (i.e. "Without opening any fridge or cupboard doors, is there any kind of confectionery in your home now displayed out in the open?") and the extent to which available foods are pre-prepared or ready to eat (i.e. "Do you have any ready to eat fresh vegetables on a shelf in the fridge or on the kitchen counter now?") (Schrempft et al., 2015). Researchers take a variety of approaches when measuring food availability and accessibility, including caregiver-reported checklists, questionnaires, or telephone interviews. While some measures are comprehensive, using multiple items to capture a wide range of foods and beverages, others use fewer items and simply focus on one food group (e.g. energy-dense foods). This variation emerges from the need to balance the richness of data against the participant burden generated by these types of studies. Longer, more comprehensive measures are time- and resource-intensive, impacting participants' willingness to respond. These measures, like many in the area of children's diets, rely on caregiver report and can be affected by social desirability biases. Caregivers might choose responses that suggest a "healthier" home food environment, because they are aware of what might be perceived as the "desirable" answer. This is arguably even more problematic when the researcher asks participants direct questions, using interview-style methodologies, than when participants complete digital or paper-based questionnaires. In contrast, observational methods, whereby the researcher visits a participant's home and visually inspects the kitchen and food storage areas, have the advantage of greater objectivity. However, such methods are labour-intensive, costly, intrusive and potentially burdensome for the participant. Another key limitation across all methodologies is that existing studies tend to collect data at a single time point. This fails to capture fluctuations in the types and/or amount of foods and beverages available in the home over extended periods, or due to seasonal changes or special occasions.

Social aspects of the home food environment include **caregiver feeding practices**, **caregiver modelling**, **caregiver support**, and **caregiver policies and rules around food** in the home. Caregiver feeding practices (also called parent feeding practices) have received the most attention in the literature and encompass specific goal-oriented behaviours, not exclusively restricted to the home setting. They comprise caregiver feeding behaviours used to influence what, when, and how much a child eats, including constructs such as (i) pressure to eat (e.g. "My child has to finish his/her plate"), (ii) use of food as reward (e.g. "I reward my child with something to

---

[1] Availability is defined as the variety and amount of foods and beverages available and the frequency with which they are available.

[2] Accessibility is defined in terms of the visibility of the food (i.e. can be seen, out in the open), whether it needs to be prepared or is ready to consume (e.g. peeled, sliced, ready-to-eat vegetables) and/or the physical location of the food (i.e. can be accessed by child, without assistance).

eat when s/he is well behaved"), (iii) restriction of food (e.g. "I have to be sure that my child does not eat too many sweets"), and (iv) emotional feeding[3] (e.g. "I give my child something to eat to make him/her feel better when he/she has been hurt"). Over the past decade, there has been a rapid increase in the development of tools designed to measure caregiver feeding practices. This has resulted in inconsistent definitions of constructs and terminology being used interchangeably (e.g. feeding styles, parenting styles, feeding behaviours, feeding practices[4]), despite having different meanings (Vaughn et al., 2013).

Caregiver modelling, like caregiver feeding practices, is not restricted to the home setting. Caregiver modelling is a mechanism by which children learn what to eat and what not to eat by observing the behaviours of their caregivers. As such, caregivers may model eating behaviours intentionally (i.e. consciously eating certain foods in front of their child) or unintentionally (i.e. a child simply observing their caregivers' natural eating behaviour). Modelling has been measured in a variety of ways, ranging from asking caregivers to report their own dietary intake (Yee et al., 2017) to asking about the intentionality of behaviours exhibited (e.g. "I model healthy eating for my child by eating healthy foods myself") (Musher-Eizenman and Holub, 2007). Simply measuring caregivers' dietary intakes is problematic as it fails to capture a key feature of the modelling process – whether the behaviour is actually observed by the child.

Like modelling, caregiver support is key in facilitating behaviour, especially amongst infants and young children. Caregiver support can be separated into two forms: (i) **practical support** (e.g. "A variety of healthy foods are made available to my child at each meal served at home") and (ii) **emotional support** (e.g. "I encourage my child to eat a variety of foods?"(Musher-Eizenman and Holub, 2007)). Support, particularly emotional support, is a subjective concept and therefore difficult to measure accurately. In contrast, caregiver policies and rules around foods and beverages in the home are more specific and easier to conceptualise. Again, measures used to capture these vary in their scope but they most commonly examine caregiver rules and limit setting in relation to food (e.g. "No snacking while watching TV/DVDs") and family mealtimes (e.g. "Must eat dinner with family") (Lytle et al., 2011). Measurement of social aspects of the home food environment most commonly rely on caregiver report, as naturalistic observation of these constructs is challenging. As with caregiver-reported measures of the physical home food environment, participants may be aware of "desirable" parenting behaviours and practices, meaning measures are potentially subject to social desirability bias.

---

[3] Otherwise known as using food to control negative emotions (i.e. when a child is upset, angry, hurt, or bored).

[4] Feeding styles capture the overall emotional climate of meals and are measured along two dimensions: responsiveness (warmth and involvement during feeding) and demandingness (parental control and supervision of feeding). Feeding behaviours can be categorised into four feeding styles: authoritarian, authoritative, indulgent, and uninvolved, characterising parents' responsiveness to the child and boundary setting during feeding interactions (Wood et al., 2020).

## 2.2 ROLE OF HOME FOOD AVAILABILITY AND ACCESSIBILITY IN CHILDREN'S DIETS

Observational and experimental studies have consistently demonstrated that the types of foods and beverages present in the home are important correlates of children's dietary intakes (Boles et al., 2019). This is unsurprising, as foods need to be both available and accessible for a child to consume them. Evidence is most consistent for fruits and vegetables, with availability identified as the strongest predictor of consumption, even among individuals with lower preference for these foods (Campbell and Crawford, 2001). Research also suggests that availability of fruits and vegetables in the home may shape children's liking for them. Repeated exposure has been consistently shown to positively influence food preferences (Cooke, 2007). Familiarity is a key determinant of a child's liking for a particular food, and liking is strongly predictive of intake in other words, children "like what they know and eat what they like" (Cooke, 2007). Various experimental and observational studies have demonstrated similar associations between availability and intake for energy-dense snack foods, dairy products, fruit juice, and sugar-sweetened beverages (Chai and Nepper, 2015). These findings have been reported in children of disparate ages and backgrounds, including rural, low-income, culturally, and ethnically diverse families (Boles et al., 2019).

Beyond availability in the home, experimental and observational research has shown that children's consumption of certain food groups increases further when those foods are accessible. For children with lower preference for fruits and vegetables, increasing the visibility of these foods within the home by placing them in easy-to-reach locations and in forms that encourage consumption (e.g. pre-prepared, ready to eat) may be particularly important for encouraging intake (Chai and Nepper, 2015). Similar findings have been observed for foods and beverages high in fat, sugar, and salt. Greater availability of, and access to, energy-dense foods has been associated with higher consumption of these foods and lower consumption of fruits and vegetables (Pearson et al., 2017). Taken together, these findings suggest making simple environmental modifications within the home, such as putting fruits and vegetables in an easy-to-reach location (e.g. a fruit bowl on the kitchen counter) and making energy-dense snack foods harder to obtain (e.g. on the top shelf, inside a cupboard), could help to improve the quality of children's diets. However, the majority of research in this field is cross-sectional which means we cannot be sure about the direction of these associations or determine true causality. Limited data from clinical trials suggest that modifications to the home food environment are associated with improvements in dietary intake (Fletcher et al., 2013). Yet, more longitudinal and experimental research is required to establish whether availability and accessibility of foods and beverages in the home causally influence children's food preferences and dietary intake. Or whether children's preferences shape their home food environment, with caregivers providing the foods and beverages their children most enjoy. In reality, the relationships between home availability and children's intakes are likely bidirectional.

## 2.3 THE ROLE OF THE SOCIAL HOME FOOD ENVIRONMENT ON CHILDREN'S DIET

Alongside providing the physical home food environment, caregivers help shape the social home food environment. Experimental and observational studies have shown that caregiver behaviours, such as caregiver feeding practices, modelling, and support, are strong predictors of children's food intake (Yee et al., 2017).

### 2.3.1 Caregiver Feeding Practices

Increasing concern about child obesity means caregiver feeding practices have received substantial attention as potential determinants of children's eating behaviours, i.e. the what, when, and how much of children's diets. Although certain practices are likely a reflection of caregivers' well-intentioned attempts to improve their children's diets, observational research has suggested the use of certain non-responsive or controlling feeding practices (including restriction and pressure to eat) may disrupt a child's ability to self-regulate their appetite and negatively impact on diet quality. "Pressure to eat", when a parent urges their child to consume a food they don't want to eat, or a greater quantity of food than they wish to, has been linked with increased selective eating behaviours (Loth, 2016). It is hypothesised that stressful feeding encounters may negatively impact food preferences or impair a child's ability to self-regulate and respond to their internal sensations of fullness (Ventura and Birch, 2008). Similarly, openly restricting access to types of foods may cause a "forbidden fruit" effect, whereby the desirability of the restricted food increases, making the child more likely to seek it out and potentially overeat when they access it (Bauer et al., 2017). However, the majority of research into caregiver feeding practices within the home is cross-sectional and survey-based, making it extremely difficult to fully adjust for confounding influences such as socioeconomic status (SES) or cultural differences, or to tease apart causation.

It is important to highlight that parenting is in part reactionary; caregivers respond to, and are influenced by, their child's characteristics and behaviours. For example, caregivers may restrict types or amounts of food in response to their child's weight status or dietary preferences. Or, a caregiver may use more pressuring practices if their child expresses fussiness around food. Several sibling studies have found support for a child-responsive model of caregiver feeding, demonstrating caregivers vary their feeding practices for children who differ in their eating behaviours or weight status. Caregivers appear to use more pressure to eat with their fussier or lighter child, and more restriction with their food responsive or heavier child (Harris et al., 2016). The limited longitudinal research in this area also supports both directionality from child characteristics to parent's use of controlling feeding practices, as well as the reverse (Rodgers et al., 2013).

### 2.3.2 Caregiver Modelling and Support

Caregivers may also shape their children's eating through intentional and unintentional modelling of behaviours in the home. We know from existing research that simply observing a caregiver passively eating a particular food is not always enough to encourage a reluctant child to eat. Infants and children are more likely to try and accept new food, or eat more of a food, when it is presented in a positive social context and the model is enthusiastic (Savage et al., 2007). Positive modelling of "healthy eating" has been consistently associated with greater consumption of fruits and vegetables in preschool (2- to 6-year olds) and primary school (7- to 11-year olds) children (Yee et al., 2017). Less positively, higher intakes of energy-dense and high sugar foods have also been observed among children whose caregivers model eating these foods (Yee et al., 2017).

Like modelling, caregiver verbal support of "healthy eating" has been associated with higher preference for and consumption of fruits and vegetables, as well as lower liking and consumption of energy-dense foods (Vollmer and Baietto, 2017). However, research into caregiver modelling and support has again been largely cross-sectional and focussed predominantly on children from higher-income and less ethically diverse backgrounds, limiting generalisability to the most vulnerable populations.

### 2.3.3 Caregiver Policies and Rules

Mealtimes are a key social feature within the home and a major component of the home food environment. Family mealtime practices, in terms of both the types of foods offered and the rules enforced, have been linked with dietary intake and obesity risk in both caregivers and children (Berge et al., 2015). Eating meals together as a family has been associated with increased consumption of fruits and vegetables (Christian et al., 2013), but the setting may also be important. Family meals consumed in front of the TV have been found to contain fewer vegetables, grains, and calcium-rich foods, and more fried foods, than those eaten away from the TV (Avery et al., 2017). Eating in front of the TV has also been associated with increases in the amount of food consumed, as well as overall energy intake at meals (Temple et al., 2007). This has been in part attributed to TV acting as a distraction which shifts a child's attention away from eating, inhibiting awareness of food intake and internal satiety cues.

A recent review emphasised children, regardless of age group, who ate whilst watching TV had poorer quality diets, consuming more energy-dense foods, more sugar-sweetened beverages, and fewer fruits and vegetables (Avery et al., 2017). In addition, children who are exposed to food advertisements are more likely to either pester their caregivers to purchase energy-dense food products or to purchase energy-dense snack foods and beverages themselves (Boyland et al., 2018). Over the past decade, children's access to a wider range of electronic devices such as mobiles, tablets, laptops, and games consoles have risen dramatically (Ofcom, 2019). Such devices are now a common feature in the home and are often present when food is eaten, whether children eat alone or with their family. Research into the home food environment is yet to catch up with the range of evolving technologies available in the home setting. But it is clear that the presence of technology acts as a distraction, potentially inhibiting awareness of food intake, internal satiety cues, and positive feeding interactions (e.g. caregiver modelling and support). More screen-time and poorer diet quality have been found to co-occur in families. Experimental research has suggested that caregiver behaviours, such as enforcing rules and limit setting around media use, may help to uncouple these behaviours and encourage healthier eating habits in children (Rutherford et al., 2015), whereas controlling and restrictive feeding practices may be counterproductive, making children more susceptible to food cues in media advertisements, leading to overconsumption of energy-dense foods (Norman et al., 2018).

## 2.4 SOCIOECONOMIC INEQUALITIES AND FOOD INSECURITY

Inequalities in diet and health exist both between and within countries. There are substantial socioeconomic differences in the rates of obesity and associated chronic diseases, including type 2 diabetes, cardiovascular disease, and dental caries. As a risk factor for these, and other conditions, diet is thought to be a key determinant of health inequalities among children as well as adults. Despite widespread acceptance that the home environment plays a key role in shaping children's diets, there is a notable lack of research examining how SES impacts food in the home. Researchers have tended to focus on disparities in neighbourhood-level food environments, such as proximity to takeaway outlets and supermarkets. This work has highlighted how people living in more deprived areas often have limited access to fresh food and groceries. In high-income countries, poorer areas tend to have greater concentrations of fast food outlets and smaller convenience stores, which offer narrower varieties of lower-quality produce at higher prices compared to larger supermarkets (Costa et al., 2019). Disparities in neighbourhood food environments can lead to inequalities in food access and may in turn influence the types of foods offered within the home. However, evidence linking neighbourhood food environments to dietary intake remains equivocal (Caspi et al., 2012). More on this topic is covered in Chapter 5 on food retail environments and in Chapter 8 on fast food environments.

The few studies exploring SES-related differences in the physical and social home food environment have revealed clear disparities (Pinard et al., 2014; Boles et al., 2019). Food insecurity, defined as limited or uncertain availability of nutritionally adequate foods, disproportionately impacts families from deprived backgrounds. For such families, decisions around food purchasing are dictated largely by price, ease of preparation, and shelf-life. More expensive healthier foods may be less accessible or affordable for deprived families, and these foods can also necessitate additional effort and equipment for preparation and storage within the home. Regular routines and family mealtimes are also harder to achieve for caregivers with limited resources and unpredictable working schedules (Jarrett et al., 2016). The coronavirus pandemic has led to a rise in food insecurity, with more households struggling to put food on the table. Low-income families, lone parents, and larger families in particular have been detrimentally impacted by the pandemic (Food Foundation, 2021). Lower-income households report having fewer family meals together, less structure around mealtimes, and fewer food supplies, equipment, and appliances (Appelhans et al., 2014). In the UK, three studies have assessed how food insecurity experienced by lower-income households may impact dietary intake (Baird et al., 2010; Pilgrim et al., 2012; Yang et al., 2018). Findings demonstrate clear differences in dietary intake, with children from food insecure households consuming fewer fruits and vegetables, and more processed meat, crisps, and sugar-sweetened beverages.

Caregivers from more deprived backgrounds are likely to find adopting recommended feeding practices particularly challenging. Lower SES has been linked to several problematic feeding strategies, including greater use of pressure to eat (Gross et al., 2012). These feeding practices likely emerge in response to the challenges experienced by people living in greater deprivation. Living in poverty is associated with increased stress, and caregiver stress has also been linked to non-optimal feeding practices, including greater use of restriction (Swyden et al., 2017). Food insecurity may also influence caregivers' feeding practices; restricting the types and quantities of foods offered at home may be necessary to ensure adequate intake while avoiding food waste. Concern about having enough food to feed the family may also result in caregivers utilising restrictive feeding practices they view as protective, such as overtly restricting intake of energy-dense foods to ensure that their child is sufficiently hungry to eat the more nutritious foods on offer (Feinberg et al., 2008). Restrictions enforced to halt the spread of COVID-19 have negatively impacted the finances of many families, but this impact is not being felt evenly across social groups. The consequences of widening social inequalities on the home food environment require urgent attention.

## 2.5 INTERVENTIONS AND IMPLICATIONS FOR FUTURE RESEARCH

As discussed, the home is a critical target for improving diet quality across the whole day but is also arguably the hardest environment to modify through intervention, due to the cost and resource-intensive nature of home-based intervention delivery. For these reasons, many existing child dietary interventions are delivered in child care or school settings. See Chapter 3 for more information on school-based policies and interventions. Interventions in these settings have the advantage of reaching a large number of children simultaneously, providing a wider reach for a lower cost. However, as most of a child's food intake is consumed within the home, and caregivers are the gatekeepers to their children's diets, interventions targeting settings outside the family home can only hope to influence a small proportion of a child's overall dietary intake.

To date, most home-based interventions have focussed on increasing fruit and vegetable consumption via methods such as repeated exposure (Hodder et al., 2019). Very few interventions have targeted other factors within the home food environment thought to contribute to overall diet quality (Johnson et al., 2016). To overcome some of the barriers of traditional home-based interventions, novel approaches such as remote delivery (including online, or by telephone) and app-based eHealth interventions have been trialled. One example of these remote interventions is *Healthy Habits*, which provides telephone-based support to caregivers of preschool children over a 4-week period, focussing on three areas of the home food environment, availability and accessibility of foods and beverages, caregiver modelling, and caregivers' policies and rules (Fletcher et al., 2013). Findings from the randomised controlled trial (RCT) of this intervention suggest it was effective in reducing children's consumption of energy-dense snack foods 2 months later, but these effects disappeared after 6 months. Modification of the home food environment through intervention is possible and may play an important role in improving children's dietary intake. However, additional research is needed to understand how these positive changes can be sustained in the long term and how interventions can best reach more diverse populations to mitigate health inequalities.

Despite the extensive body of literature exploring the negative impacts of less responsive, more controlling caregiver feeding practices, very few intervention programs have encouraged caregivers to be more responsive to their children's eating cues within the home. The Australian-based *NOURISH* intervention has provided promising results in this area (Daniels et al., 2015). *NOURISH* provided first-time mothers with infants aged 4 months *anticipatory guidance*[5] on early caregiver feeding practices (including structured food choice, positive role modelling, avoidance of emotional feeding). The intervention led to reductions in non-responsive feeding practices (including pressure to eat and restriction). These reductions were associated with improvements in child diet quality, including increased liking of fruits and exposure to a wider range vegetables, and limited exposure to energy-dense snacks and beverages (Daniels et al., 2015). Building on the success of *NOURISH*, a Norwegian intervention *Early Food for Future Health* targeted caregiver feeding practices through short video clips (3–5 minutes in duration) addressing infant feeding topics, parent–child feeding situations, and making healthy food from easily available ingredients. Children in the intervention group were more likely to consume fruits and vegetables, eat meals as a family, and less likely to engage in screen-time during meals compared to children in the control group (Helle et al., 2019). Such early interventions may help lay the foundation for healthy eating in childhood. However, it is unclear whether these findings translate to lower SES, ethnically diverse samples. Strategies for modifying the home food environment, which take into account the potential barriers (e.g. cost, time pressures, shift work, lack of resources) and facilitators (e.g. financial aid, food parcels) experienced by more deprived families, are desperately needed.

## 2.6 CONCLUSIONS

Over the last few decades a large body of research has examined the physical and social aspects of the home food environment and how they relate to children's diets, eating behaviours, and weight. Although great strides have been made in our understanding, it is important to acknowledge the limitations of the existing literature. Heterogeneity in methodological approaches and a lack of agreement on terminology and definitions has restricted progress. Research to date has been largely cross-sectional, preventing conclusions about the direction of associations between the home food environment and children's dietary intake or weight. Studies have also predominantly been conducted in high-income countries, and families from higher-income and less ethnically diverse backgrounds, limiting our understanding of how these constructs differ for other groups. Longitudinal and interventional studies, collecting detailed data at multiple time points, are needed to elucidate causality in the relationship between the home food environment and children's diet quality. Importantly,

[5] Anticipatory guidance is a proactive and preventive approach which provides parents with information about behaviours they can expect and positive ways to manage these.

guidance is needed on the optimal approaches for modifying the home food environment to improve the quality of children's diets and reduce obesity risk, particularly in the most vulnerable populations.

## REFERENCES

Appelhans, B.M., Waring, M.E., Schneider, K.L. and Pagoto, S.L. 2014. Food preparation supplies predict children's family meal and home-prepared dinner consumption in low-income households. *Appetite*. **76**, pp. 1–8.

Avery, A., Anderson, C. and McCullough, F. 2017. Associations between children's diet quality and watching television during meal or snack consumption: A systematic review. *Maternal & Child Nutrition*. **13**(4), e12428, pp. 1–20.

Bailey-Davis, L., Poulsen, M.N., Hirsch, A.G., Pollak, J., Glass, T.A. and Schwartz, B.S. 2017. Home food rules in relation to youth eating behaviors, body mass index, waist circumference, and percent body fat. *Journal of Adolescent Health*. **60**(3), pp. 270–276.

Baird, J., Lawrence, W., Jarman, M., Black, C., Inskip, H., Cooper, C. and Barker, M. 2010. 067 Food insecurity, well-being and inequalities in diet in UK women. *Journal of Epidemiology & Community Health*. **64**(Suppl 1), pp. A26–A27.

Bauer, K.W., Haines, J., Miller, A.L., Rosenblum, K., Appugliese, D.P., Lumeng, J.C. and Kaciroti, N.A. 2017. Maternal restrictive feeding and eating in the absence of hunger among toddlers: A cohort study. *International Journal of Behavioral Nutrition and Physical Activity*. **14**(1), pp.1–10..

Berge, J.M., Wall, M., Hsueh, T.F., Fulkerson, J.A., Larson, N. and Neumark-Sztainer, D. 2015. The protective role of family meals for youth obesity: 10-year longitudinal associations. *Journal of Pediatrics*. **166**(2), pp.296–301.

Bjelland, M., Brantsæter, A.L., Haugen, M., Meltzer, H.M., Nystad, W. and Andersen, L.F. 2013. Changes and tracking of fruit, vegetables and sugar-sweetened beverages intake from 18 months to 7 years in the Norwegian mother and child cohort study. *BMC Public Health*. **13**(1), pp. 1–12.

Blissett, J., Bennett, C., Fogel, A., Harris, G. and Higgs, S. 2016. Parental modelling and prompting effects on acceptance of a novel fruit in 2–4-year-old children are dependent on children's food responsiveness. *British Journal of Nutrition*. **115**(3), pp. 554–564.

Boles, R.E., Johnson, S.L., Burdell, A., Davies, P.L., Gavin, W.J. and Bellows, L.L. 2019. Home food availability and child intake among rural families identified to be at-risk for health disparities. *Appetite*. **134**, pp. 135–141.

Boyland, E., Whalen, R., Christiansen, P., Mcgale, L., Duckworth, J., Halford, J., Clark, M., Rosenberg, G., Vohra, J. 2018 and Vohra, J. 2018. *See It, Want It, Buy It, Eat It How Food Advertising Is Associated with Unhealthy Eating Behaviours in 7–11 Year Old Children* [Online]. [Accessed 17 April 2020]. Available from: http://www.cancerresearchuk.org/.

Campbell, K. and Crawford, D. 2001. Family food environments as determinants of preschool-aged children's eating behaviours: Implications for obesity prevention policy. A review. *Australian Journal of Nutrition and Dietetics*. **58**(1), pp. 19–25.

Caspi, C.E., Sorensen, G., Subramanian, S. V. and Kawachi, I. 2012. The local food environment and diet: A systematic review. *Health and Place*. **18**(5), pp. 1172–1187.

Chai, W. and Nepper, M.J. 2015. Associations of the home food environment with eating behaviors and weight status among children and adolescents. *J Nutr Food Sci*., p. 12.

Christian, M.S., Evans, C.E.L., Hancock, N., Nykjaer, C. and Cade, J.E. 2013. Family meals can help children reach their 5 a day: A cross-sectional survey of children's dietary intake from London primary schools. *Journal of Epidemiology and Community Health*. **67**(4), pp. 332–338.

Cooke, L. 2007. The importance of exposure for healthy eating in childhood: A review. *Journal of Human Nutrition and Dietetics*. **20**(4), pp. 294–301.

Costa, B.V.L., Menezes, M.C., Oliveira, C.D.L., Mingoti, S.A., Jaime, P.C., Caiaffa, W.T. and Lopes, A.C.S. 2019. Does access to healthy food vary according to socioeconomic status and to food store type? An ecologic study. *BMC Public Health*. **19**(1), p. 775.

Daniels, L.A., Mallan, K.M., Nicholson, J.M., Thorpe, K., Nambiar, S., Mauch, C.E. and Magarey, A. 2015. An early feeding practices intervention for obesity prevention. *Pediatrics*. **136**(1), pp. e40–e49.

Feinberg, E., Kavanagh, P.L., Young, R.L. and Prudent, N. 2008. Food insecurity and compensatory feeding practices among urban black families. *Pediatrics*. **122**(4), pp. e854–e860.

Fletcher, A., Wolfenden, L., Wyse, R., Bowman, J., McElduff, P. and Duncan, S. 2013. A randomised controlled trial and mediation analysis of the 'Healthy Habits', telephone-based dietary intervention for preschool children. *The International Journal of Behavioral Nutrition and Physical Activity*. **10**(1), pp. 1–11.

Food Foundation. 2021. *A Crisis within a Crisis: The Impact of Covid-19 on Household Food Security* [Online]. [Accessed 18 March 2021]. Available from: https://foodfoundation.org.uk/wp-content/uploads/2021/03/FF_Impact-of-Covid_FINAL.pdf.

Gross, R.S., Mendelsohn, A.L., Fierman, A.H., Racine, A.D. and Messito, M.J. 2012. Food insecurity and obesogenic maternal infant feeding styles and practices in low-income families. *Pediatrics*. **130**(2), pp. 254–261.

Harris, H.A., Fildes, A., Mallan, K.M. and Llewellyn, C.H. 2016. Maternal feeding practices and fussy eating in toddlerhood: A discordant twin analysis. *International Journal of Behavioral Nutrition and Physical Activity*, **13**(81), pp. 1–9.

Helle, C., Hillesund, E.R., Wills, A.K. and Øverby, N.C. 2019. Evaluation of an eHealth intervention aiming to promote healthy food habits from infancy - The Norwegian randomized controlled trial Early Food for Future Health. *International Journal of Behavioral Nutrition and Physical Activity*. **16**(1), pp. 1–16.

Hodder, R.K., O'Brien, K.M., Stacey, F.G., Tzelepis, F., Wyse, R.J., Bartlem, K.M., Sutherland, R., James, E.L., Barnes, C. and Wolfenden, L. 2019. Interventions for increasing fruit and vegetable consumption in children aged five years and under. *Cochrane Database of Systematic Reviews*. **2019**(11), pp. 1–407.

Jarrett, R.L., Bahar, O.S. and Kersh, R.T. 2016. When we do sit down together. *Journal of Family Issues*. **37**(11), pp. 1483–1513.

Johnson, B.J., Hendrie, G.A. and Golley, R.K. 2016. Reducing discretionary food and beverage intake in early childhood: A systematic review within an ecological framework. *Public Health Nutrition*. **19**(9), pp. 1684–1695.

Loth, K.A. 2016. Associations between food restriction and pressure-to-eat parenting practices and dietary intake in children: A selective review of the recent literature. *Current Nutrition Reports*. **5**(1), pp. 61–67.

Lytle, L.A., Hearst, M.O., Fulkerson, J., Murray, D.M., Martinson, B., Klein, E., Pasch, K. and Samuelson, A. 2011. Examining the relationships between family meal practices, family stressors, and the weight of youth in the family. *Annals of Behavioral Medicine*. **41**(3), pp. 353–362.

Musher-Eizenman, D. and Holub, S. 2007. Comprehensive feeding practices questionnaire: Validation of a new measure of parental feeding practices. *Journal of Pediatric Psychology*. **32**(8), pp. 960–972.

Norman, J., Kelly, B., McMahon, A.T., Boyland, E., Baur, L.A., Chapman, K., King, L., Hughes, C. and Bauman, A. 2018. Children's self-regulation of eating provides no defense against television and online food marketing. *Appetite*. **125**, pp. 438–444.

Ofcom. 2019. *Children and Parents Media Use and Attitudes: Annex 1* [Online]. [Accessed 7 June 2019]. Available from: https://www.ofcom.org.uk/__data/assets/pdf_file/0027/134892/Children-and-Parents-Media-Use-and-Attitudes-Annex-1.pdf.

Pearson, N., Griffiths, P., Biddle, S.J.H., Johnston, J.P. and Haycraft, E. 2017. Individual, behavioural and home environmental factors associated with eating behaviours in young adolescents. *Appetite.* **112**, pp. 35–43.

Pilgrim, A., Barker, M., Jackson, A., Ntani, G., Crozier, S., Inskip, H., Godfrey, K., Cooper, C. and Robinson, S. 2012. Does living in a food insecure household impact on the diets and body composition of young children? Findings from the Southampton Women's Survey. *Journal of Epidemiology and Community Health.* **66**(6), p. e6.

Pinard, C.A., Yaroch, A.L., Hart, M.H., Serrano, E.L., McFerren, M.M. and Estabrooks, P.A. 2014. The validity and reliability of the Comprehensive Home Environment Survey (CHES). *Health Promotion Practice.* **15**(1), pp. 109–117.

Rodgers, R.F., Paxton, S.J., Massey, R., Campbell, K.J., Wertheim, E.H., Skouteris, H. and Gibbons, K. 2013. Maternal feeding practices predict weight gain and obesogenic eating behaviors in young children: A prospective study. *International Journal of Behavioral Nutrition & Physical Activity.* **10**, pp. 1–10.

Rutherford, L., Brown, J.E., Skouteris, H., Fuller-Tyszkiewicz, M. and Bittman, M. 2015. Screen media, parenting practices, and the family environment in Australia: A longitudinal study of young children's media use, lifestyles, and outcomes for healthy weight. *Journal of Children and Media.* **9**(1), pp. 22–39.

Savage, J.S., Fisher, J.O. and Birch, L.L. 2007. Parental influence on eating behavior: Conception to adolescence. *The Journal of Law, Medicine & Ethics.* **35**(1), pp. 22–34.

Schrempft, S., Van Jaarsveld, C.H.M., Fisher, A. and Wardle, J. 2015. The obesogenic quality of the home environment: Associations with diet, physical activity, TV viewing, and BMI in preschool children. *PLoS ONE.* **10**(8), p. e0134490.

Swyden, K., Sisson, S.B., Morris, A.S., Lora, K., Weedn, A.E., Copeland, K.A. and DeGrace, B. 2017. Association between maternal stress, work status, concern about child weight, and restrictive feeding practices in preschool children. *Maternal and Child Health Journal.* **21**(6), pp. 1349–1357.

Temple, J.L., Giacomelli, A.M., Kent, K.M., Roemmich, J.N. and Epstein, L.H. 2007. *Television Watching Increases Motivated Responding for Food and Energy Intake in Children 1–3* [Online]. [Accessed 16 June 2020]. Available from: https://academic.oup.com/ajcn/article-abstract/85/2/355/4649500.

Terry, K. and Beck, S. 1985. Eating style and food storage habits in the home: Assessment of obese and nonobese families. *Behavior Modification.* **9**(2), pp. 242–261.

Vaughn, A.E., Tabak, R.G., Bryant, M.J. and Ward, D.S. 2013. *Measuring Parent Food Practices: A Systematic Review of Existing Measures and Examination of Instruments* [Online]. [Accessed 9 March 2020]. Available from: http://www.ijbnpa.org/content/10/1/61.

Ventura, A.K. and Birch, L.L. 2008. Does parenting affect children's eating and weight status? *The International Journal of Behavioral Nutrition and Physical Activity.* **5(1)**, pp. 1–12.

Vollmer, R.L. and Baietto, J. 2017. Practices and preferences: Exploring the relationships between food-related parenting practices and child food preferences for high fat and/or sugar foods, fruits, and vegetables. *Appetite.* **113**, pp. 134–140.

Wood, A.C., Blissett, J.M., Brunstrom, J.M., Carnell, S., Faith, M.S., Fisher, J.O., Hayman, L.L., Khalsa, A.S., Hughes, S.O., Miller, A.L., Momin, S.R., Welsh, J.A., Woo, J.G. and Haycraft, E. 2020. Caregiver influences on eating behaviors in young children. *Journal of the American Heart Association.* **8**(e014520), pp. 1–15.

Yang, T.C., Sahota, P., Pickett, K.E. and Bryant, M. 2018. Association of food security status with overweight and dietary intake: Exploration of White British and Pakistani-origin families in the Born in Bradford cohort. *Nutrition Journal.* **17**(1), pp. 1–11.

Yee, A.Z.H., Lwin, M.O. and Ho, S.S. 2017. The influence of parental practices on child promotive and preventive food consumption behaviors: A systematic review and meta-analysis. *International Journal of Behavioral Nutrition and Physical Activity.* **14**(1), pp. 1–14.

# 3 The School Food Environment

*Suzanne Spence and Grace Gardner*
Newcastle University

*Dorota Zarnowiecki*
Flinders University

*Katie Adolphus, Clare L. Lawton, and Louise Dye*
University of Leeds

*Emma Patterson*
Karolinska Institutet

*Charlotte E.L. Evans*
University of Leeds

**CONTENTS**



DOI: 10.1201/9781003043720-3

## 3.1 INTRODUCTION

With large numbers of children attending school and school food contributing to 30% of children's dietary intake (Nelson et al., 2007), the school environment is an opportune setting to impact what children eat and drink. Scientific evidence supports the use of the school environment to improve children's diets; systematic reviews show positive impacts of dietary interventions (van Cauwenberghe et al., 2010), policy evaluations highlight the impact of school food standards (Spence et al., 2013, Evans et al., 2015), and research studies employing food choice architecture interventions demonstrate potentially positive findings, though these have mainly focused on fruit and vegetables (Broers et al., 2017).

The first section of this chapter considers key events relating to school meals and school standards in England, as this is where the lead author is based. Globally, school meal provision and standards vary by country and within countries. The second part examines practices in a selection of countries (Japan, Sweden, and Australia) where policies have been introduced, evaluated, and published in the scientific literature. Whilst school meals are a vital component of school food, school food incorporates more than the food served at lunchtime. This chapter briefly explores practices from school breakfasts and school gardens to whole-school approaches.

## 3.2 SCHOOL MEALS IN THE UK: PROVISION AND STANDARDS

Each region of the UK (England, Wales, Scotland, and Northern Ireland) has its own governing body responsible for school food, and although all have food standards for lunch and wider school food provision, there is variation in content, implementation, and requirements (Adamson et al., 2013). This section focuses on school food provision in England which constitutes 86% of the UK population.

There have been substantial changes to school meals and school food standards in the last 100 years (Figure 3.1). Initially, school meals were implemented to address undernutrition in children and extended to include children from more deprived families (Webster, 1985); potentially initiating the continued stigma associated with free school meals. In 1944, the Education Act legislated all children were entitled to free school meals, but this ended in 1950 (Evans and Harper, 2009). Currently in the UK, children can have free or paid school meals, or bring a home-packed lunch into school (referred to as a bag lunch in the US and a packed lunchbox in Australia). Eligibility for free school meals is based on criteria related to income (GOV.UK, 2020). The first nutrient-based standards (energy, fats, and protein) were introduced in 1941 (https://www.cwt.org.uk/). Standards are applicable to school lunches provided in schools; home-packed lunches are excluded from national mandated standards although individual schools may have their own policies. The removal of nutrient-based standards in the 1980s and the introduction of compulsory competitive tendering adversely impacted on school food provision, regulation, and quality (Evans and Harper, 2009). In 2001, after failed requests in the 1990s, food-based standards were re-introduced (School Meals Review Panel, 2005). The formation of the School Meals Review Panel (SMRP) (2005), a media broadcast of celebrity chef

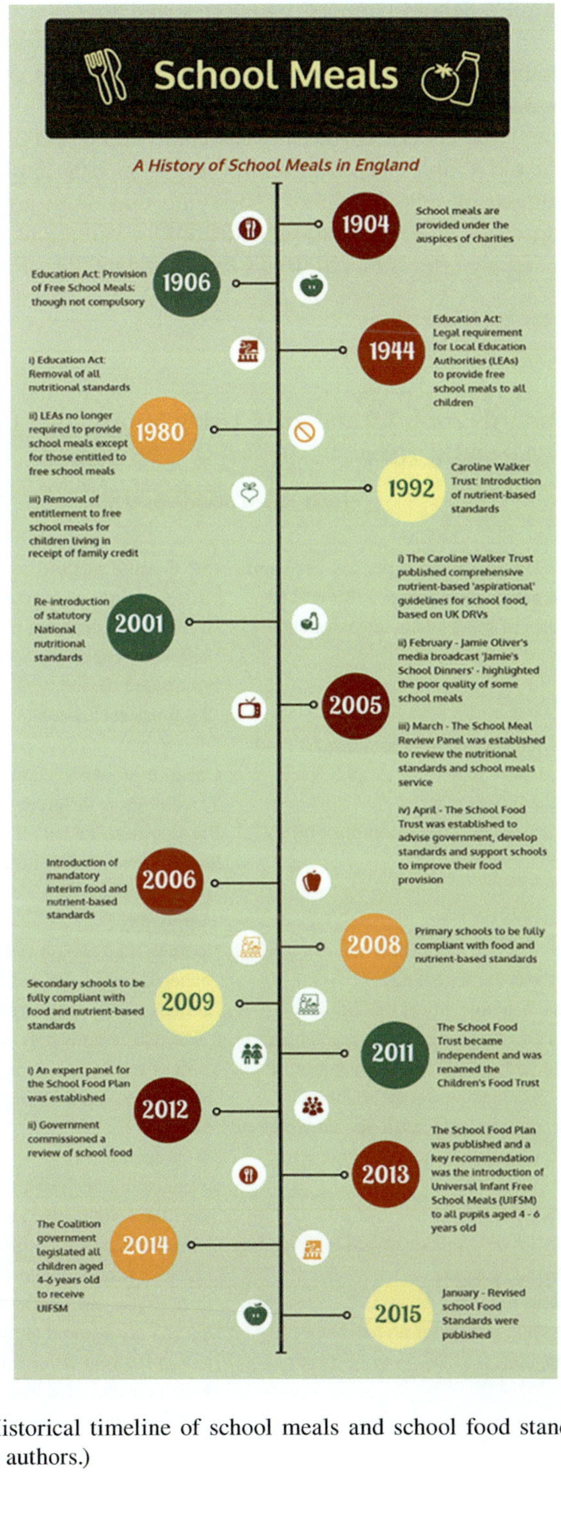


**FIGURE 3.1** Historical timeline of school meals and school food standards in England. (Designed by the authors.)

Jamie Oliver's 'Jamie's School Dinners' which received attention from both parents and the government (Spence, 2005), and the establishment of the School Food Trust led to a transformation of the school food system with nutrient as well as food-based standards (Figure 3.1) (the Education Act, 2008).

Food-based standards specified which foods could and could not be served over a 3-week menu cycle (Table 3.1). Nutrient-based standards applied to the average nutritional content of school lunches specifying minimum and maximum levels for planned provision (The Education Act, 2008). Evaluations of the standards reported positive dietary effects on children's lunchtime intakes (Pearce et al., 2011,

**TABLE 3.1**
**Food-Based Standards 2008/09 and 2014 Using Information from the Department of Education, 2014**

| | Food-Based Standards (UK) | |
|---|---|---|
| | 2008/09 | 2014 |
| Fruit and vegetables | Not less than two portions per day per pupil must be provided; at least one should be vegetables or salad and at least one should be fruit | One or more portions of fruit and one or more portions of vegetables/per day<br>At least three different fruits and three different vegetables/weekly<br>Fruit-based dessert containing ≥50% fruit 2+ times each week |
| Starchy food | Starchy food cooked in fat or oil must not be provided more than three times a week across the school day<br>Bread with no added fat or oil must be provided every day | One or more portions per day<br>One or more wholegrain varieties/per week<br>Three or more different starchy foods/week<br>Bread with no added fat or oil daily<br>Starchy food cooked in fat or oil must not be provided more than 2 days/week across the school day |
| Food's high in fat, sugar, salt | No more than two deep-fried items in a single week across the school day<br>Cakes and biscuits only at lunchtime<br>No snacks, except nuts, seeds, vegetables, and fruit with no added salt, sugar, or fat may be provided across the school day<br>Savoury crackers or breadsticks can be served at lunch with fruit or vegetables or dairy food<br>No confectionery<br>Salt must not be available to add to food after the cooking process<br>Condiments may only be available in sachets or individual portion of no more than 10 g or one teaspoon | No more than two portions of deep-fried, battered or breaded products or foods that contain pastry each week<br>Cakes and biscuits only at lunchtime<br>Savoury crackers/ breadsticks served at lunchtime with fruit, vegetables, or dairy food<br>No confectionery<br>Salt must not be available to add to food after the cooking process is complete<br>Condiments may only be available in sachets or individual portion of no more than 10 g or one teaspoon<br>Desserts are allowed at lunchtime only except for yoghurt of fruit-based desserts with a content of at least 50% fruit are permitted at any time of the day |

(*Continued*)

**TABLE 3.1 (*Continued*)**
**Food-Based Standards 2008/09 and 2014 Using Information from the Department of Education, 2014**

| | Food-Based Standards (UK) | |
|---|---|---|
| | 2008/09 | 2014 |
| Meat, fish, eggs, beans, and other non-dairy sources of protein | Oily fish must be provided one or more every 3 weeks<br>A meat product (manufactured or homemade) from each of the four groups below may be provided no more than once per fortnight across the school day, providing the meat product also meets the standards for minimum meat content and does not contain any prohibited offal:<br>Group 1: burger, hamburger, chopped meat, corned beef<br>Group 2: sausage, sausage meat, link, chipolata, luncheon meat,<br>Group 3: individual meat pie, meat pudding, Melton Mowbray pie, game pie, Scottish (or Scotch) pie, pasty or pastie, bridie, sausage roll,<br>Group 4: any other shaped or coated meat product | Oily fish must be provided once or more every 3 weeks<br>A portion of meat, fish, eggs, beans, and other non-dairy sources of protein must be provided daily<br>A portion of meat or poultry must be provided 3 or more days/week<br>Vegetarians: portion of non-dairy protein must be provided 3 or more days/week<br>Meat or poultry product may not be provided more than once a week in primary schools and twice each week in secondary schools |
| Milk and dairy | **No standard** | A portion of dairy food must be provided daily<br>Lower fat milk must be available daily during school sessions |

Nicholas et al., 2013) and in their total daily intakes (Spence et al., 2013). To simplify the standards, they were replaced by the School Food Plan in 2013 (www.schoolfoodplan.com) based on foods (not nutrients) and free school meals for all young children aged 4–6 years (Department for Education, 2014). A recent report suggests the quality of school food is worsening again (Food for Life, 2019) due to rising costs of ingredients and overheads, increased grab 'n' go options compared with hot meals, and healthier items, for example, fruit and salmon being replaced with desserts and biscuits due to financial constraints. Monitoring of standards also remains an issue. In 2019, the Time to Solve Childhood Obesity Chief Medical Officer's report recognised the school environment as important and made several recommendations for schools, including consideration of approaches to improve free school meal uptake, increasing free school meal allowance to ensure it covers the full cost of a healthy meal, implementation of robust monitoring to ensure current food standards are adhered to in all schools, adoption of water and milk-only policies, and developing a national approach supporting schools and local authorities to commission healthier catering procurement (Davies, 2019).

In the UK, lunches prepared at home and brought to school are excluded from the standards. Research exploring the nutritional quality of home-packed lunches highlight that on average these provide children with less nutritious food both at lunchtime and over the whole day compared with children having a school meal (Evans et al., 2010). Some schools do have their own home-packed lunch policies, there is no national policy. School food policies therefore only influence the diets of children who consume a school meal and approximately half of children bring in their own food to school. Potential opportunities to improve children's diets across the wider school environment require more inclusive approaches.

## 3.3 SCHOOL MEALS GLOBALLY: PROVISION AND STANDARDS

### 3.3.1 School Lunch Programme: Japan

One of the most highly regarded school food systems in the world is the Japanese school food programme known as Kyu-shoku. It is part of a wider programme of food education called Shoku-Iku (Shoku means food and Iku means education) which is aimed at the whole community to encourage an appreciation of tasty nutritious food. Shoku-Iku was enshrined in law in 2005 to help people make good food choices related to health, culture, safety, and appreciation across the country (Tanaka and Miyoshi, 2012). Central to the school food programme is the understanding that lunchtime is an extension of the children's education; therefore, children eat together in their classroom with their teacher. Schools that are part of the school food programme do not offer children the choice of having the school meal or bringing in food; all children in participating schools eat the lunch that the school provides. In non-participating schools, parents provide a bento box. Approximately 90% of elementary schools and two thirds of junior high schools (children aged 12–15 years) participate in Kyu-shoku (Miyawaki et al., 2019). There is only one daily meal choice and children are encouraged (but not forced) to try all foods offered. There is usually a 1-month cycle of menus which range from traditional meals of rice, fish, and vegetables to curries, bread, and noodles. Generally, three different foods are served which are all savoury (Figure 3.2). Fruit is served at least once per week, but puddings and desserts high in sugars are rarely served, perhaps once or twice a month. Children are 'active' participants in the school lunch process than in many programmes elsewhere, they take turns to serve food to their classmates and wait until everyone is served before eating. A carton of milk is usually served with the meal and no other drinks other than water are served, although many children bring green tea. Many schools have an in-house dietitian who carries out the menu planning and ensures the meals meet the stringent nutritional standards (Meeyoung et al., 2017). In elementary schools, there are standards for three different age groups taking into account age requirements. This is achieved by ordering fish and bread rolls of different sizes to ensure that the youngest children receive a balanced meal. Despite the lack of choice compared with that more commonly seen in schools in other wealthy countries, anecdotal evidence suggests food waste is much lower than in other countries at around 7%. The cost of the programme is subsidised by the government. The cost to parents is 140 yen (US$1.30, €1.20, £1.00) per meal, which pays for

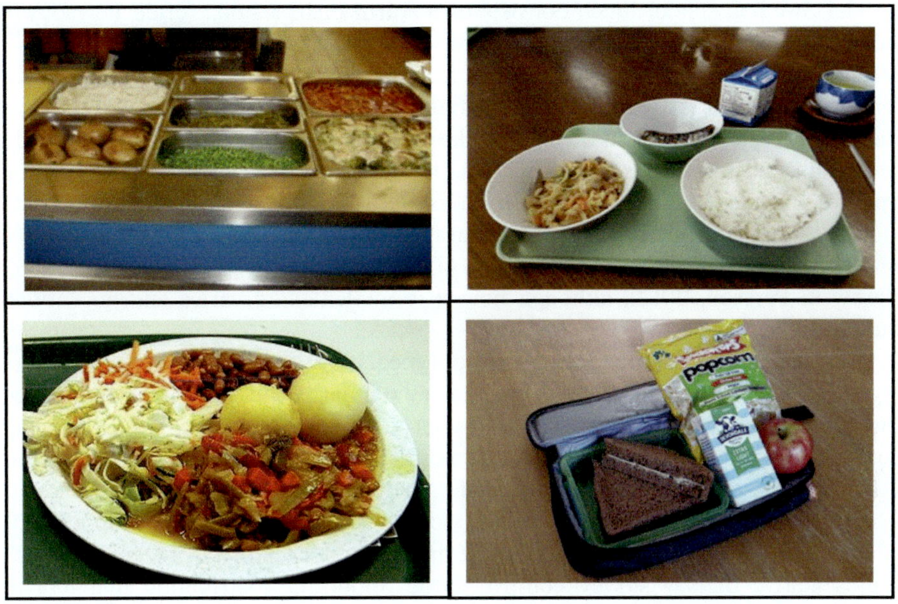


**FIGURE 3.2** Examples of school food available in England, Japan, Sweden, and Australia. Photos attributed to authors for England (top left), Japan (top right), and Australia (bottom right). Swedish school lunch in 2008 (bottom left) by Casey Lehman. (Available at https://commons.wikimedia.org/wiki/File:School_lunch.jpg and licensed under CC BY_SA 2.0; https://creativecommons.org/licenses/by-sa/2.0/.)

the ingredients, and a 140-yen government subsidy goes to schools to pay for staff. Children in low-income households are eligible for free school meals. Evaluation of the Japanese school food programme has highlighted positive benefits of participating, both in terms of fruits and vegetable intakes (Yamaguchi et al., 2018) and obesity (Miyawaki et al., 2019).

### 3.3.2 School Meal System: Sweden

Sweden is almost unique in legislating free school lunches to all school pupils aged 6–16 years. Free school lunches are not means-tested, and to all schools whether publicly or privately run, making this system rare. As in many countries, school food was introduced as a form of charity and a means to encourage poor children to continue to attend school in the late 18th century. Subsidised lunches were introduced in 1946, with a focus on improving nutritional status but also on enabling parents to work. By the 1970s, the practice was widespread, although it was not enshrined in national law until the Education Act in 1997. This act states among other things that all education is to be provided free of charge, including tuition, materials, and meals. The majority of primary schools (83%) are run by local authorities. Schools are financed predominantly through local authority income tax. All schools follow the same law and national curriculum, including those that are privately run. In 2011, a new education act came into force and stipulated that school meals should also be 'nutritious'.

The Swedish school lunch consists of a warm dish, a salad (often nowadays a salad buffet), bread, and milk/water. In the majority of schools, a choice of dishes is offered. Children may not bring lunches from home. Food is either prepared on-site or comes from a nearby school/central municipal kitchen. Children generally serve themselves, and they eat in a canteen-like setting. This is often nowadays called a restaurant and the title 'school chef' has replaced 'dinner ladies' to help promote positive attitudes to school meals. Teachers are usually present for the lunch, especially for younger pupils, and are encouraged to use the mealtime as an opportunity to interact with pupils. This concept of the 'pedagogical lunch' – is deep-rooted (Osowski Persson, 2012), although how it is implemented varies and no national guidance exists.

Food and nutrient guidelines for school meals are issued by the Swedish Food Agency (2019). Whilst there are no mandatory standards, meals are expected to meet the Nordic Nutrition Recommendations over a 4-week period. The guidelines suggest foods to promote and limit, but do not dictate, instead the guidelines encourage schools to take a common-sense and holistic approach. This lack of restrictions is possible in part because of the long tradition of relatively healthy school meals, where deep-fried foods, desserts, or soft drinks do not feature. A recent nationally representative dietary survey confirmed the important contribution that lunches make (Eustachio Colombo et al., 2020). Although intakes of certain nutrients such as iron, vitamin D, and fibre tend to be slightly lower than the recommendations, school lunches provide around half of children's daily vegetable intake and have a higher nutrient density than other meals. The guidelines also emphasise the need to consider other aspects of meal quality, such as the environment, and the potential for school meals to be integrated into pedagogical activities.

Despite the long history of Swedish school meals, little is known about the impacts. One long-term study, using register data, of adults who received a free lunch for a varying numbers of years, suggested it led to gains in earning potential (Alex-Petersen et al., 2018). Similar to other countries, little monitoring of school meal quality has taken place (Lucas et al., 2017). A web-based evaluation tool was developed in 2010 to help schools and local authorities (Patterson et al., 2013). This evaluation tool is now used by nearly half of schools and data suggests improvements in nutritional quality since the 2011 policy change (Patterson and Elinder, 2015).

### 3.3.3 School Lunch Provision: Australia

In Australia, most children bring a packed 'lunchbox' from home, which provides food and drink for consumption at school during scheduled mid-morning/afternoon breaks 'recess' and lunch (Sutherland et al., 2020). Many schools have canteens or 'tuckshops', which are a small shop where children can purchase cold foods and drinks (Lawlis et al., 2016). The types of foods provided and nutritional quality of lunchboxes have remained relatively stable (Sanigorski et al., 2005, Sutherland et al., 2020). Contemporary data shows that the most common lunch item continues to be sandwiches (provided in 81% of lunchboxes) and common snack foods are fruit, sweet and savoury biscuits, crisps, muesli/fruit bars, and cakes/muffins (Sutherland et al., 2020). The provision of fruit and vegetables appears to have slightly increased, perhaps due to initiatives such as Crunch&Sip (Section 3.4.2), 85% of lunchboxes contain at least one serving, and on average 2.5 servings, of 'unhealthy' foods (Sutherland et al., 2020). For over half of children, their school-time 'unhealthy' food intake exceeds the recommended intake of 'unhealthy' foods for the whole day (https://www.eatforhealth.gov.au/guidelines) and is unrelated to socio-economic factors, (Sutherland et al., 2020) highlighting the need to improve all children's lunchboxes.

Parents report that they make compromises in nutrition to address other challenges when packing lunchboxes, including convenience, cost, food safety, and providing food their children will consume (Bathgate and Begley, 2011). With lunchbox provision from home not regulated by guidelines or policies, the question remains as to the best way to support parents to provide healthier lunchboxes. Interventions targeting parents and children have tested a range of strategies to improve the nutritional quality of lunchboxes, such as education, physical resources (e.g. lunch packs), incentives for children, and developing policies (Nathan et al., 2019). These interventions have had a modest impact on increasing vegetable provision but less success in reducing provision of 'unhealthy' foods (Nathan et al., 2019).

With a rise in digital technology, online platforms such as apps or websites, that reach parents at home, provide a promising approach to supporting parents to improve the healthfulness of lunchboxes (Zarnowiecki et al., 2020). Digital interventions targeting parents have been shown to be effective for improving dietary intake and nutrition knowledge but need to be co-designed with parents to include components that parents want, for example, practical tools, interactive content, and support from other parents and health professionals (Zarnowiecki et al., 2020).

Unlike lunchboxes, the types of foods that can be sold in Australian school canteens are regulated by policies. Under the Australian Government structure (Australia is a federation of states), school food provision is regulated by State and Territory Governments rather than the Federal Government, and therefore policies and programmes vary across jurisdictions. Most states and territories employ mandatory canteen standards, which are based on jurisdiction-specific guidelines and guided by National 'Healthy School Canteen' voluntary guidelines (Lucas et al., 2017). Compliance varies (Woods et al., 2014). Most canteen standards use a 'traffic light system' that categorises foods according to their nutritional quality (see Table 3.2).

## 3.4 BEYOND SCHOOL MEALS: THE WIDER SCHOOL FOOD ENVIRONMENT

School food standards at lunchtime play a vital role in improving children's diets; however, to address the many factors influencing children's diets across the school day, alternative solutions are needed.

### 3.4.1 School Breakfasts

A substantial body of evidence demonstrates the short- and long-term positive effects of breakfast consumption on a range of outcomes including diet quality, macro- and micronutrient intake, weight status, social interaction and development, cognitive

**TABLE 3.2**
**Food Categories for Foods and Drinks Sold in Australian School Canteens Using Information from the Australian Government Department of Health (2014)**

| | | |
|---|---|---|
| **GREEN** | Always available on the canteen menu | Contain a wide range of nutrients and are generally low in saturated fat, added sugar, and/or sodium. For example, vegetables, fruit, grain foods, milk and dairy products, lean meat, fish, poultry, and alternatives. |
| **AMBER** | Select carefully, restricted provision (e.g. nutrient and portion criteria) | Contain some valuable nutrients, but higher in added sugar, fat, and/or sodium. For example, flavoured milk drinks, breakfast cereals, meat products, and savoury hot foods. |
| **RED** | Not recommended on canteen menu | Low in nutritional value and high in fat, added sugar and/or sodium. For example, soft drinks, confectionery, cakes, deep-fried foods. |

*Source:* Guidelines for healthy foods and drinks supplied in school canteens, Commonwealth of Australia, Canberra ACT. Accessed 25 June 2021, Reprinted under licence CC 4.0 (https://creativecommons.org/licenses/by/4.0/). Available at https://www.health.gov.au/resources/publications/national-healthy-school-canteens-guidelines-for-healthy-foods-and-drinks-supplied-in-school-canteens.

function, and educational outcomes in schoolchildren. However, many schoolchildren omit breakfast. The Healthy Lifestyle in Europe by Nutrition in Adolescence (HELENA) study reported that 38% of European adolescents aged 13–17 years agreed with the statement 'I often skip breakfast' (Hallström et al., 2011). The Health Behaviour in School-aged Children (HBSC) study also reported similarly high rates of breakfast skipping in 11- to 15-year olds from 41 countries. The proportion of adolescents reporting that they habitually ate breakfast (7 days per week) ranged from 33% to 75% between the countries included (Vereecken et al., 2009).

School breakfast programmes are a type of school food provision that takes place on the school premises prior to the start of the formal school day. Whilst there are a variety of breakfast programme models, typical breakfast programmes provide schoolchildren with the opportunity to consume breakfast in an adult-supervised environment with their peers. School breakfast programmes also typically offer schoolchildren opportunities to participate in structured activities before the start of the formal school day. There has been a fairly rapid growth of school breakfast programmes in England over the past 20 years. An audit of school breakfast club provision in 2014 (www.kelloggs.co.uk) indicated that over 85% of UK schools now have some form of breakfast provision.

Numerous scientific studies have demonstrated the positive effect of breakfast consumption on a range of educational outcomes in children and adolescents including cognitive function, in-class behaviour, and academic performance (Adolphus et al., 2016). Cognitive function is assessed by objective cognitive function tasks of memory, attention, reaction time, and executive function. The evidence from acute intervention studies comparing breakfast vs. no breakfast suggests that consuming breakfast has a transient beneficial effect on cognitive function measured within 4 hours post-ingestion (Adolphus et al., 2016). The chronic effects of school breakfast programme interventions on cognitive function also generally show that school breakfast programmes can have a positive effect on cognitive function in children and adolescents, although the evidence is mixed (Adolphus et al., 2016). Studies examining the effects of breakfast on behaviour in children and adolescents by utilising classroom observations or teacher-completed behavioural rating scales generally demonstrate a positive acute effect of breakfast on on-task behaviour in children (Adolphus et al., 2013). This effect was apparent in children irrespective of whether they were considered well-nourished, undernourished, or low socio-economic status (Adolphus et al., 2013). Several studies have considered the effects of breakfast on academic performance in terms of school grades and achievement test scores, which reflect typical performance indicators used within the education system. This evidence demonstrates that both habitual breakfast consumption frequency and school breakfast programmes are positively associated with academic performance in children and adolescents (Adolphus et al., 2013).

Regular breakfast consumption is also associated with many positive diet-quality indices. Children and adolescents who habitually consume breakfast are more likely to have favourable macronutrient intakes including higher intakes of dietary fibre, total carbohydrate, and lower total fat intake (Deshmukh-Taskar et al., 2010). Evidence also suggests that daily micronutrient intakes are higher in breakfast consumers compared with breakfast skippers (Coulthard et al., 2017). Of note, a recent study using data from the National Diet and Nutrition Survey (NDNS) demonstrated that breakfast consumption is associated with higher-quality dietary intake in a large sample of 1,686 school-age children aged 4–18 years. The findings demonstrated that fibre, folate, vitamin C, calcium, iron, and iodine intakes were higher in frequent breakfast consumers (Coulthard et al., 2017). Consequently, school breakfast initiatives represent an opportunity to improve the diet and health of young people.

School breakfast clubs may offer an avenue by which to increase breakfast consumption by providing an opportunity to eat breakfast immediately before school with peers. A cluster randomised controlled trial evaluated the effect of the Welsh Primary School Free Breakfast Initiative on breakfast consumption along with immediate verbal memory in 9- to 11-year olds (Murphy et al., 2011). However, the intervention had little impact on breakfast-eating or on cognitive outcomes at 1-year follow-up. The proportion of children eating breakfast everyday remained unchanged whilst the proportion of children eating breakfast at home decreased, suggestive of a shift in consumption from at home to at school. Similarly, a systematic review of the efficacy of interventions aimed at increasing breakfast-eating frequency showed that only 3 of the 11 included trials were successful in changing breakfast eating (Kothe and Mullan, 2011). The lack of efficacy of these trials highlights the need to increase understanding of the personal and motivational factors affecting breakfast consumption. Furthermore, changes in cognitive performance, academic achievement, and behaviour reported in intervention studies that do not affect breakfast intake or have low participation rates are an artefact of other factors. Interventions which adopt an evidence-based theoretical framework to produce change in breakfast-eating behaviour may be more effective in changing breakfast eating and The Theory of Planned

Behaviour may offer a promising theoretical model for predicting high-quality breakfast consumption (Mullan et al., 2013).

### 3.4.2 Fruit and Vegetable Initiatives

In England, as part of the government's strategy to encourage children to eat more fruit and vegetables a national School Fruit and Vegetable Scheme (SFVS) exists in all state-funded primary schools (Hughes et al., 2012). This scheme provides a free piece of fruit or vegetable daily for every child in Reception, Year 1, and Year 2. Children usually receive this either during morning or afternoon break. Evaluation indicated that children who participated in the SFVS consumed more fruits and vegetables. However, children from more deprived families continued to consume less fruits and vegetables (Hughes et al., 2012).

A voluntary programme implemented in Australia, Crunch&Sip (www.crunchandsip.com.au/), encourages a set break time during the school day for students to consume vegetables or fruit and drink water they have brought from home. This programme is now running in schools across Australia and encourages a whole-school approach including free fruit for children in disadvantaged areas (Dana et al., 2019). Evaluation indicates that the programme has successfully increased fruits and vegetables. In a pilot vegetable promotion project, the proportion of children bringing vegetables for Crunch&Sip more than doubled (21% vs. 46%) and the programme improved teachers' knowledge of the nutritional benefits of vegetables and confidence to teach these (Myers et al., 2018).

Another initiative in England is the Food for Life school partnership that works with schools to make healthy, sustainable eating the norm and a pleasant experience for children (Food for Life, 2019). The Food for Life partnership encompasses strands such as food quality – procurement of local, seasonal, and organic products and food education – to include environmental and sustainability topics through gardening and farm visits (Weitkamp et al., 2013). Findings show children attending schools participating in the Food for Life partnerships are twice as likely to eat their 5-a-day compared to children in matched comparison schools (Jones et al., 2015). A systematic review and meta-analysis also supports the use of initiatives in school settings to improve fruit intakes (Evans et al., 2012).

### 3.4.3 School Gardens

School gardens are an experiential learning approach which involves gardening classes in combination with cooking classes, nutrition education, and integration of garden-related learning into the curriculum, for example, through science experiments (Ohly et al., 2016). They provide a 'hands on' experience of planting, caring for and harvesting produce, through which children learn actively (Davis et al., 2015). School gardening has risen in popularity due to their benefits for a range of health and well-being outcomes. Several studies have shown that school gardening can increase children's consumption of fruit and vegetables (Davis et al., 2015; Ohly et al., 2016). Increases in consumption of fruit and vegetables have been attributed to repeated exposure to and opportunities to taste a variety of different fruit and vegetables during gardening programmes (Ohly et al., 2016). School gardening can also improve other nutrition-related outcomes that support healthy eating in children, including nutrition knowledge and willingness to try fruit and vegetables (Davis et al., 2015; Ohly et al., 2016). Cooking and nutrition activities help children to develop life skills, which can be particularly important for children from families with poor cooking skills and nutrition knowledge (Ohly et al., 2016). More broadly, garden programmes enable students to learn about other cultures, increase knowledge about food origins and the supply chain, water conservation, seasonality, and sustainability (Ohly et al., 2016).

### 3.4.4 Whole-School Approach

The concept of a health promoting school has been around for three decades and is defined as a school that '*constantly strengthens its capacity as a healthy setting for living, learning and working*' (WHO, 2014). The concept of a 'whole school approach' is perhaps now more of a focus. A whole-school approach to food and drink combines the macro level (leadership, policy) through to the individual level (pupil, parent voices). Figure 3.3 provides an adaptation of an example to highlight some aspects included in a whole-school approach from the School Food Plan. There is limited evidence on the effect of whole-school approaches; however, a Cochrane review reported positive effects for some interventions, for example, fruit and

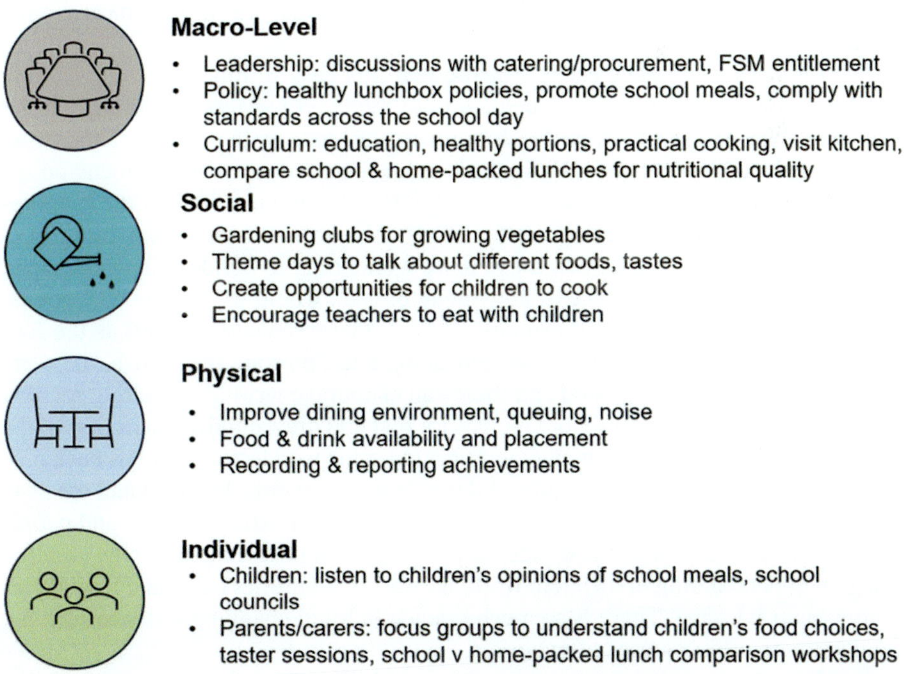


**FIGURE 3.3** An example of a whole-school approach from the School Food Plan. (Reprinted with permission from the School Food Plan and available at www.schoolfoodplan.com.)

vegetable intakes (Langford et al., 2014). The review also advocated for increased collaboration between health and education professionals to examine related outcomes and suggests secondary schools require more attention (Langford et al., 2014). Evaluations considering the longer-term impacts are required to understand the mechanisms of what is effective for individuals and populations (Langford et al., 2017). Although there is limited evidence, it is reasonable to suggest adopting a whole-school approach potentially enables a more consistent system to address children's diets across the school day and develop knowledge and behaviours relevant for their everyday lives (Case Study).

## 3.5 CASE STUDY: A HEAD TEACHERS' RESOLVE TO INCLUDE FOOD ACROSS THE SCHOOL DAY

(By Mr Timothy Baker: Head teacher Charlton Manor school, London, UK)

To include food education as a discrete subject, in an already packed curriculum, is difficult. However, food education is crucial, particularly for young children, so how do we ensure it is something that children learn and is embedded as part of their everyday experience? Food education and healthy eating need to have the same emphasis as English and maths. After all, if you find that maths is not a strength it need not disadvantage you as you can rely on someone else's ability at maths to support you, such as an accountant. On the other hand, making the right choices around eating healthily can only be done by you, and to do this you need to have a good understanding.

Food is part of so many aspects of life that it is easy to link to the curriculum. At Charlton Manor, we link the curriculum to food and use food as the vehicle for including food education. A curriculum area often used with food is maths, fractions of a pizza, for example. With a little more time, we can also put focus on the pizza. We can make the base and ensure it is healthy. We can look at the toppings and discuss the benefits of using certain foods. We can also include how many pepper slices or mushrooms we could use if we were going to divide it between eight, or if only four decided to have it, how many of each would they get now. Cooking in maths can include ratio and proportion, area, measurements, as well as the four operations (addition, subtraction, multiplication, and division). In English, there are many fictional books using food and these can encourage writing. Revolting recipes, for example, can be used to act out recipes for real and draw children in as part of the story. This has encouraged reluctant writers, and some wonderful work has been produced. In history, food can transport children to different eras, from Roman meals to Tudor feasts, the children can understand the influence of different times and people on food choices as well as the divide between rich and poor. In geography, children can gain understanding of different world flavours and families can share food representing their heritage. There is so much science in food: changing states to melting, conduction to different uses of materials.

Food can be included in so many topics, and it is important to do so. It is like writing. By spending time teaching children to hold a pencil properly and write, after a while the focus changes, we expect them to use these skills throughout all the subjects to communicate. In the same way by teaching cutting, grating, and mixing skills as well as other cooking skills, we can develop their confidence so that eventually the focus is not on the individual skill, as it is accepted that they are able to do it but instead on the curriculum area being covered. In this way, it is really teaching children valuable skills and equipping them to make informed choices and have the ability to carry out these choices in their lives outside school.

## 3.6 CONCLUSIONS

This chapter has considered the substantial changes to school food in England, and the different approaches in Japan, Sweden, and Australia. These examples highlight opportunities to learn from different approaches globally to develop best practice in schools, for example, Japan highlights the value given to the school meal as an extension of their education and a time for developing social interaction skills, as well as the potential to offer two savoury courses rather than a mixture of savoury and sweet. Improving school food reduces inequalities in diet through the provision of free or subsidised school food but requires commitment from numerous stakeholders: procurement, catering, teachers, head teachers, parents, and pupils. Globally, more action is required for monitoring, optimising, and evaluating school-based policies to ensure equitable improvements in children's diets and health.

## REFERENCES


Adamson, A., Spence, S., Reed, L., Conway, R., Palmer, A., Stewart, E., Mcbratney, J., Carter, L., Beattie, S. & Nelson, M. 2013. School food standards in the UK—Implementation and evaluation. *Public Health Nutrition*, 16, pp. 968–981.

Adolphus, K., Lawton, C. L., Champ, C. L. & Dye, L. 2016. The effects of breakfast and breakfast composition on cognition in children and adolescents—A systematic review. *Advances in Nutrition*, 7, pp. 590s–612s.

Adolphus, K., Lawton, C. L. & Dye, L. 2013. The effects of breakfast on behavior and academic performance in children and adolescents. *Frontiers in Human Neuroscience*, 7, pp. 425.

Alex-Petersen, J., Lundborg, P. & Rooth, D.-O. 2018. *Long-term effects of childhood nutrition—Evidence from a school lunch reform*. IZA Discussion Paper No. 11234.

Australian Government Department of Health. 2014. *Guidelines for healthy foods and drinks supplied in school canteens*, Commonwealth of Australia, Canberra ACT [Online]. Available https://www.health.gov.au/resources/publications/national-healthy-school-canteens-guidelines-for-healthy-foods-and-drinks-supplied-in-school-canteens [Accessed 25th June 2021].

Bathgate, K. & Begley, A. 2011. 'It's very hard to find what to put in the kid's lunch'—What Perth parents think about food for school lunch boxes. *Nutrition & Dietetics*, 68, pp. 21–26.

Broers, V. J. V., De Breucker, C., Van Den Broucke, S. & Luminet, O. 2017. A systematic review and meta-analysis of the effectiveness of nudging to increase fruit and vegetable choice. *European Journal of Public Health*, 27, pp. 912–920.

Coulthard, J. D., Palla, L. & Pot, G. K. 2017. Breakfast consumption and nutrient intakes in 4–18-year-olds—UK National Diet and Nutrition Survey Rolling Programme (2008–2012). *British Journal of Nutrition*, 118, pp. 280–290.

Dana, L., Jongenelis, M., Sapountsis, N. & Pettigrew, S. 2019. *Implementation of classroom fruit and vegetable breaks in Western Australian Primary Schools.* WA Cancer Prevention Research Unit (WACPRU), Curtin University, Perth.

Davies, S. 2019. *Time to solve childhood obesity.* Department of Health Social Care.

Davis, J., Spaniol, M. & Somerset, S. 2015. Sustenance and sustainability—Maximizing the impact of school gardens on health outcomes. *Public Health Nutrition*, 18, pp. 2358–2367.

Department for Education. 2014. *Revised standards for food in schools—Government response to the consultation on revised school food standards* [Online]. Available https://www.gov.uk/government/consultations/revised-standards-for-food-in-schools--2 [Accessed 18th June 2021].

Deshmukh-Taskar, P. R., Nicklas, T. A., O'Neil, C. E., Keast, D. R., Radcliffe, J. D. & Cho, S. 2010. The relationship of breakfast skipping and type of breakfast consumption with nutrient intake and weight status in children and adolescents—The National Health and Nutrition Examination Survey 1999–2006. *Journal of the American Dietetic Association,* 110, pp. 869–878.

Eustachio Colombo, P., Patterson, E., Elinder, L. S. & Lindroos, A. K. 2020. The importance of school lunches to the overall dietary intake of children in Sweden—A nationally representative study. *Public Health Nutrition*, 23, pp. 1705–1715.

Evans, C. E. L., Christian, M. S., Cleghorn, C. L., Greenwood, D. C. & Cade, J. E. 2012. Systematic review and meta-analysis of school-based interventions to improve daily fruit and vegetable intake in children aged 5 to 12y. *The American Journal of Clinical Nutrition,* 96, pp. 889–901.

Evans, C. E. L., Greenwood, D. C., Thomas, J. D. & Cade, J. E. 2010. A cross-sectional survey of children's packed lunches in the UK—Food- and nutrient-based results. *Journal of Epidemiology and Community Health*, 64, pp. 977–983.

Evans, C. E. L. & Harper, C. 2009. A history and review of school meal standards in the UK. *Journal of Human Nutrition and Dietetics*, 22, pp. 89–99.

Evans, C. E. L., Mandl, V., Christian, M. S. & Cade, J. E. 2015. Impact of school lunch type on nutritional quality of English children's diets. *Public Health Nutrition*, 19, pp. 36–45.

Food for Life. 2019. *State of the Nation—Children's food in England.* London. Available https://www.foodforlife.org.uk/whats-happening/state-of-the-nation [Accessed 10 November 2021].

GOV.UK. 2020. *Apply for free school meals* [Online]. Available https://www.gov.uk/apply-free-school-meals [Accessed 8 May 2020].

Hallström, L., Vereecken, C. A., Ruiz, J. R., Patterson, E., Gilbert, C. C., Catasta, G., Díaz, L.-E., Gómez-Martínez, S., González Gross, M., Gottrand, F., Hegyi, A., Lehoux, C., Mouratidou, T., Widham, K., Aström, A., Moreno, L. A. & Sjöström, M. 2011. Breakfast habits and factors influencing food choices at breakfast in relation to socio-demographic and family factors among European adolescents. The HELENA Study. *Appetite*, 56, pp. 649–657.

Hughes, R., Edwards, K., Clarke, G., Evans, C., Cade, J. & Ransley, J. 2012. Childhood consumption of fruit and vegetables across England—A study of 2306 6–7-year-olds in 2007. *British Journal of Nutrition*, 108, pp. 733–742.

Jones, M., Pitt, H., Oxford, L., Bray, I., Kimberlee, R. & Orme, J. 2015. *Pupil survey in local commission areas—Food for Life's impact on primary school children's consumption of fruit and vegetables.* UWE, Bristol.

Kothe, E. & Mullan, B. 2011. Increasing the frequency of breakfast consumption. *British Food Journal*, 113, pp. 784–796.

Langford, R., Bonell, C., Komro, K., Murphy, S., Magnus, D., Waters, E., Gibbs, L. F. & Campbell, R. 2017. The Health promoting schools framework—Known unknowns and an agenda for future research. *Health Education & Behavior*, 44, pp. 463–475.

Langford, R., Bonell, C. P., Jones, H. E., Pouliou, T., Murphy, S. M., Waters, E., Komro, K. A., Gibbs, L. F., Magnus, D. & Campbell, R. 2014. The WHO health promoting school framework for improving the health and well-being of students and their academic achievement. Cochrane Database of Systematic Reviews. Issue 4. Art. No.: CD008958. doi: 10.1002/14651858.CD008958.pub2.

Lawlis, T., Knox, M. & Jamieson, M. 2016. School canteens—A systematic review of the policy, perceptions and use from an Australian perspective. *Nutrition & Dietetics*, 73, pp. 389–398.

Lucas, P. J., Patterson, E., Sacks, G., Billich, N. & Evans, C. E. L. 2017. Preschool and school meal policies—An overview of what we know about regulation, implementation, and impact on diet in the UK, Sweden, and Australia. *Nutrients*, 9, p. 736.

Meeyoung, K., Satoko, A., Chengyu, Z., Soyoung, K., Jiyu, C., Emely, H., Miho, N. & Jihyun, Y. 2017. Comparison of the nutrient-based standards for school lunches among South Korea, Japan, and Taiwan [online]. *Asia Pacific Journal of Clinical Nutrition*, 26, pp. 160–168.

Miyawaki, A., Lee, J. S. & Kobayashi, Y. 2019. Impact of the school lunch program on overweight and obesity among junior high school students—A nationwide study in Japan. *Journal of Public Health*, 41, pp. 362–370.

Mullan, B., Wong, C. & Kothe, E. 2013. Predicting adolescent breakfast consumption in the UK and Australia using an extended theory of planned behaviour. *Appetite*, 62, pp. 127–132.

Murphy, S., Moore, G. F., Tapper, K., Lynch, R., Clarke, R., Raisanen, L., Desousa, C. & Moore, L. 2011. Free healthy breakfasts in primary schools—A cluster randomised controlled trial of a policy intervention in Wales, UK. *Public Health Nutrition*, 14, pp. 219–226.

Myers, G., Wright, S., Blane, S., Pratt, I. S. & Pettigrew, S. 2018. A process and outcome evaluation of an in-class vegetable promotion program. *Appetite*, 125, pp. 182–189.

Nathan, N., Janssen, L., Sutherland, R., Hodder, R. K., Evans, C. E., Booth, D., Yoong, S. L., Reilly, K., Finch, M. & Wolfenden, L. 2019. The effectiveness of lunchbox interventions on improving the foods and beverages packed and consumed by children at centre-based care or school—A systematic review and meta-analysis. *International Journal of Behavioral Nutrition and Physical Activity*, 16, 38.

Nelson, M., Lowes, K. & Hwang, V. 2007. The contribution of school meals to food consumption and nutrient intakes of young people aged 4–18 years in England. *Public Health Nutrition*, 10, pp. 652–662.

Nicholas, J., Wood, S., Harper, C. & Nelson, M. 2013. The impact of the food-based and nutrient-based standards on lunchtime food and drink provision and consumption in secondary schools in England. *Public Health Nutrition*, 16, pp. 1052–1065.

Ohly, H., Gentry, S., Wigglesworth, R., Bethel, A., Lovell, R. & Garside, R. 2016. A systematic review of the health and well-being impacts of school gardening—Synthesis of quantitative and qualitative evidence. *BMC Public Health*, 16, p. 286.

Osowski Persson, C. 2012. The Swedish school meal as a public meal—Collective thinking, actions and meal patterns. PhD, Uppsala University.

Patterson, E. & Elinder, L. S. 2015. Improvements in school meal quality in Sweden after the introduction of new legislation-a 2-year follow-up. *European Journal of Public Health*, 25, pp. 655–660.

Patterson, E., Quetel, A.-K., Lilja, K., Simma, M., Olsson, L. & Elinder, L. S. 2013. Design, testing and validation of an innovative web-based instrument to evaluate school meal quality. *Public Health Nutrition*, 16, pp. 1028–1036.

Pearce, J., Harper, C., Haroun, D., Wood, L. & Nelson, M. 2011. Key differences between school lunches and packed lunches in primary schools in England in 2009. *Public Health Nutrition*, 14, pp. 1507–1510.

Sanigorski, A., Bell, A., Kremer, P. & Swinburn, B. 2005. Lunchbox contents of Australian school children—Room for improvement. *European Journal of Clinical Nutrition*, 59, pp. 1310–1316.

School Meals Review Panel. 2005. Turning the Tables. Transforming School Food—A report on the development and implementation of nutritional standards for school lunches. Department for Education and Skills.

Spence, D. 2005. Jamie's School Dinners. *British Medical Journal,* 330, 678.

Spence, S., Delve, J., Stamp, E., Matthews, J. N. S., White, M. & Adamson, A. J. 2013. The impact of food and nutrient-based standards on primary school children's lunch and total dietary intake—A natural experimental evaluation of government policy in England. *PLOS ONE*, 8(10), e78298.

Sutherland, R., Nathan, N., Brown, A., Yoong, S., Reynolds, R., Walton, A., Janssen, L., Desmet, C., Lecathelinais, C. & Gillham, K. 2020. A cross-sectional study to determine the energy density and nutritional quality of primary-school children's lunchboxes. *Public Health Nutrition*, 23, pp. 1108–1116.

Swedish Food Agency. 2019. *Bra måltider I skolan [Good meals in school]* [Online]. Available https://www.livsmedelsverket.se/globalassets/publikationsdatabas/broschyrer-foldrar/bra-maltider-i-skolan.pdf [Accessed 2019].

Tanaka, N. & Miyoshi, M. 2012. School lunch program for health promotion among children in Japan. *Asia Pacific Journal of Clinical Nutrition*, 21, pp. 155–158.

The Education Act. 2008. *The education (nutritional standards and requirements for school food) (England) (amendment) regulations 2008* [Online]. Available http://www.opsi.gov.uk/si/si2008/pdf/uksi_20081800_en.pdf [Accessed 28 March 2012].

van Cauwenberghe, E., Maes, L., Spittaels, H., Van Lenthe, F., Brug, J., Oppert, J. & De Bourdeaudhuij, I. 2010. Effectiveness of school-based interventions in Europe to promote healthy nutrition in children and adolescents—Systematic review of published and 'grey' literature. *British Journal of Nutrition*, 103, pp. 781–797.

Vereecken, C., Dupuy, M., Rasmussen, M., Kelly, C., Nansel, T. R., Al Sabbah, H., Baldassari, D., Jordan, M. D., Maes, L., Niclasen, B. V. & Ahluwalia, N. 2009. Breakfast consumption and its socio-demographic and lifestyle correlates in schoolchildren in 41 countries participating in the HBSC study. *International Journal of Public Health*, 54 Suppl 2, pp. 180–190.

Webster, C. 1985. Health, welfare and unemployment during the depression. *Past & Present*, 109, pp. 204–230.

Weitkamp, E., Jones, M., Salmon, D, Kimberlee, R. & Orme, J. 2013. Creating a learning environment to promote food sustainability issues in primary schools? Staff perceptions of implementing the food for life partnership programme. *Sustainability*, 5, pp. 1128–1140.

WHO. 2014. *School and youth health—What is a health promoting school?* [Online]. Available https://www.who.int/health-topics/health-promoting-schools#tab=tab_1 [Accessed 10 November 2021].

Woods, J., Bressan, A., Langelaan, C., Mallon, A. & Palermo, C. 2014. Australian school canteens—Menu guideline adherence or avoidance? *Health Promotion Journal of Australia*, 25, pp. 110–115.

Yamaguchi, M., Kondo, N. & Hashimoto, H. 2018. Universal school lunch programme closes a socioeconomic gap in fruit and vegetable intakes among school children in Japan. *European Journal of Public Health*, 28, pp. 636–641.

Zarnowiecki, D., Mauch, C. E., Middleton, G., Matwiejczyk, L., Watson, W. L., Dibbs, J., Dessaix, A. & Golley, R. K. 2020. A systematic evaluation of digital nutrition promotion websites and apps for supporting parents to influence children's nutrition. *International Journal of Behavioral Nutrition and Physical Activity*, 17, 17.

# 4 The Workplace Food Environment

*Heather M. Padilla*
University of Georgia

*Enid C. Roemer*
Johns Hopkins Bloomberg School of Public Health

*Rachel E. McCardel and David M. DeJoy*
University of Georgia

**CONTENTS**



## 4.1 INTRODUCTION

Work and food have always been connected. Throughout human history, people have worked in order to eat, either by growing, gathering, or bartering for foodstuffs, or by performing various tasks in return for payment with which to purchase food. With widespread industrialisation and urbanisation, more and more people entered the paid labour force and went off to work. As people began spending large portions of their waking hours at their work locations, these locations became food environments, that is, workers needed to eat during the workday. Prior to the early 20th

DOI: 10.1201/9781003043720-4

century, workdays of 10–12 hours were quite common, as was the 6-day workweek. In the U.S., it was not until the *Fair Labor Standards Act of 1938* was amended in 1940 that the 40-hour workweek became the "law of the land" (U.S. Wage and Hour Division 2011).

Certain employment sectors, such as health care and public safety, have long operated 24 hours a day, 7 days per week. In these settings, employees typically work shifts (e.g., day, evening, or night shifts), sometimes rotating among the different shifts. Technological advances, from the steam engine to the light bulb, to the internet, have boosted productivity and altered when, how, and where people work, but they have not substantially reduced the amount of time people spend working. Even today, most adults spend the majority of their waking hours at work and consume about 1/3 of their daily caloric intake at work (Hartline-Grafton et al. 2010; Lima, Costa & Rocha 2018).

The most basic element of the workplace food environment is time: time to eat free from job duties. In many instances, this is unpaid time; in other instances, it is paid time. Having some physical place to eat is also basic. Some worksites provide facilities for storing and/or preparing food, while others feature onsite cafeterias or other food venues. Cafeterias are frequently associated with remote work locations, large workforces, multiple work shifts, and work settings where it is advantageous to keep employees on location.

The 1970s marked the advent of workplace health promotion programmes in the U.S. that coincided with increasing awareness of the burden of preventable disease and deaths attributable to lifestyle factors and the creation of the Office of Disease Prevention and Health Promotion (ODPHP). In the years following, worksite wellness studies began to appear in the peer-reviewed and published literature. These studies reported that comprehensive worksite wellness programmes resulted in health care costs savings and improved productivity (e.g., Bly, Jones & Richardson 1986; Bertera 1990). Early programmes tended to focus on informational or educational offerings, frequently combined with health risk assessments and/or biometric screenings but did not pay much direct attention to the food environment. As these programmes have expanded and matured, more attention has been given to formalised behaviour change initiatives in areas such as physical activity and nutrition/weight management (DeJoy et al. 2014) and to the implementation of comprehensive or multi-component programming, including the use of policy and environmental actions to facilitate and support programme objectives (Kent et al. 2016; Pelletier 2005; Terry et al. 2008).

Comprehensive and multi-component programmes often make use of social-ecological or multi-level conceptual models to guide programme development (McLeroy et al. 1988). Story et al. (2008) have proposed an ecological framework specific to food environments (see Chapter 1).

In this chapter, we adapt Story's model to be specific to workplace food environments (see Figure 4.1). This modified framework provides a useful basis for examining the complex interrelationships between the behavioural and environmental factors that interact and comprise the workplace food environment. Figure 4.1 includes the individual worker, the demands or requirement of specific jobs or work assignments, and three environmental contexts linked to eating behaviours: social environments, physical environments, and macro-level or extra-organisational environments.

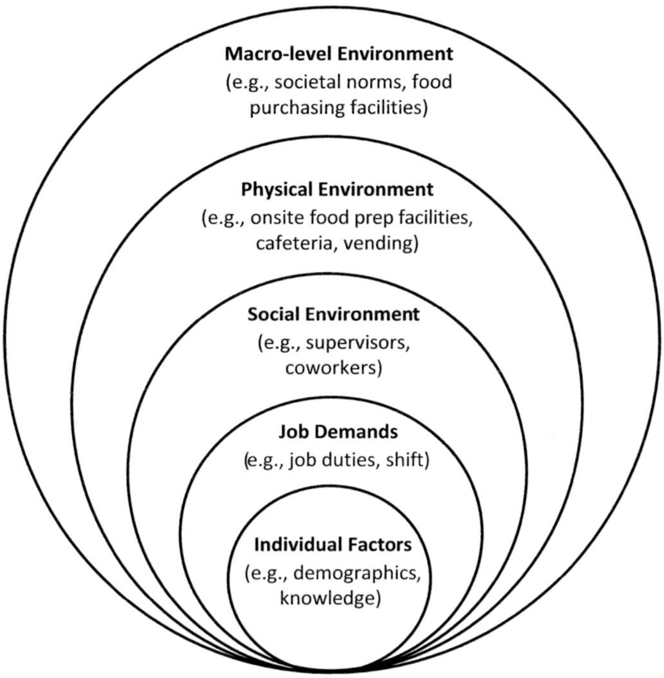


**FIGURE 4.1** Ecological model of the workplace food environment. (Adapted from Story et al. 2008 (see Figure 1.2).)

We define the workplace food environment as foods and beverages in the worksite including vending machines, cafeterias, foods offered at meetings/special occasions, snack bars, canteens, and kitchens along with the physical and social supports in the environment that affect an employee's ability to choose and consume healthy options. The remainder of this chapter discusses and critiques research and practice pertinent to food access at work, food, and dietary-related programming in work settings and current best practice guidelines. The chapter concludes by addressing future trends in workplace food-related research and policy.

## 4.2 FOOD PROVISION AT WORK

The workplace has various avenues through which foods and beverages may be obtained. Some of those are onsite and presumably controlled by the employer such as vending, cafeteria, foods served at events, and onsite markets. However, these provisions often require the worksite to coordinate what, when, and how foods are provided with vendors and contractors. Additionally, there are other sources of foods and beverages in the workplace that are not under direct control of the employer but may be influenced by the worksite culture including coworkers bringing food to share, employees bringing in their own food, and various business dinners or shared meals. In addition to providing food, worksites may be equipped with facilities for food preparation or consumption (e.g., microwave ovens, sinks,

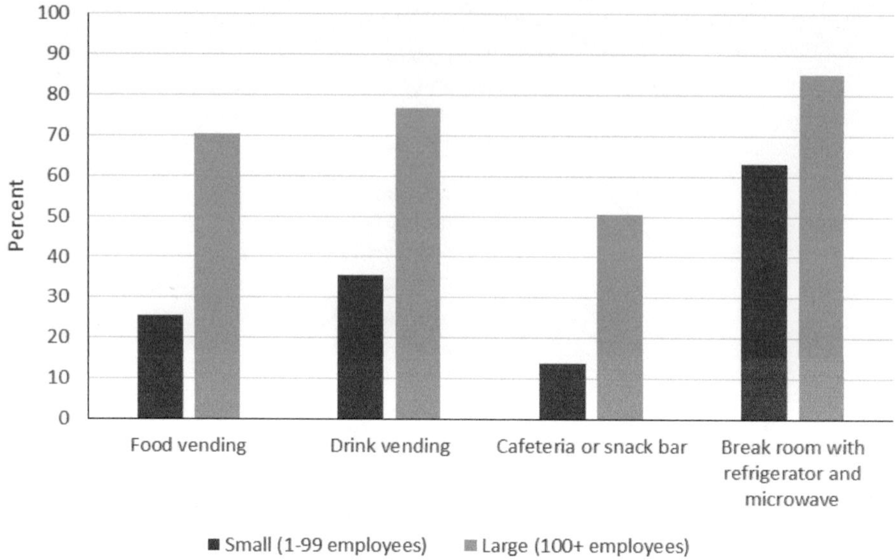


**FIGURE 4.2** Availability of food provisions in U.S. worksites reported by employees in the 2013 Consumer Styles Survey. (Data from Onufrak et al. 2018.)

refrigerators, tables, and chairs) and access to water through water fountains or bottle filling stations.

Not all resources are available to all workers. Access to food, beverages, and preparation facilities varies by worksite, employer, and, in some cases, by work shift and job category or classification. In the U.S., the most commonly provided provision for employees is access to a breakroom with a refrigerator and microwave (Onufrak et al. 2018). A majority of workers (61%) also report water access through a fountain, cooler, or filtered water station. Drink vending machines are reportedly available to about half of employed adults (54%), with access to food/snack/candy vending machines less common (45%) and even fewer worksites providing access to cafeterias or snack bars (30%). All provisions are more frequently reported by employees who work for worksites with more than 100 employees. Figure 4.2 shows the availability of food sources in U.S. worksites by small and large employers. In the U.S., nearly half of employed adults work for small businesses leaving significant gaps in access to food provisions for many workers (U.S. Small Business Administration Office of Advocacy 2019).

With the variability in food availability in the workplace, it is not surprising that workers often bring food from home, obtain food from nearby restaurants or stores, or, in some cases, return home for meals. Where food is obtained and consumed is influenced by geographic culture and location (macro-level environment) in addition to job demands and the social and physical environment of the worksite. A significant factor in both where food is obtained and consumed is the length of the meal break. In a survey of European workers from ten different countries, the mean lunch break was 37 minutes and varied significantly from 30 to 56 minutes (Corvo, Fontefrancesco & Matacena 2020). The timing of the break can vary across and within organisations as those with more flexible work arrangements often have more control over the timing and length of their meals break. In the same survey of European workers, 31% reported the ability to completely control the timing and length of lunch breaks while 28% reported no control of their meal breaks (Corvo, Fontefrancesco & Matacena 2020). Women, young persons, people belonging to lower income groups, and shift workers in factories, warehouses, and call-centres were more likely to report lack of control over meal breaks, highlighting disparities and inequities in having adequate time to source and consume food at work (Corvo, Fontefrancesco & Matacena 2020). For example, 34% of females surveyed by Corvo and colleagues (2020) reported no control over the timing or length of their meal breaks compared to 24% of males.

In the U.S., approximately 16.5 million people obtain food at work three or more times per week (Onufrak et al. 2019). More workers (20%) report receiving free food and beverages than those who reported purchasing food and beverages at work (10%) (Onufrak et al. 2019). College graduates were twice as likely to receive free food at work as employees with less than a high school education (Onufrak et al. 2019). While free food at work is associated with increased feelings of value and appreciation, employees also report that free foods make it harder to control their weight (Baskin et al. 2016).

According to a study by Corvo, Fontefrancesco, and Matacena (2020) on the food environment in Europe, a large portion of workers bring their lunch from home (42%) while fewer (20%) obtain their food from an onsite restaurant or cafeteria though there are variations by country. For example, 30% of workers in France indicated that they typically obtained their lunch from a restaurant or cafeteria compared to only 12% of workers in the United Kingdom. Price was the most influential factor in where lunch is purchased followed by value for money, quality/freshness of food, convenience of location, and variety and choice offered. Fewer than 10% of workers surveyed indicated that the provision of healthy options was important in where they chose to purchase their meal. When choosing what to eat, the healthiness becomes more important but taste, price, and value for money remain top factors for what working adults choose to eat (Corvo, Fontefrancesco & Matacena 2020).

Lunch and snacks are the most commonly consumed food in the workplace (Onufrak et al. 2019). Although food may be frequently brought from home, many employees eat in the workplace – in a break area (31%), at their desk (17%), or in an onsite cafeteria (16%) (Corvo, Fontefrancesco & Matacena 2020). A majority of employees eat with friends at work or their colleagues (Corvo, Fontefrancesco & Matacena 2020). As such, worksite cafeterias are much more than places to purchase food. In fact, they can be viewed as places that foster camaraderie and wellbeing at work by providing opportunities for socialisation, informal problem-solving, and work efficiency (Corvo, Fontefrancesco & Matacena 2020).

In many places, healthy foods in the workplace are the exception rather than the rule. In U.S.-based surveys conducted by Onufrak and colleagues (2018, 2019), fewer than 20% of employees reported that their employer provided opportunities to eat healthy. Nearly half of the foods obtained at work were coffee, regular soft drinks, sandwiches, tap water, tea, diet soft drinks, cookies and brownies, lettuce salad, French fries, and potato chips. These foods are low in nutritional quality and high in calories, particularly calories from solid fats and sugars. Additionally, many of these foods are high in sodium. For employees who reported access to cafeterias, slightly more than half (56.5%) reported healthy items comprising anywhere between 10% and 50% of offerings. As was the case with access to food provisions at work, employees working for companies with 100+ employees were more likely to indicate that their employer provided healthy choices (26.3%) compared to workers at companies with fewer than 100 employees (14.3%). Free drinking water on every floor was quite common with both large (71%) and smaller employers (52.2%). However, nearly 2/3 of employees reported few or no healthy items in vending machines and fewer than 5% reported that more than 50% of vending options were healthy (Onufrak et al. 2018).

## 4.3 HEALTHY WORK-BASED PROGRAMMES

Employers can promote employee health by providing healthy food options that are accessible, affordable, and convenient. Providing healthy foods often starts with a worksite policy that sets the expectation for such offerings in the worksite. Policies, when effectively implemented, influence both the physical and social environments of the worksite, and when combined with environmental interventions ensure that healthy foods are available, affordable, and easy to identify. When these strategies are combined with educational materials and programmes that promote and teach healthy eating, they impact the individual level in addition to the social and physical environments of the workplace (Figure 4.1; Nicholls et al. 2017). This comprehensive workplace approach of combining policy, environmental, and individual strategies for healthy eating has stronger evidence for effectiveness than policy and environmental interventions alone (Kahn-Marshall & Gallant 2012).

### 4.3.1 Trends in Workplace Programmes in the United States

The 2017 Workplace Health in America survey reports that, in the U.S., healthy eating programmes are the second most common type of health promotion programme offered at worksites (Centers for Disease Control and Prevention [CDC] 2018). Workplace programmes typically encourage employees to increase fruit and vegetable consumption, decrease fat or sugar, and reduce salt (Kahn-Marshall & Gallant 2012; Geaney et al. 2011). Workplace strategies to improve the food environment have included point-of-purchase calorie labelling, increased availability of healthy options in vending machines, price reductions of healthy options, catering policies to increase healthy foods and beverages at business events, and nutrition messaging to encourage purchase or consumption of healthy items (Kahn-Marshall & Gallant 2012). However, most programmes offered in the workplace are informational-only (43%) or a combination of information and skill-building (53%) and unfortunately, only a small percentage of worksites (10%) report policies for making healthier foods and beverages available (CDC 2018).

Generally, workplace programmes that target the workplace food environment in terms of access or price have resulted in positive effects. Access to fruits and vegetables; coworker support for a low-fat diet; and increased intake of healthy foods including whole grains, fruits, and vegetables; and low-fat milk products has been reported (Kahn-Marshall & Gallant 2012) and price reductions of 25%–50% for

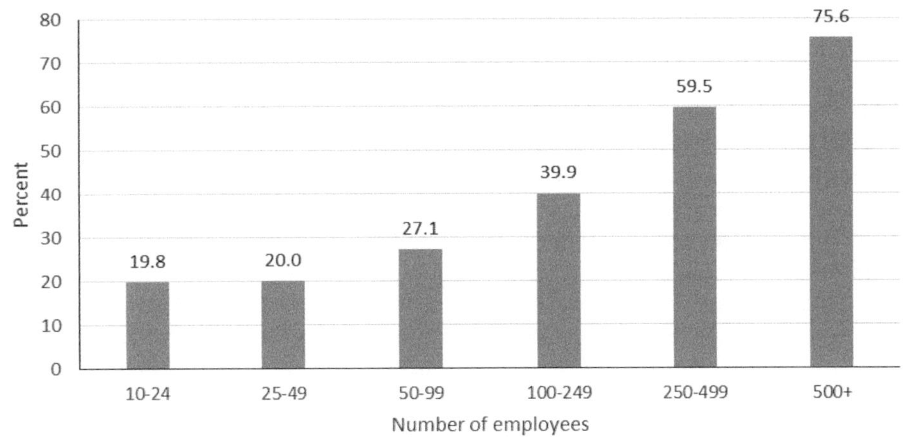


**FIGURE 4.3** Percentage of worksites in the U.S. (based on weighted estimates) that reported a nutrition programme in the 2017 Workplace Health in America survey, by worksite size. (Adapted from CDC 2018.)

healthy foods in vending machines have been associated with increased low-fat snack sales (Kahn-Marshall & Gallant 2012). Interventions informed by choice architecture, where snacks were placed in less convenient locations away from beverage stations, were shown to reduce consumption of free snacks that are usually high in fats, sugars, and salt (Baskin et al. 2016). Such interventions provide promising strategies for employers who want to offer free foods to increase employee satisfaction but want to minimise the likelihood of increasing consumption of calories among employees. More information on choice architecture is provided in Chapter 15.

As is the case with access to foods, there is significant variation in the availability of programmes by worksite size, with a higher proportion of the largest employers (>500 employees) reporting that they offer programmes (76%) and significantly fewer small employers (10–49 employees) doing so (20%) (CDC 2018). Figure 4.3 shows the proportion of employers offering various nutrition programmes by worksite size. For example, signs and labels in cafeterias and vending areas were reported by 21% of large employers compared to only 10% of small employers. Similar patterns were observed with healthy food and drink choices at meetings – 24% of larger companies provided healthy choices compared to only 14% of smaller companies. Twenty-four percent of large employers provided information on nutrition and healthy eating in the form of posters, flyers, brochures, and classes compared to 7% of small employers.

In addition to worksite size, there are disparities by industry with a higher percentage of worksites in the hospital and public administration sectors offering nutrition programmes (CDC 2018).

### 4.3.2 Trends in Workplace Programmes in Japan

Japan is unique in that it requires employers to take on an active role in delivering public health interventions that range from administering health exams to behavioural programmes (Organisation for Economic Cooperation and Development

[OECD] 2019). These expectations are set forth in the *Japanese Industrial Safety and Health Act of 1972* that requires health promotion in the workplace to be developed in cooperation with employees and takes into account both physical and mental health. Additionally, employers are incentivised to offer workplace-based programmes that are voluntary (OECD 2019). Similar to the U.S., there is variation in interventions across employers with larger employers more likely to implement a comprehensive program (OECD 2019). In particular, employees who work for companies with fewer than 50 employees may not have access to the same benefits. Employers are required to provide full-time employees with a health exam and, likewise, employees are required to participate. As such, participation in health exams is quite high. Workplace health promotion programmes include physical environment changes in the workplace to improve diet; however, there is significant variability among these programmes based on the size of the organisation and the type of environment including whether canteens are on premises (OECD 2019). Also, employee participation in the voluntary programmes is largely unknown.

### 4.3.3 Trends in Workplace Programmes in Ireland

In an example of a comprehensive programme in Ireland, an intervention that altered food preparation procedures in the canteen, limited oil and salt, provided substitutes for high fat and salt products (e.g., processed meats), offered fruit-based desserts, and posted messages encouraging salt reduction and healthy eating was successful in reducing the consumption of sugars, total fat, saturated fat, and salt (Geaney et al. 2011).

### 4.3.4 Worksite Programmes in Low- and Middle-Income Countries

Only more recently (in the past decade) are we beginning to see published evaluation of worksite-based nutrition interventions and food choices of various of types of workers in low/middle-income countries.

Similar to more industrialised countries, there is evidence that worksites in South Africa that have wellness facilities and intervention programmes targeting employee dietary habits have a higher proportion of employees meeting dietary recommendations of eating five or more servings of fruits and vegetables per day compared with companies without such supportive food environments (Kolbe-Alexander et al. 2014). One recent study involving South African construction workers found multiple factors beyond nutritional knowledge that influence food choice, including cultural background (e.g., familiar, "traditional" foods), economics (e.g., affordability), environment (e.g., marketing/packaging), psychological (e.g., mood), and physiological (e.g., taste) factors (Okoro, Musonda & Agumba 2017). In another study on organisational and individual-level facilitators and barriers to provision and consumption of healthier foods at worksite canteens in China, researchers found again that several other factors influenced food choice more than nutritional value, including taste, trust of food quality, and cost (Li et al. 2018). More interesting is that the study found that workers differentiated the concepts of "eating well" and "eating healthy", and that traditional, familiar foods, and unhealthy foods that were perceived as tastier proved to be stronger influencers on dietary behaviours at work. Li et al. (2018) created a conceptual framework based on the ecological model that highlights the balance between the individual, organisational, and regional factors that influence the social and physical workplace food environment in China.

Best practices established in industrialised countries may not apply to low- or middle-income countries. In short, it is important to understand cultural context, values, and unique work environments to be able to better target opportunities to improve the nutritional health of all employees through tailored messages and education strategies.

## 4.4 BEST PRACTICE CASE STUDY EXAMPLE

Below, we present an example of an organisation that has taken a best practice approach to creating workplace food environments where the healthy choice is also the easy choice. The example is a comprehensive, socio-ecological approach in a U.S. company that targets different levels of the workplace food environment addressing the individual worker with consideration to their job demands and the social and physical environment.

### 4.4.1 Case Study: Edwards Lifesciences, U.S.

Edwards Lifesciences (Edwards) is a manufacturing company that produces patient-focused medical innovations for structural heart disease, critical care, and surgical monitoring. Headquartered in Irvine, California, U.S., Edwards has more than 40 offices and manufacturing centres in North America, Europe, Africa, and Asia. There are approximately 4,000 employees at headquarters and 12,000 globally.

*Total Health* is the company's wellness programme that focuses on six pillars of health and has received multiple workplace health awards.[1] Nutrition is one of the pillars. The food environment includes best practices in the areas of education, strategic communications, access and availability of healthy food choices, social and physical environmental supports, and measurement and evaluation. In addition to providing point of decision health information and using multiple modalities to inform employees about programme offerings, events, and resources, *Total Health* has tailored the access and availability of healthy foods to the specific needs and interests of its employees. To accommodate a variety of diets, the onsite café has numerous healthy options, including vegetarian, vegan, gluten-free, and organic options, salad and soup, hot food, and sandwich stations. Furthermore, the prices are affordable. Unhealthy options such as fries and soda are strategically placed at the back of the café.

The physical environment includes breakrooms that provide coffee, tea, water, refrigerators, and microwaves. There are also plenty of inviting indoor café seating, and outdoor shaded tables and benches to encourage employees to fully enjoy their meal breaks away from their workstations. In terms of the social environment,

[1] For more information on Edwards Lifesciences' program see: https://www.cdc.gov/workplacehealthpromotion/initiatives/resource-center/case-studies/case-study-edwards-lifesciences.html.

managers hold weekly dialogues with employees to share wellness updates. Employees also receive motivational messages from senior executives to stay healthy. Finally, the company routinely keeps track of health risks, participation rates, and satisfaction to see how programmes can be improved. For example, based on employee feedback, breakfast salad options were added to the menu to meet demands of the night shift for more lunch-like foods when they clock out. They also offer healthy grab-and-go dinner options to take home at the end of the workday. These strategies represent a comprehensive approach to addressing the food environment and make the healthy choice the easy choice.

## 4.5 IMPLICATIONS FOR FUTURE OF WORKPLACE FOOD ENVIRONMENT RESEARCH AND POLICY

The workplace landscape is rapidly changing in terms of the make-up of the workforce and how and where work is performed. The workforce is aging and becoming more diverse in most developed societies. Flexible work and nonstandard work arrangement are becoming more common. Workplace policies and practices specific to the food environment will need to follow these trends and adapt to encourage all workers to consume healthy foods and beverages and support their efforts to do so. The ecological model presented in Figure 4.1 can guide interventions to address multiple levels of the workplace food environment in this changing landscape.

### 4.5.1 Aging Workforce

In most industrialised countries, the workforce is aging. According to the U.S. Bureau of Labor Statistics (2016), labor force participation by those 55+ has been on the rise since 1996. Globally, those 65 and older are the fastest growing age group and one in six people in the world will be over age 65 by 2050 (United Nations n.d.) (Figure 4.4). Older workers tend to have higher numbers of health/disease risk factors (e.g., weight gain) and co-morbid conditions (e.g., type 2 diabetes, obesity, hypertension) (Hymel et al. 2011). Studies of workplace wellness programmes supporting employee health have demonstrated that weight management and multiple chronic health conditions (e.g., cardiovascular disease) can be controlled with healthy diets (Anderson et al. 2009; Groeneveld et al. 2010). However, little research currently exists examining which workplace wellbeing programmes and policies are of greatest benefit to older employees. There is a need for integrating knowledge about the ageing process and pertinent behavioural theories to research on workplace interventions, including nutrition/food environmental supports tailored for the older workforce that can effectively support their health and wellbeing (Truxillo, Cadiz & Hammer 2015).

### 4.5.2 Flexible Work Arrangements: Remote and Shift Work

Globally, 62% of employers offer some form of a flexible workplace policy, which may include one or more of the following flexibilities: *scheduling* of hours worked regarding alternative work schedules (e.g., compressed workweek) and arrangement of schedule (e.g., shift and break schedule), *number* of hours worked (e.g., part

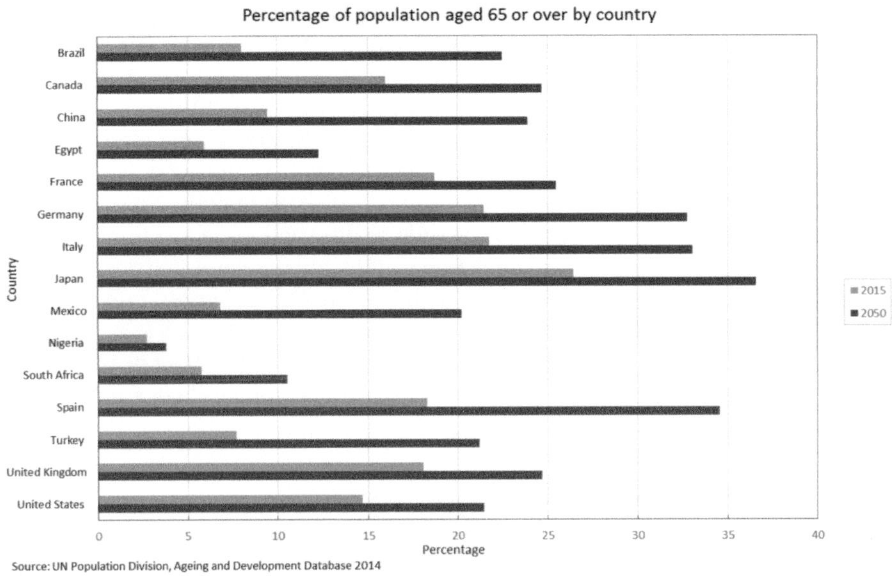


**FIGURE 4.4** Current and projected increases in population aged 65 and older by country. (National Institute for Occupational Safety and Health [NIOSH] 2015.)

time, job sharing), and *place* of work (e.g., home or satellite location). Additionally, 77% of businesses are using flexible workplace policies to attract and retain talent (International Workplace Group 2019). In the U.S., it is estimated that as many as 25% of workers are able to work from home (Baker 2020). Trends towards teleworking have accelerated in the age of the Covid-19 pandemic of 2020/21. Workers who can work from home may not be returning to the workplace full time or at all. This change removes the worker from most of the physical workplace food environment interventions; none of these onsite features are relevant to the remote worker. There will be an increased need for interventions targeting the macro-level environment to support healthy food choices for remote workers. Such interventions would be in addition to the use of strategies onsite as there are many workers who cannot work remotely or take advantage of flexible work arrangements, often even within the same work organisations due to differences in job tasks.

Remote working and other flexible work arrangements create additional barriers to reaching employees with traditional workplace health promotion programmes. As such, there may be an increased reliance on technology-based health promotion programmes and interventions (e.g., websites, apps, telephone-based nutrition consultations) to help employees create healthier food environments and habits. Implementation research will be important for discerning how technological approaches are most effective to support the remote worker.

Work demands and technology have not only made it possible but also increased the need for more shift workers. Shift workers are at a higher risk for a variety of health conditions including chronic fatigue, anxiety, and cardiovascular disease compared to individuals working more typical daytime hours (Morgan et al. 2011).

Moreover, shift work has been found to be an independent predictor of increased body mass index and prevalence of obesity (Atkinson et al. 2008). Shift workers' meal patterns may contribute to these health risks as shift workers eat more, eat their last meal later in the day, and have fewer meals (Nicholls et al. 2017).

A number of organisational barriers exist that make healthy eating more challenging for shift workers. Often onsite food outlets are open only during typical business hours which leave evening and night shift workers with fewer options to purchase food. Thus, it will be even more important to provide healthy options in vending machines, have environmental supports for storage and preparation such as refrigerators and microwaves, and offer tailored individual nutrition/weight loss programmes that are convenient to shift workers' schedule. For shift workers on the go (e.g., share-car drivers, long-haul truckers, delivery service workers), education about healthy preparations and nutritious options in the retail environment to support better eating habits is also an area to be considered growing as part of workplace wellness programming.

## 4.6 EQUITY AND HEALTH DISPARITIES

In the above sections, we have highlighted disparities that exist in access to both food provisions and health promotion programming. Particularly, disparities exist between large and small worksites. In the U.S., small worksites employ nearly half of the U.S workforce (U.S. Small Business Administration Office of Advocacy 2018). Similar trends are found in Europe where more than 50% of workers work for small- or medium-sized organisations (Federal Institute for Occupational Safety and Health 2001). Small worksites in the U.S are more likely than larger worksites to employ workers who earn low wages, and employees who earn low wages are more likely to have low levels of education, identify as a minority race or ethnicity, and have higher levels of health risk (Baron et al. 2014). Implementation research is needed to increase the number of small worksites offering programmes and will likely require financial resources and infrastructure support (Ryan 2017).

## 4.7 CONCLUSIONS

Work organisations are in a unique position to reach a large segment of the adult working population to positively influence adult nutrition behaviours through programmes, policies, and supportive environments. Indeed, the workplace may be the only place some adults are exposed to opportunities for nutrition education, healthy food access and availability, and individual behaviour change programmes. A multilevel, ecological approach is important for understanding the complex relationship between individual behaviour and environmental factors and informing strategies to improve food choices.

Large worksites, in comparison to small worksites, typically have more outlets for food access but not necessarily more healthy foods. However, large worksites are more likely to offer nutrition programmes. Such programmes are often individually focused and lack organisational initiatives to improve the food environment. Policies to promote healthy eating are reported in fewer than 10% of work organisations in the U.S. but may be more or less in other countries. Policies are important for setting the expectation across the organisation and creating a culture of health that is reflected in the social and physical environments as well as programmes that promote individual behaviour change. Multi-component programmes that target the social and physical environments while also providing individual-level programmes have been more effective for improving nutrition in employed adults.

The workplace is uniquely positioned to create a healthy food environment that can mitigate inequities employees may experience within their communities such as food deserts. As the landscape of the workplace changes with increasingly higher numbers of older adults, people with chronic disease, and remote working, implementation research will be critical for advancing our knowledge of what programmes work for employees with varying demographics and needs as well as how to better expand programming to small worksites to make the workplace food environment as equitable as possible.

## REFERENCES

Anderson, LM, Quinn, TA, Glanz, K, Ramirez, G, Kahwati, LC, Johnson, DB, Buchanan, LR, Archer, WR, Chattopadhyay, S, Kalra, GP, & Katz, DL 2009, 'The effectiveness of worksite nutrition and physical interventions for controlling employee overweight and obesity: A systematic review', *American Journal of Preventive Medicine*, vol. 37, no. 4, pp. 340–357.

Atkinson, G, Fullick, S, Grindey, C, & Maclaren, D 2008, 'Exercise, energy balance and the shift worker', *Sports Medicine*, vol. 38, no. 8, pp. 671–685.

Baker, MG 2020, 'Nonrelocatable occupations at increased risk during pandemics--United States, 2018', *American Journal of Public Health*, vol. 110, no. 8, pp. 1126–1132.

Baron, SL, Beard, S, Davis, LK, Delp, L, Forst, L, Kidd-Taylor, A, Liebman, AK, Linnan, L, Punnett, L, & Welch, LS 2014, 'Promoting integrated approaches to reducing health inequities among low-income workers: Applying a social ecological framework', *American Journal of Industrial Medicine*, vol. 57, no. 5, pp. 539–556.

Baskin, E, Gorlin, M, Chance, Z, Novemsky, N, Dhar, R, Huskey, K, & Hatzis, M 2016, 'Proximity of snacks to beverages increases food consumption in the workplace: A field study', *Appetite*, vol. 103, pp. 244–248, doi: 10.1016/j.appet.2016.04.025

Bertera, R 1990, 'The effects of workplace health promotion on absenteeism and employment costs in a large industrialized population', *American Journal of Health Promotion*, vol. 80, no. 9, pp. 1101–1105.

Bly, JL, Jones, RC, and Richardson, JE 1986 'Impact of worksite health promotion on health care costs and utilization: Evaluation of Johnson & Johnson Live for Health program', *Journal of the American Medical Association*, vol. 256, no. 23, pp. 3235–3240.

Centers for Disease Control and Prevention (CDC) 2018, *Workplace health in America 2017*, https://www.cdc.gov/workplacehealthpromotion/data-surveillance/docs/2017-Workplace-Health-in-America-Summary-Report-FINAL-updated-508.pdf.

Corvo, P, Fontefrancesco, MF, & Matacena, R 2020, 'Eating at work: The role of the lunch-break and canteens for wellbeing at work in Europe', *Social Indicators Research*, vol. 150, pp. 1043–1076. doi: 10.1007/s11205-020-02353-4

DeJoy, DM, Dyal, MA, Padilla, HM, & Wilson, MG 2014, 'National workplace health promotion surveys: The Affordable Care Act and future surveys', *American Journal of Health Promotion*, vol. 28, no. 3, pp. 142–145.

Federal Institute for Occupational Safety and Health 2001, *Healthy employees in healthy organizations: The European network for workplace health promotion*, https://www.baua.de/DE/Angebote/Publikationen/Praxis/A29.pdf?__blob=publicationFile.

Geaney, F, Harrington, J, Fitzgerald, AP, & Perry, IJ 2011, 'The impact of a workplace catering initiative on dietary intakes of salt and other nutrients: A pilot study', *Public Health Nutrition,* vol. 14, no. 8. pp. 1345–1349.

Groeneveld, IF, Proper, KI, van der Beek, AJ, Hildebrandt, VH, & van Mechelen, W 2010, 'Lifestyle-focused interventions at the workplace to reduce the risk of cardiovascular disease – a systematic review', *Scandinavian Journal of Work Environment and Health,* vol. 36, no. 3, pp. 202–215, doi: 10.5271/sjweh.2891

Hartline-Grafton, HL, Rose, D, Johnson, CC, Rice, JC, & Webber, LS 2010, 'The Influence of weekday eating patterns on energy intake and BMI among female elementary school personnel', *Obesity*, vol. 18, no. 4, pp. 736–742.

Hymel, PA, Loeppke, RR, Baase, CM, Burton, WN, Hartenbaum, NP, Hudson, TW, McLellan, RK, Mueller, KL, Roberts, MA, Yarborough, CM, Konicki, DL, & Larson, PW 2011, 'Workplace health protection and promotion: A new pathway for a healthier—and safer—workforce', *Journal of Occupational and Environmental Medicine*, vol. 53, no. 6, pp. 695–702, doi: 10.1097/JOM.0b013e31822005d0.

International Workplace Group 2019, *The IWG global workspace survey: Welcome to generation flex-the employee power shift*, https://assets.regus.com/pdfs/iwg-workplace-survey/iwg-workplace-survey-2019.pdf.

Japan 1972, *Japanese Industrial Safety and Health Act 1972, No. 57.*

Kahn-Marshall, JL, & Gallant, MP 2012, 'Making healthy behaviors the easy choice for employees: A review of the literature on environmental and policy changes in worksite health promotion', *Health Education & Behavior*, vol. 39, no. 6, p. 752.

Kent, K, Goetzel, RZ, Roemer, EC, Prasad, A, & Freundlich, N 2016, 'Promoting healthy workplaces by building cultures of health and applying strategic communications', *Journal of Occupational and Environmental Medicine*, vol. 58, no. 2, pp. 114–122.

Kolbe-Alexander, T, Greyling, M, da Silva, R, Milner, K, Patel, D, Wyper, L, Beckowski, M, Lambert, EV, & Goetzel, R 2014, 'The relationship between workplace environment and employee health behaviors in a South African workforce', *Journal of Occupational and Environmental Medicine*, vol. 56, no. 10, pp. 1094 1099, doi: 10.1097/JOM.0000000000000236.

Li, R, Wu, Y, Jing, L, & Jaacks, LM 2018, 'Enablers and barriers to improving worksite canteen nutrition in Pudong, China: A mixed-methods formative research study', *BMJ Open*, vol. 8, no. 4, doi: 10.1136/bmjopen-2017-020529.

Lima, J, Costa, S, & Rocha, A 2018, 'How do university workers eat at the workplace?', *Nutrition & Food Science,* vol. 48, no. 2 pp. 194–205.

McLeroy, KR, Bibeau, D, Steckler, A, & Glanz, K 1988, 'An ecological perspective on health promotion programs', *Health Education & Behavior*, vol. 15, no. 4, pp. 351–377.

Morgan, PJ, Collins, CE, Plotnikoff, RC, Cook, AT, Berthon, B, Mitchell, S, & Callister, R 2011, 'Efficacy of a workplace-based weight loss program for overweight make shift workers: The workplace POWER (Preventing Obesity Without Eating like a Rabbit) randomized controlled trial', *Preventive Medicine,* vol. 52, no. 5, pp. 317–325.

National Institute for Occupational Safety and Health (NIOSH) 2015, *Productive ageing and work*, https://www.cdc.gov/niosh/topics/productiveaging/dataandstatistics.html.

Nicholls, R, Perry, L, Duffield, C, Gallagher, R, & Pierce, H 2017, 'Barriers and facilitators to healthy eating for nurses in the workplace: An integrative review', *Journal of Advanced Nursing*, vol. 73, no. 5, p. 1051, doi: 10.1111/jan.13185.

Organisation for Economic Cooperation and Development (OECD) 2019, *OECD Reviews of Public Health: Japan: A Healthier Tomorrow*, OECD Publishing, Paris. doi: 10.1787/9789264311602-en.

Okoro, CS, Musonda, I, & Agumba, J 2017, 'Evaluating the influence of nutrition determinants on construction workers' food choices', *American Journal of Men's Health*, vol. 11, no. 6, pp. 1713–1727, doi: 10.1177/1557988315625775.

Onufrak, SJ, Watson, KB, Kimmons, J, Pan, L, Khan, LK., Lee-Kwan, SH, & Park, S 2018, 'Worksite food and physical activity environments and wellness supports reported by employed adults in the United States, 2013', *American Journal of Health Promotion*, vol. 32, no. 1, pp. 96–105.

Onufrak, SJ, Zaganjor, H, Pan, L, Lee-Kwan, SH, Park, S, & Harris, DM 2019, 'Foods and beverages obtained at worksites in the United States', *Journal of the Academy of Nutrition & Dietetics*, vol. 119, no. 6, pp. 999–1008, doi: 10.1016/j.jand.2018.11.011.

Pelletier, KR 2005, 'A review and analysis of the clinical and cost-effectiveness studies of comprehensive health promotion and disease management programs at the worksite: Update VI 2000–2004', *Journal of Occupational and Environmental Medicine*, vol. 47, no. 10, pp. 1051–1058.

Ryan, M 2017, 'Special challenges and opportunities for small business', In MP O'Donnell (ed.), *Health Promotion in the Workplace*, 5th edn, CreateSpace Independent Publishing Platform, Troy, MI, pp. 649–661.

Story, M, Kaphingst, KM, Robinson-O'Brien, R, & Glanz, K 2008, 'Creating healthy food and eating environments: Policy and environmental approaches', *Annual Review of Public Health*, vol. 29, pp. 253–272.

Terry, PE, Seaverson, ELD, Grossmeier, J, & Anderson, DR 2008, 'Association between nine quality components and superior worksite health management program results', *Journal of Occupational and Environmental Medicine*, vol. 50, no. 6, pp. 633–641.

Truxillo, DM, Cadiz, DM, & Hammer, LB 2015, 'Supporting the aging workforce: A review and recommendations for workplace intervention', *Annual Review of Organizational Psychology & Organizational Behavior*, vol. 2, pp. 351–381.

United Nations n.d., *Ageing*, https://www.un.org/en/global-issues/ageing.

U.S. Bureau of Labor Statistics 2016, *A look at the future of the U.S. labor force to 2060*, viewed 16 June 2020, https://www.bls.gov/spotlight/2016/a-look-at-the-future-of-the-us-labor-force-to-2060/pdf/a-look-at-the-future-of-the-us-labor-force-to-2060.pdf.

U.S. Wage and Hour Division 2011, *The Fair Labor Standards Act of 1938, as amended*, http://purl.fdlp.gov/GPO/gpo24709.

U.S. Small Business Administration Office of Advocacy 2018, *2018 Small business profile*, https://www.sba.gov/sites/default/files/advocacy/2018-Small-Business-Profiles-US.pdf.

U.S. Small Business Administration Office of Advocacy 2019, *2019 Small business profile*, https://cdn.advocacy.sba.gov/wp-content/uploads/2019/04/23142719/2019-Small-Business-Profiles-US.pdf.

# 5 The Retail Food Environment

*Christina Vogel*
University of Southampton

*Carmen Piernas*
University of Oxford

**CONTENTS**



## 5.1 INTRODUCTION

Food retailers, particularly supermarkets, are a primary source of food for millions of households across high-income countries (Department for Environment Food and Rural Affairs, 2020; Global Agricultural Information Network, 2019), as well as increasing numbers of families in transitioning countries (Hawkes, 2008). Research investigating the influence that food retailers and supermarkets have on diet-related behaviours has burgeoned over the past 15 years because there is growing understanding that food retailers offer suitable, and potentially important, settings to improve population diet. In this chapter, we conducted a synthesis of semi-systematic and systematic reviews, following Cochrane methodology (Pollock et al., 2020) to obtain the latest knowledge on the relationship between the food retail environment and diet. We identified which interventions are most effective at producing better dietary-related behaviours, namely diet, purchasing and sales.

DOI: 10.1201/9781003043720-5

All systematic reviews included in this overview were published between 2012 and 2020. The evidence to date has focused on two distinct areas: (i) access to supermarkets and other food retailers, and (ii) components of the in-store and online retail food environment that can influence food choice including product availability, price, positioning, price promotions and signage. The evidence focuses on research conducted with adult populations; however, a brief summary of findings from studies with children/adolescents is provided. There is some evidence that unhealthy retail food environments, both spatially and within stores, may be exacerbating dietary inequalities and that efforts to improve retail food environments could reduce disparities in population health (Vogel et al., 2016; Burgoine et al., 2017; Vogel et al., 2017). A narrative summary of the evidence for the impact of food retail influences on dietary inequalities is also presented as well as an informative case study.

## 5.2 SPATIAL ACCESS TO SUPERMARKETS AND FOOD RETAILERS

A previous synthesis of literature, published in 2014 (Black et al., 2014), incorporating ten systematic reviews, which covered 102 articles examining food outlet access according to area deprivation. The review identified consistent trends for disparities in food environments in the US, where residents of low-income or ethnic minority neighbourhoods showed disproportionately poorer access to healthier food outlets, namely supermarkets and grocery stores, than those living in more affluent neighbourhoods. Studies conducted in other high-income countries including Canada, Australia and the UK, however, have shown no consistent differences in supermarket access according to the level of neighbourhood deprivation or ethnic composition. There was, however, consistent international evidence for inequalities in access to takeaway and fast food outlets which appeared in high numbers in neighbourhoods of greater disadvantage and ethnicity across countries. See Chapters 8 and 9 for more details about the eating out of home food environment.

Two review articles have assessed the international observational evidence, from 42 articles published between 2002 and 2013, investigating associations between access to food outlets and diet among adults (Caspi et al., 2012; Black et al., 2014). Overall, syntheses showed only weak evidence of a trend for increased density of, or proximity to, food stores selling healthy foods in residential neighbourhoods being associated with better dietary outcomes. Research from the US was more consistent than evidence from other high-income countries. Approximately half of the 21 US studies showed that better access to supermarkets related to healthier dietary behaviours; but less than a quarter of findings from all countries showed significant positive results. Two recent systematic reviews of literature from Canada and China (Stevenson et al., 2019; An et al., 2020), covering 13 articles published between 2012 and 2018, support these earlier reviews indicating limited evidence for a relationship between spatial access to healthier food outlets (i.e. supermarkets, fruit and vegetables stores, wet markets) and dietary behaviours. Turning to intervention literature may provide more conclusive evidence about the causal relationship between access to healthier retail food outlets and dietary outcomes.

Three systematic reviews have examined the effect that opening a new healthy food retail opportunity in socioeconomically disadvantaged communities, with previously poor healthy food access, has on fruit and vegetable intake (Abeykoon et al., 2017; Woodruff et al., 2017; Hollis-Hansen et al., 2019). All interventions were conducted in the last two decades, containing a total of 51 articles published between 2002 and 2018; 19 studies were reported in more than one review. Most evidence comes from the US, with a few studies conducted in the UK or Australia. Collectively, across all three reviews, there is some evidence that opening a new healthy food retail outlet in areas with low healthy food access increases fruit and vegetable consumption among adults; changes in portions per day varied across studies from approximately one third fewer portions per day to approximately half an additional portion per day. The evidence for dietary benefits from opening a new supermarket is weakest, with almost all studies reporting no or unexpected results (i.e. less healthy dietary intakes at follow-up). Supermarket studies with the strongest experimental designs consistently showed no effect. The few supermarket studies that measured body mass index (BMI) also found no change in weight status among participants. Sensitivity analyses in some studies, however, identified greater dietary benefits for those living in closer proximity to the new supermarket than for those living further away.

The evidence for mobile produce markets, which delivered fresh fruit and vegetables directly to the target community, was most consistent and positive. Two cluster randomised controlled trials (RCTs), involving more than a dozen communities, found statistically significant increases in fruit and vegetable consumption among interventions compared to control participants of between 0.3 and 0.4 cups (approximately half a portion) of fruits and vegetables per day. Mobile produce market studies with weaker experimental designs also showed consistent benefits for fruit and vegetable intake. Evidence for opening new farmers markets to improve healthy food access in socioeconomically disadvantaged communities is equivocal because many published evaluations provide insufficient data for a conclusion to be made, or study designs have high risk of bias.

### 5.2.1 Children/Adolescents

Only one intervention study examined the effects of a new healthy food retailer on dietary behaviours of children across the three systematic reviews. This study found that the daily fruit and vegetable intake of children aged 3–13 years increased by 0.48 cups per day (over half a portion) after five months exposure to a mobile produce market in their local community (Gorham et al., 2015). The study was conducted in six different communities; however, it had a high risk of bias because no comparison group was used. Evidence from observational literature examining associations between food outlet access and diet among children and adolescents synthesised from three systematic reviews (Zhou et al., 2019; Xin et al., 2019; Engler-Stringer et al., 2014), covering 10 studies of supermarkets and 11 of convenience stores published between 2007 and 2017, revealed inconclusive evidence for supermarket access but consistent evidence that greater access to convenience stores is associated with poorer dietary behaviours. Studies from the US, UK, Australia and Kenya all showed that increased access to supermarkets was associated with poorer dietary behaviours while others from the US and Canada showed better dietary behaviours with improved supermarket access (Engler-Stringer et al., 2014; Zhou et al., 2019).

One study from the UK showed that young children with greater exposure to healthy specialty stores (e.g. fruit and vegetables stores, fishmongers, butchers) around their home and school have better quality diets (Barrett et al., 2017). Further high-quality research incorporating longitudinal exposure and outcome measures is needed to identify whether new, or increased numbers of, healthy food retailers in lower access areas influence the diet-related behaviours of children and adolescents.

### 5.2.2 Overview of Impact on Inequalities

The intervention literature described above mainly focused on improving healthy food accessibility in deprived neighbourhoods by opening one new healthier food retailer in the target community. The lack of clear improvement in dietary outcomes, particularly for new supermarkets, may in part be explained by previous observational literature. Mackenbach et al. (2019) examined the evidence for socioeconomic differences in associations between food environment exposures and dietary behaviours from 12 studies conducted in the US, UK, Canada, New Zealand and Brazil, published from 2008 to 2018. Half of the studies showed that: (i) a higher proportion of convenience stores or fast food outlets, (ii) lower density of supermarkets or fresh produce outlets, or (iii) shopping at less healthful supermarkets was associated with poorer diet behaviours among those of lower socioeconomic position (SEP) but not among those of high SEP. When considering these results, particularly in light of the new store intervention studies' findings, it is interesting to note that many adopted relative measures of food environment exposures rather than absolute measures. Relative measures can provide a more comprehensive conceptualisation of the food environment because they consider the competing choices with which customers are presented (Stevenson et al., 2019; Cobb et al., 2015). Research from the UK, for example, shows that food outlet access is dominated by unhealthy food outlets, with only 1% of a population sample of women being exposed to healthy overall food environments while conducting their daily activities (Vogel et al., 2017). In such settings, one new supermarket may not provide sufficient change against a back drop of several unhealthy stores. In Brazil, research shows that in areas with low densities of supermarkets and fresh produce markets individuals with low incomes had poorer fruit and vegetable consumption than those with high incomes. In neighbourhoods with higher density of supermarkets and fresh produce markets, however, no differential association was observed (Duran et al., 2016).

Supermarket environments, unlike fresh produce outlets or markets, offer an array of unhealthy products to customers alongside healthy products (Hollis-Hansen et al., 2019; Abeykoon et al., 2017). This product variety and the accompanying marketing strategies used to promote unhealthy foods may make it more challenging for customers to only purchase healthy foods from a new store. Research from a large population sample of residents from two low-income US neighbourhoods found that individuals who report frequently shopping at large supermarkets have higher intakes of fats from unhealthy foods, while those who shop more often at fresh produce stores eat more fruit and vegetables (Vaughan et al., 2017). Policy incentives to increase numbers of healthy food retailers, such as fruit and vegetable stores or mobile produce markets (see Figure 5.1), could help to provide residents with fewer obstacles to purchasing

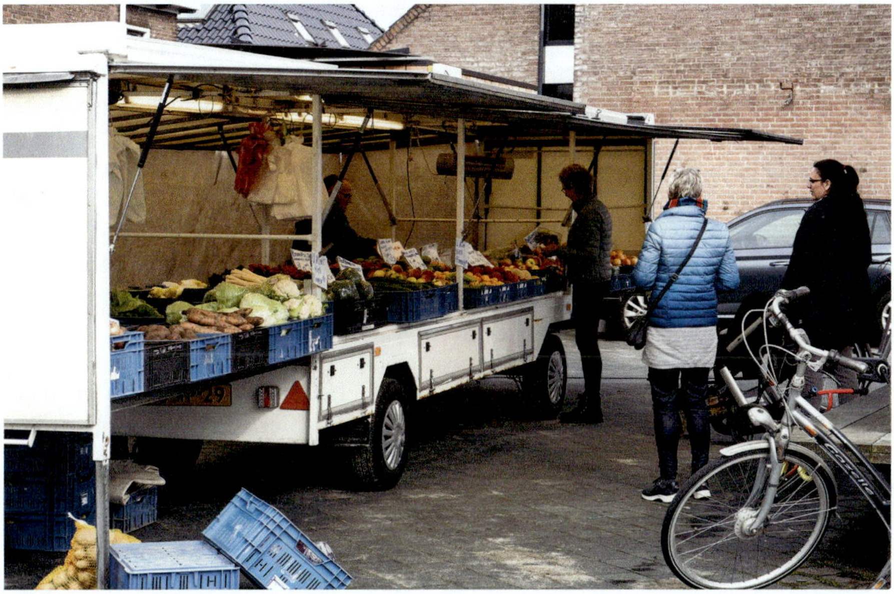

**FIGURE 5.1** Image of fresh produce van. (Reprinted with permission from Shutterstock, available at https://www.shutterstock.com/image-photo/koudum-netherlands-april-29-2021-people-1965878800.)

more healthy foods, particularly if fruit and vegetables are sold at reduced prices or below retail values as was the case in most mobile produce market studies (Hollis-Hansen et al., 2019). Such action, however, could be hindered by financial constraints of local authorities or small business owners. Interventions that focus on making the in-store environments of existing food retailers healthier may provide a more appropriate strategy for improving population diet and addressing dietary inequalities.

The next section reviews evidence from interventions that alter the environment within supermarkets and which are implemented by supermarket staff. We focus on intervention literature because it generally produces more reliable evidence; however, observational evidence was reviewed where gaps in intervention evidence exist.

## 5.3 IN-STORE AND ONLINE SUPERMARKET ENVIRONMENTS AND DIET

A total of 11 systematic reviews of intervention studies were used to synthesise the literature regarding in-store and online supermarket environments and diet-related outcomes. These systematic reviews covered a total of 301 articles, with 110 appearing in at least two reviews. The majority of studies synthesized were conducted in high-income countries, mainly in the US, with the vast majority of evidence emerging over the last decade.

The nature of the studies reviewed has developed over time. Earlier interventions targeted individual behaviour change through signage (e.g. shelf tags, recipe cards), while more recent interventions have focused on structural changes to the in-store environment, namely product availability, price and positioning. Other types of interventions including food industry reformulation, food packaging and portion size and nudging are discussed in Chapters 6, 15 and 16, respectively. Overall, the evidence is overwhelmingly derived from multicomponent interventions which target several aspects of the in-store food environment concurrently, as opposed to single component interventions. Although many review authors highlight the challenges of identifying single intervention strategies which are likely to be most effective from the existing literature, we present the evidence for the key intervention components in an effort to provide insight and direction for policy intervention and future research.

### 5.3.1 Signage and Swaps

Six systematic reviews assessed evidence for the effectiveness of in-store interventions using point-of-purchase signage to prompt healthier food choices (e.g. shelf tags, recipe cards). These interventions were typically implemented over short time periods (weeks to months) with few running for more than one year. Earlier systematic reviews, including studies conducted in the 1980–1990s, reported there was insufficient or mixed evidence that stand-alone signage interventions were effective at promoting sales of targeted healthy items (van't Riet, 2013; Escaron et al., 2013). Two later reviews reported more positive effects on diet-related outcomes from interventions using signage to identify healthier food options, even in the absence of other intervention components (Adam and Jensen, 2016; Cameron et al., 2016). More recent reviews, one including only RCTs (Hartmann-Boyce et al., 2018), however, reported only limited evidence that interventions using signage strategies are effective (Karpyn et al., 2020). van't Riet (2013) reported that interventions which used signage to highlight the absence of unhealthy nutrients (e.g. calories, fats, sodium, cholesterol, or sugars), alone or in combination with presence of healthy nutrients, showed greater levels of effectiveness at producing healthier purchasing patterns than interventions which only highlighted healthy foods or nutrients. A Cochrane review of strategies targeting sugar-sweetened beverage consumption identified low-certainty evidence that shelf tags reduced intake (von Philipsborn et al., 2020).

Another intervention strategy to highlight healthier products to customers at the point of purchase is to offer healthier swaps to less healthy products originally selected by an individual. Evidence for this strategy comes from a limited number of real and experimental online supermarket RCTs examined in one review (Hartmann-Boyce et al., 2018). Results show potentially beneficial, albeit small, effects.

Overall, this synthesis of evidence for signage and swap strategies suggests their effectiveness is limited, though several reviews reported improved dietary-related outcomes when interventions incorporated signage components alongside strategies targeting structural components of the in-store environment (van't Riet, 2013; Escaron et al., 2013; Adam and Jensen, 2016; Cameron et al., 2016).

### 5.3.2 Availability

Five systematic reviews of in-store interventions examined the effectiveness of availability, covering studies from 1978 to 2020, mostly in high-income countries

(Escaron et al., 2013; Cameron et al., 2016; Hartmann-Boyce et al., 2018; Karpyn et al., 2020; Shaw et al., 2020). These interventions spanned different strategies including increased varieties of healthier foods, decreased availability of unhealthy options or changes to the amount of space allocated for display.

The body of evidence testing the effectiveness of increasing the availability or variety of healthier foods, such as increased shelf space of fruits and vegetables or stocking a low-salt substitute, was limited yet mostly showed beneficial effects on dietary-related behaviours (Hartmann-Boyce et al., 2018; Karpyn et al., 2020). A more recent review (Shaw et al., 2020) reported that greater availability of healthier foods did not consistently result in better diet-related behaviours, yet no studies concurrently reduced the availability of unhealthy foods. Evidence from observational studies generally indicated that greater shelf space dedicated to healthier products and less space for unhealthier products was associated with healthier outcomes; with stronger evidence for sales and purchasing outcomes than for diet (Shaw et al., 2020).

Most reviews reported the effect of availability in the context of multicomponent interventions, typically in conjunction with signage, price and/or positioning interventions. Three reviews covering literature across high-income countries (Escaron et al., 2013; Adam and Jensen, 2016; Cameron et al., 2016) indicated a beneficial effect on fresh produce sales or dietary quality when more shelf space was provided together with signage and/or price interventions. However, the review which assessed only US studies showed mixed evidence for similar interventions (Karpyn et al., 2020). These differences may be attributed to the geographical areas covered by the reviews. Two reviews reported good evidence that availability interventions have stronger and more consistent beneficial effects when combined with positioning strategies (Shaw et al., 2020; Karpyn et al., 2020).

Overall, there is some evidence that increasing the availability of healthy foods can improve diet-related behaviours, particularly when implemented alongside positioning strategies to enhance their prominence. Further evidence is needed to understand the effect of reducing unhealthy food availability alone and in combination with increasing health food availability. Such combinations were tested in a recent study from the UK which demonstrated important population-level improvements in dietary-related outcomes among customers shopping at discount supermarkets (Vogel et al., 2021).

### 5.3.3 Price

Price interventions within supermarkets have been evaluated in six systematic reviews (Escaron et al., 2013; Adam and Jensen, 2016; Gittelsohn et al., 2017; Karpyn et al., 2020; von Philipsborn et al., 2020; Hartmann-Boyce et al., 2018), spanning studies conducted in North America, Europe and Australasia, published from 1978 up to 2018. A broader discussion on financial incentives and disincentives can be found in Chapter 17. Stand-alone interventions targeting the price or affordability of healthier foods (e.g. vouchers/rebates or prolonged price discounts for fruits and vegetables, whole grains or water) showed consistent evidence of positive effects on sales, purchasing or consumption of healthier options across four reviews (Adam and Jensen, 2016; Hartmann-Boyce et al., 2018; Karpyn et al., 2020; Gittelsohn et al., 2017).

One review importantly highlights that none of the studies which decreased prices of healthy foods reported unintended consequences, namely increased purchasing of unhealthy items. RCTs show inconsistent effects of price discounts on low-calorie beverages in stores but the evidence base is small (von Philipsborn et al., 2020). Overall, the evidence indicates a dose-response, whereby the higher the discount, the more substantial the effect on healthier diet-related behaviours.

The evidence for price interventions aiming to disincentivise unhealthy foods in retail outlets is limited. Two studies, from the US and France (Gittelsohn et al., 2017), evaluated the impact of subsidies/incentives on healthier foods, while concurrently increasing the price or restricting availability of unhealthier items. Both studies found that purchases or consumption of healthier foods increased, while unhealthy food or energy intake decreased.

Across reviews, price discounts on healthy food items were reported to have been frequently coupled with additional intervention strategies which builds on findings of pathway modelling of the determinants of dietary behaviours (Vogel et al., 2019). Recent reviews indicate that price interventions in combination with signage strategies or healthy eating information/behaviour change materials generally result in healthier food purchases and consumption, with some studies showing a small enhancement of stand-alone price effects (Gittelsohn et al., 2017; Adam and Jensen, 2016; Hartmann-Boyce et al., 2018; Karpyn et al., 2020).

### 5.3.4 Positioning

Two systematic reviews examined the evidence for in-store product positioning interventions influencing diet-related behaviours (Karpyn et al., 2020; Shaw et al., 2020), covering studies from the US and five European countries from 2009 to 2019. Across both reviews, there is reasonably consistent evidence that healthy positioning strategies produce results in the expected direction for health benefit. The strength of evidence is comparable for studies that focused solely on positioning healthy foods in more prominent locations, such as store entrance, check-outs or aisle ends (see Figure 5.2), and for those which concurrently positioned healthy foods in prominent locations and unhealthy foods in less prominent locations; but evidence is weaker for studies testing co-positioning of healthy and unhealthy foods in prominent locations. A recent exemplar study from the US (Liu et al., 2018) tested the differential effects of positioning at aisle ends (i) only healthy, (ii) only unhealthy and (iii) both healthy and unhealthy products. Results showed that prominent positioning of only healthy foods increased featured product sales without affecting unhealthy food sales, but prominent positioning of only unhealthy foods produced a larger increase in sales of featured products plus a marginal decrease in sales of healthy items. Prominent positioning of both products types led to large sales increases for unhealthy products but only marginal sales increases for healthy items.

The effect of positioning is stronger for sales/purchasing outcomes than for dietary outcomes, and also for store positioning than shelf positioning strategies; though only limited literature exists for diet and shelf positioning interventions (e.g. positioning healthy products at eye level) (Shaw et al., 2020). Multicomponent studies incorporating signage alongside positioning strategies showed little additional benefit

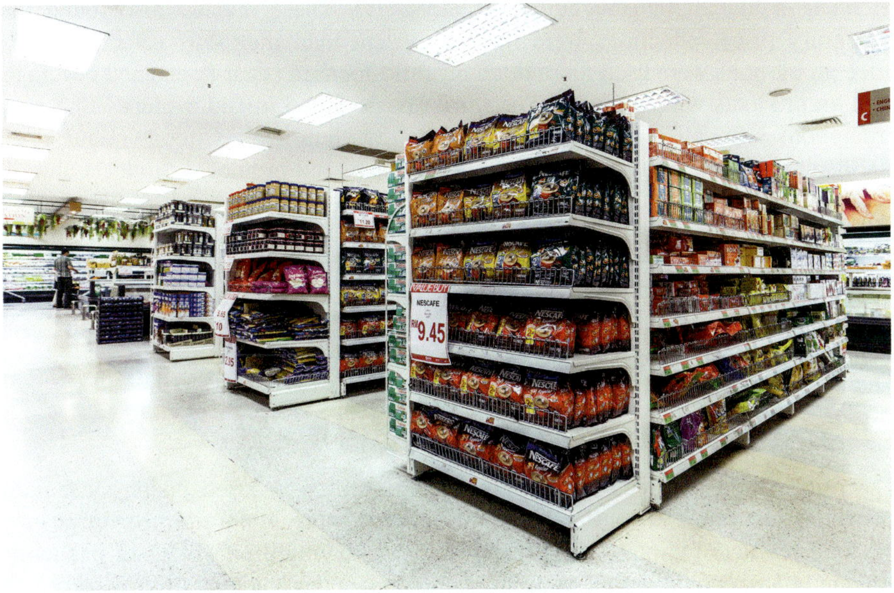


**FIGURE 5.2** End of retail aisle with promotions in a supermarket. (Reprinted with permission from Shutterstock, available at https://www.shutterstock.com/image-photo/kuala-lumpur-malaysia-june-16-sogo-164736608.)

from positioning alone (Karpyn et al., 2020; Shaw et al., 2020). In contrast, the vast majority of studies that combined positioning and availability strategies produced consistently beneficial results regardless of whether the intervention targeted healthy, unhealthy or both types of products, or measured sales/purchases or dietary outcomes (Shaw et al., 2020). This finding highlights the intrinsic link between product availability and positioning as marketing strategies, whereby positioning products in prominent in-store locations is typically additional to their usual in-aisle location, thus increasing availability/shelf space.

### 5.3.5 Price Promotions

None of the 11 systematic reviews examining supermarket intervention literature tested the effectiveness of price promotions at altering dietary-related behaviours. The term 'price promotions' includes strategies such as temporary price reduction, multi-buy offers, larger packaging volumes or meal deal offers (Chandon and Wansink, 2012). Three systematic reviews assessed observational literature to identify the prevalence of price promotions on healthy and unhealthy foods and beverages within retail food outlets (Bennett et al., 2020; Kaur et al., 2020; Houghtaling et al., 2019), and one additionally examined the association between price promotions and diet-related behaviours (Bennett et al., 2020). All studies were published between 2009 and 2020 and were conducted in high-income countries. Two reviews reported consistent observational evidence that price promotions in food retailers are more prevalent on unhealthy foods and beverages, compared with healthier items

(Bennett et al., 2020; Houghtaling et al., 2019). These reviews also found that temporary price reductions were more prevalent than multi-buy offers, and that price promotions were used more often on child-focused sugar-sweetened beverages than on products without sugar. The third review found mixed evidence that price promotions were more prevalent on less healthy, than healthy, foods (Kaur et al., 2020). This review excluded studies that only assessed promoted products and did not provide data on food availability, which may partly account for the difference in its overall results. The single review assessing associations with diet-related behaviour concluded that price promotions appear to increase consumer food and beverage purchases by between 18% and 53%, with greater magnitude of association for unhealthy options. These results need to be viewed with some caution because causal relationships cannot be inferred from observational evidence.

## 5.4 ONLINE FOOD RETAIL ENVIRONMENT

The information provided in this chapter has mostly focused on physical retail environments; however, online grocery shopping is an important growth channel for food retailers (Mintel, 2018); particularly following-the COVID-19 pandemic. Among other benefits, online grocery shopping has the potential to provide greater access to healthier foods, including in 'food deserts' as seen in the US (Brandt et al., 2019; Pitts et al., 2018). Shopping online has also been found to restrict consumers' purchases of unhealthy alternatives, compared to shopping in store (Huyghe et al., 2017). Recent evidence from RCTs within an online experimental supermarket platform have tested the effectiveness of swaps and prominent positioning of lower saturated fat foods (Koutoukidis et al., 2019), as well as labelling and increased availability of lower-energy density products, with promising results (Marty et al., 2020). Additional approaches to improve food choice while shopping online are covered in Chapter 13 on food labelling.

## 5.5 OVERVIEW OF IMPACT ON INEQUALITIES

It has been argued that environmental (rather than individual level) approaches, and interventions that target automatic behavioural responses, have greater likelihood of addressing health inequalities than those engaging active decision-making processes (Adams et al., 2016; Marteau et al., 2011). If so, the pricing, positioning and availability interventions described above may be approaches that can reduce, rather than, exacerbate dietary inequalities (Hollands et al., 2016; Adams et al., 2016; Vogel et al., 2016). However, further evidence is needed to assess the impact of in-store interventions on dietary inequalities (Hartmann-Boyce et al., 2018; Shaw et al., 2020; Escaron et al., 2013).

Several studies that tested healthier availability and positioning strategies were conducted among populations of lower SEP and showed reasonable consistency in producing better diet and sales outcomes (Shaw et al., 2020). However, no intervention studies in this review were identified that explicitly assessed differential intervention effects by SEP, although such studies are underway (Vogel et al., 2020). Another review identified a small number of swap and price studies that tested if intervention effectiveness varied by SEP, showing no clear difference in effect by level income, education or employment (Hartmann-Boyce et al., 2018). Subsequent research also showed no evidence of differential effects of swaps or labelling and increased availability of lower-energy density products by SEP (Koutoukidis et al., 2019; Marty et al., 2020).

Little difference by individual SEP has been observed for use of price promotions, but discount supermarkets appear to employ price promotions more heavily on unhealthy foods than standard supermarkets (Bennett et al., 2020). A recent scoping review of the retail food environment and diet among vulnerable indigenous populations showed that price discounts on healthy foods generally had beneficial effects on food purchasing (by up to approximately one quarter of a fruit/vegetable portion per day), but limited effects for signage interventions (Luongo et al., 2020). The authors importantly highlight that the success in some of the emerging intervention literature stems from close involvement of indigenous communities to co-design their food stores in ways that respond directly to community needs and priorities (Luongo et al., 2020). One intervention study recently implemented in food stores in indigenous communities is particularly noteworthy because of its comprehensiveness in tackling several unhealthy food marketing strategies, robust evaluation design and co-production approach (see case study).

## 5.6 CASE STUDY

Healthy Stores 2020: Restricting promotional and marketing strategies on unhealthy food and beverages in Australian supermarkets (Brimblecombe et al., 2020)

*Evidence before this study*

There is limited evidence on the effect of restricting promotional activities on less healthy food and beverages, particularly in real-world grocery settings.

*Intervention*

This community-based pragmatic RCT involved 20 supermarkets located in remote areas of Australia. The intervention was co-designed with the retailer to optimise the environment as a 'health-enabling' setting.

Intervention stores implemented a number of strategies targeting unhealthy foods and beverages which contribute to high intakes of free sugars, including (i) removal of promotions (e.g. price promotions, price discounts, volume-based promotions); (ii) no signage or misleading signage activities (e.g. fresh produce fridge containing confectionery); (iii) removal of unhealthy foods from prominent locations (e.g. end of aisle, check-outs); (iv) reduced shelf space and fewer varieties of high sugar products within aisles; (v) removal of large sugary drinks >600 mL from fridges; (vi) floor signage highlighting sugar in drinks and promoting water.

*Findings and implications of this study*

The intervention significantly reduced sales of all free sugars (−2.8%). Sales of sugary drinks (−13.2%) and confectionery (−4.3%, non-significant) also decreased. Supermarket profit was not affected by the intervention.

Healthy Stores 2020 constitutes a real-world example of an effective intervention conducted in close collaboration with a retailer which achieved relevant public health impacts without affecting business priorities.

## 5.7 CONCLUSIONS

Within supermarkets, price reductions on healthy foods alone, or in combination with price increases on unhealthy foods, show the strongest, most consistent evidence for improving diet-related behaviours and in a dose–response manner (see Figure 5.3). Strategies that combine increased availability and prominent positioning of healthy foods (i.e. aisle ends, entrance, check-outs) plus reduced prominence of unhealthy foods show moderately consistent results at producing healthier sales patterns. Co-locating healthy and unhealthy products in prominent positions does not improve sales of healthy products. Price promotions are generally more prevalent on unhealthy than healthy foods and exert influence greater on unhealthy than healthy products, though existing evidence is observational. Signage strategies promoting healthy foods at point of purchase show little benefit when implemented alone, but personalised swap suggestions show some promise at improving diet-related outcomes. Mobile fresh produce vans also show promise; however, most studies sold produce at reduced prices, below retail value.

The existing evidence provides policy makers with sufficient evidence for government action to shape food retail outlets to be healthier. In particular, policies to discount fruit and vegetables, increase unhealthy food prices, improve the availability and prominence of healthy foods and reduce the availability and prominence of unhealthy foods. More robust evidence in this area is needed in different countries as the bulk of studies included in the reviews were conducted in high-income countries.

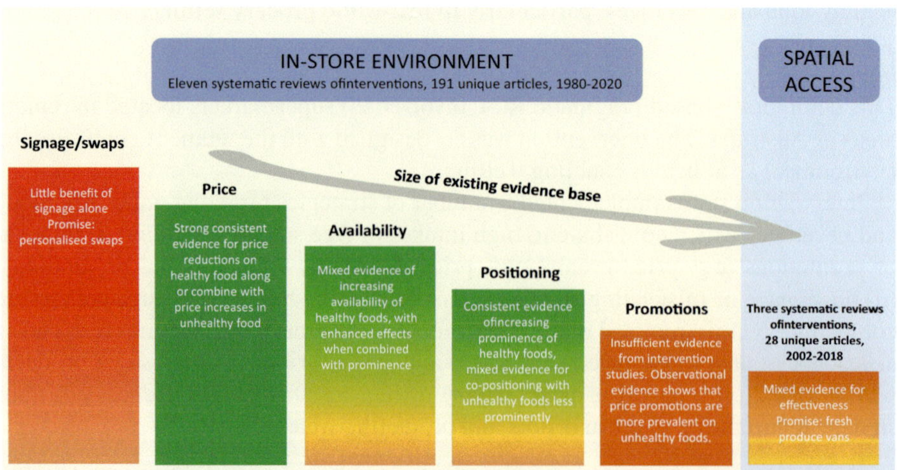


**FIGURE 5.3** Synthesis of evidence in retail food environments. Larger bars indicate larger evidence base. Colour coding: red = little evidence of effectiveness; amber = moderate evidence of effectiveness or small existing evidence base; green = strong evidence of effectiveness.

Policy strategies to increase access to healthy specialty stores, combined with robust evaluations, could be explored to improve the imbalance in access to healthy and unhealthy food outlets such as takeaways.

## REFERENCES


Abeykoon, A. H., Engler-Stringer, R. & Muhajarine, N. 2017. Health-related outcomes of new grocery store interventions: a systematic review. *Public Health Nutr,* 20, 2236–2248.

Adam, A. & Jensen, J. D. 2016. What is the effectiveness of obesity related interventions at retail grocery stores and supermarkets? A systematic review. *BMC Public Health,* 16, 1247.

Adams, J., Mytton, O., White, M. & Monsivais, P. 2016. Why are some population interventions for diet and obesity more equitable and effective than others? The role of individual agency. *PLOS Med,* 13, e1001990.

An, R., He, L. & Shen, M. J. 2020. Impact of neighbourhood food environment on diet and obesity in China: A systematic review. *Public Health Nutr,* 23, 457–473.

Barrett, M., Crozier, S., Lewis, D., Godfrey, K., Robinson, S., Cooper, C., Inskip, H., Baird, J. & Vogel, C. 2017. Greater access to healthy food outlets in the home and school environment is associated with better dietary quality in young children. *Public Health Nutr,* 20(18): 3316–3325.

Bennett, R., Zorbas, C., Huse, O., Peeters, A., Cameron, A. J., Sacks, G. & Backholer, K. 2020. Prevalence of healthy and unhealthy food and beverage price promotions and their potential influence on shopper purchasing behavior: a systematic review of the literature. *Obes Rev,* 21, e12948.

Black, C., Moon, G. & Baird, J. 2014. Dietary inequalities: what is the evidence for the effect of the neighbourhood food environment? *Health & Place,* 27, 229–242.

Brandt, E. J., Silvestri, D. M., Mande, J. R., Holland, M. L. & Ross, J. S. 2019. Availability of grocery delivery to food deserts in states participating in the online purchase pilot. *JAMA Network Open,* 2, e1916444.

Brimblecombe, J., Mcmahon, E., Ferguson, M., De Silva, K., Peeters, A., Miles, E., Wycherley, T., Minaker, L., Greenacre, L. & Gunther, A. 2020. Effect of restricted retail merchandising of discretionary food and beverages on population diet: a pragmatic randomised controlled trial. *Lancet Planet Health,* 4, e463–e473.

Burgoine, T., Mackenbach, J. D., Lakerveld, J., Forouhi, N. G., Griffin, S. J., Brage, S., Wareham, N. J. & Monsivais, P. 2017. Interplay of socioeconomic status and supermarket distance is associated with excess obesity risk: a UK cross-sectional study. *Int J Environ Res Public Health,* 14, 1290.

Cameron, A. J., Charlton, E., Ngan, W. W. & Sacks, G. 2016. A systematic review of the effectiveness of supermarket-based interventions involving product, promotion, or place on the healthiness of consumer purchases. *Curr Nutr Rep,* 5, 129–138.

Caspi, C. E., Sorensen, G., Subramanian, S. V. & Kawachi, I. 2012. The local food environment and diet: a systematic review. *Health Place,* 18, 1172–1187.

Chandon, P. & Wansink, B. 2012. Does food marketing need to make us fat? A review and solutions. *Nutr Rev,* 70, 571–593.

Cobb, L. K., Appel, L. J., Franco, M., Jones-Smith, J. C., Nur, A. & Anderson, C. A. 2015. The relationship of the local food environment with obesity: a systematic review of methods, study quality, and results. *Obesity (Silver Spring),* 23, 1331–1344.

Department for Environment Food and Rural Affairs. 2020. Food statistics in your pocket: food Chain. New York, UK.

Duran, A. C., De Almeida, S. L., Latorre Mdo, R. & Jaime, P. C. 2016. The role of the local retail food environment in fruit, vegetable and sugar-sweetened beverage consumption in Brazil. *Public Health Nutr,* 19, 1093–1102.

Engler-Stringer, R., Le, H., Gerrard, A. & Muhajarine, N. 2014. The community and consumer food environment and children's diet: a systematic review. *BMC Public Health,* 14, 522.

Escaron, A. L., Meinen, A. M., Nitzke, S. A. & Martinez-Donate, A. P. 2013. Supermarket and grocery store-based interventions to promote healthful food choices and eating practices: a systematic review. *Prev Chronic Dis,* 10, E50.

Gittelsohn, J., Trude, A. C. B. & Kim, H. 2017. Pricing strategies to encourage availability, purchase, and consumption of healthy foods and beverages: a systematic review. *Prev Chronic Dis,* 14, E107.

Global Agricultural Information Network 2019. *Retail Food Sector Report 2019.* Canberra, Australia.

Gorham, G., Dulin-Keita, A., Risica, P. M., Mello, J., Papandonatos, G., Nunn, A., Gorham, S., Roberson, M. & Gans, K. M. 2015. Effectiveness of fresh to you, a discount fresh fruit and vegetable market in low-income neighborhoods, on children's fruit and vegetable consumption, Rhode Island, 2010–2011. *Prev Chronic Dis,* 12, E176.

Hartmann-Boyce, J., Bianchi, F., Piernas, C., Payne Riches, S., Frie, K., Nourse, R. & Jebb, S. A. 2018. Grocery store interventions to change food purchasing behaviors: a systematic review of randomized controlled trials. *Am J Clin Nutr,* 107, 1004–1016.

Hawkes, C. 2008. Dietary implications of supermarket development: a global perspective. *Dev Policy Rev,* 26, 657–692.

Hollands, G. J., Marteau, T. M. & Fletcher, P. C. 2016. Non-conscious processes in changing health-related behavior: a conceptual analysis and framework. *Health Psychol Rev,* 10, 381–394.

Hollis-Hansen, K., Vermont, L., Zafron, M. L., Seidman, J. & Leone, L. 2019. The introduction of new food retail opportunities in lower-income communities and the impact on fruit and vegetable intake: a systematic review. *Transl Behav Med,* 9, 837–846.

Houghtaling, B., Serrano, E. L., Kraak, V. I., Harden, S. M., Davis, G. C. & Misyak, S. A. 2019. A systematic review of factors that influence food store owner and manager decision making and ability or willingness to use choice architecture and marketing mix strategies to encourage healthy consumer purchases in the United States, 2005–2017. *Int J Behav Nutr Phys Act,* 16, 5.

Huyghe, E., Verstraeten, J., Geuens, M. & Van Kerckhove, A. 2017. Clicks as a healthy alternative to bricks: how online grocery shopping reduces vice purchases. *J Marketing Res,* 54, 61–74.

Karpyn, A., Mccallops, K., Wolgast, H. & Glanz, K. 2020. Improving consumption and purchases of healthier foods in retail environments: a systematic review. *Int J Environ Res Public Health,* 17(20), 7524. https://doi.org/10.3390/ijerph17207524

Kaur, A., Lewis, T., Lipkova, V., Fernando, S., Rayner, M., Harrington, R. A., Waterlander, W. & Scarborough, P. 2020. A systematic review, and meta-analysis, examining the prevalence of price promotions on foods and whether they are more likely to be found on less-healthy foods. *Public Health Nutr,* 23, 1281–1296.

Koutoukidis, D. A., Jebb, S. A., Ordonez-Mena, J. M., Noreik, M., Tsiountsioura, M., Kennedy, S., Payne-Riches, S., Aveyard, P. & Piernas, C. 2019. Prominent positioning and food swaps are effective interventions to reduce the saturated fat content of the shopping basket in an experimental online supermarket: a randomized controlled trial. *Int J Behav Nutr Phys Act,* 16, 50.

Liu, P. J., Dallas, S. K., Harding, M. & Fitzsimons, G. J. 2018. The sales impact of featuring healthy foods, indulgent foods, or both: findings from a large-scale retail field study. *J Assoc Consum Res,* 3, 346–363.

Luongo, G., Skinner, K., Phillipps, B., Yu, Z., Martin, D. & Mah, C. L. 2020. The retail food environment, store foods, and diet and health among indigenous populations: a scoping review. *Curr Obes Rep* 9, 288–306. https://doi.org/10.1007/s13679-020-00399-6

Mackenbach, J. D., Nelissen, K. G. M., Dijkstra, S. C., Poelman, M. P., Daams, J. G., Leijssen, J. B. & Nicolaou, M. 2019. A systematic review on socioeconomic differences in the association between the food environment and dietary behaviors. *Nutrients,* 11, 2215.

Marteau, T. M., Ogilvie, D., Roland, M., Suhrcke, M. & Kelly, M. P. 2011. Judging nudging: can nudging improve population health? *BMJ,* 342, d228.

Marty, L., Cook, B., Piernas, C., Jebb, S. A. & Robinson, E. 2020. Effects of labelling and increasing the proportion of lower-energy density products on online food shopping: a randomised control trial in high-and low-socioeconomic position participants. *Nutrients,* 12, 3618.

Mintel. 2018. UK online grocery retailing industry report (updated 2018) [Online]. Mintel.com. Available https://store.mintel.com/uk-online-grocery-retailing-market-report [Accessed].

Pitts, S. B. J., Ng, S. W., Blitstein, J. L., Gustafson, A. & Niculescu, M. 2018. Online grocery shopping: Promise and pitfalls for healthier food and beverage purchases. *Public Health Nutr,* 21, 3360–3376.

Pollock, M., Fernandes, R., Becker, L., Pieper, D. & Hartling, L. 2020. Chapter V, Overviews of reviews. In Jpt, H., Thomas, J., Chandler, J., Cumpston, M., Li, T., Page, M. & Welch, V. (eds.) Cochrane Handbook for Systematic Reviews of Interventions, 2nd ed. Chichester, UK: John Wiley & Sons.

Shaw, S. C., Ntani, G., Baird, J. & Vogel, C. A. 2020. A systematic review of the influences of food store product placement on dietary-related outcomes. *Nutr Rev,* 78, 1030–1045.

Stevenson, A. C., Brazeau, A. S., Dasgupta, K. & Ross, N. A. 2019. Neighbourhood retail food outlet access, diet and body mass index in Canada: a systematic review. *Health Promot Chronic Dis Prev Can,* 39, 261–280.

van'T Riet, J. 2013. Sales effects of product health information at points of purchase: a systematic review. *Public Health Nutr,* 16, 418–429.

Vaughan, C. A., Collins, R., Ghosh-Dastidar, M., Beckman, R. & Dubowitz, T. 2017. Does where you shop or who you are predict what you eat? The role of stores and individual characteristics in dietary intake. *Prev Med,* 100, 10–16.

Vogel, C., Abbott, G., Ntani, G., Barker, M., Cooper, C., Moon, G., Ball, K. & Baird, J. 2019. Examination of how food environment and psychological factors interact in their relationship with dietary behaviours: test of a cross-sectional model. Int J Behav Nutr Phys Act, 16, 12.

Vogel, C., Crozier, S., Dhuria, P., Shand, C., Lawrence, W., Cade, J., Moon, G., Lord, J., Ball, K., Cooper, C. & Baird, J. 2020. Protocol of a natural experiment to evaluate a supermarket intervention to improve food purchasing and dietary behaviours of women (WRAPPED study) in England: a prospective matched controlled cluster design. BMJ Open, 10, e036758.

Vogel, C., Crozier, S., Penn-Newman, D., Ball, K., Moon, G., Lord, J., Cooper, C. & Baird, J. 2021. Altering product placement to create a healthier layout in supermarkets: Outcomes on store sales, customer purchasing, and diet in a prospective matched controlled cluster study. *PLoS Med,* 18, e1003729.

Vogel, C., Ntani, G., Inskip, H., Barker, M., Cummins, S., Cooper, C., Moon, G. & Baird, J. 2016. Education and the relationship between supermarket environment and diet. *Am J Prev Med,* 51, e27–e34.

Vogel, C., Lewis, D., Ntani, G., Cummins, S., Cooper, C., Moon, G. & Baird, J. 2017. The relationship between dietary quality and the local food environment differs according to level of educational attainment: A cross-sectional study. *PLoS One,* 12, e0183700.

Von Philipsborn, P., Stratil, J. M., Burns, J., Busert, L. K., Pfadenhauer, L. M., Polus, S., Holzapfel, C., Hauner, H. & Rehfuess, E. A. 2020. Environmental interventions to reduce the consumption of sugar-sweetened beverages: Abridged cochrane systematic review. *Obes Facts,* 13, 397–417.

Woodruff, R., Raskind, I., Harris, D., Gazmararian, J., Kramer, M., Haardörfer, R., & Kegler, M. 2018. The dietary impact of introducing new retailers of fruits and vegetables into a community: Results from a systematic review. *Public Health Nutrition*, 21(5), 981–991. https://doi.org/10.1017/S1368980017003226

Xin, J., Zhao, L., Wu, T., Zhang, L., Li, Y., Xue, H., Xiao, Q., Wang, R., Xu, P., Visscher, T., Ma, X. & Jia, P. 2019. Association between access to convenience stores and childhood obesity: a systematic review. *Obes Rev*, 22, e12908.

Zhou, Q., Zhao, L., Zhang, L., Xiao, Q., Wu, T., Visscher, T., Zhao, J., Xin, J., Yu, X., Xue, H., Li, H., Pan, J. & Jia, P. 2019. Neighborhood supermarket access and childhood obesity—A systematic review. *Obes Rev*, 22, 1–12.

# 6 Role of the Food Industry in Improving the Food Environment

## *Reformulation and Logistical Considerations*

*Nastasia Belc*
National R&D Institute for Food Bioresources (IBA)

*Eleonora Morganti*
University of Leeds

*Denisa E. Duță and Teodora-Alexandra Iordache*
National R&D Institute for Food Bioresources (IBA)

*Katherine Flynn*
ISEKI-Food Association

**CONTENTS**



DOI: 10.1201/9781003043720-6

## 6.1 INTRODUCTION

Consumption decisions and eating habits around the world have changed in recent decades due to the technological and economic developments of globalization: from staple grains, legumes, and fruits and vegetables to mostly processed foods, away-from-home foods, refined carbohydrates, animal-source foods, edible oils, and sugar-sweetened beverages (Popkin, 2015; Turnera et al, 2018). With globalization has come reductions in food costs and food spending which now accounts for 10%–20% of household income in most high-income countries compared to about a third of spending in the 1980s (DEFRA, 2020).

Most of this spending takes place in supermarkets, smaller stores, and food outlets, where the food industry is responsible for providing safe, palatable, and affordable food that meets consumer preferences (Yang et al., 2019). More than 80% of food in supermarkets is processed, and some are highly processed (ultra-processed foods). In addition to increased processing and ready-to-eat foods over the last decades, consumers in many countries have also come to expect year-round availability of a wide variety of imported foods including fruits and vegetables.

Although most consumers can access and purchase a healthy diet with sufficient fruits and vegetables and moderate amounts of energy-dense foods, many people do not achieve this. WHO, EU, and individual governments are introducing more regulation around food processing and developing health and nutrition action plans to encourage healthier diets (World Health Organization, 2018). The three main approaches include targeting and educating the consumer, providing voluntary targets to industry, or providing mandatory targets. In most high-income countries, focus has been on consumer awareness rather than reformulation. This has had little impact on food choice overall, and may have impacted wealthier and more educated consumers, thereby widening inequalities in diet and health (The European Consumer Organisation, 2015). Thus, measures to improve food quality through reformulation have been introduced along with other measures such as a tax on sugary drinks (see Chapter 17). Other related chapters in this book also discuss the role of food marketing by food producers (Chapter 14) and why the food industry is not doing more to improve diet and health (Chapter 7).

In addition to challenges around reformulation of foods, the logistical considerations of delivering food to consumers are considered. Food is delivered, not just to supermarkets but also to cafés, restaurants, recreational centres (Morganti, 2019), and shops whose main business is non-food items (see Chapter 9). Urban freight transport, otherwise defined as "last mile for food", plays a vital role in ensuring a fast and continuous replenishing of food supplies. Even during the exceptional times of the COVID-19 pandemic in 2020–2021, which led to a rise in stockpiling behaviour and supply chains having to respond to increased demand for home consumption, urban freight operations have been a key element to secure provision of food to communities with minimal disruption. However, access to nutrient-rich foods is hampered by the fact that processed products high in fats, sugars, and/or salt are easier to ship, handle, store, and display than fresh produce such as fruit and vegetables. This section of the chapter discusses how transport and logistics have an impact on available foods, as well as related environmental issues.

## 6.2 FOOD REFORMULATION

It is universally recognized that the quality of food is the sum of the quality of the ingredients and the processing technologies, which must be considered in order to improve public health (Popkin, Adair, & Ng, 2012). Although food processing is associated with negative effects on the quality of foodstuffs such as increasing fats, sugars, and salt, food processing also plays a role in extending food shelf-life and making some foods more palatable (EUFIC, 2010; Albuquerque et al., 2018). Food reformulation aims to decrease fats, sugars, and/or salt in processed foods. It is a strategy that changes the original recipe of a food by replacing, adding, and/or removing some ingredients to improve the overall nutritional profile (Domenech-Asensi et al., 2016; Luo et al., 2019). Recommended nutrient levels include trans-fats contributing less than 1% of total energy intake (World Health Organization, 2015a, 2019), salt intakes of less than 5 g/day for adults and 2 g/day for children (World Health Organization, 2013), and free sugars of less than 10% of daily energy intake, and ideally, less than 5% (World Health Organization, 2015b; Luo et al, 2019) all of which are currently considerably higher in a typical diet in many countries. Furthermore, interest is now focused on foods more likely to be consumed by vulnerable groups, such as children and those on lower incomes.

### 6.2.1 Regulation of Food Reformulation

In addition to targeting individuals to improve food choice, voluntary recommendations for food producers and action plans on health and nutrition have been in existence long before the EU framework in Europe. These early initiatives were generally not very successful in improving food choices, which highlighted the need for more regulation.

In most EU countries, food reformulation is developed based on monitored voluntary agreements between food industry/associations and authorities (Belc et al., 2019) rather than mandatory regulations. The reductions are gradual, to enable consumers to adapt to, for example, a less salty product, and ultimately bring about changes in consumer eating behaviour. Different European reformulation schemes are listed in Table 6.1. Most of these started on a voluntary basis, with the earliest in France in 2002.

Food reformulation acceptance by consumers is influenced by the pathway used, that is, different technologies or replacers for fats, sugars, and salt. These are considered in turn.

### 6.2.2 Fats

According to the European Strategy for Prevention and Control of Noncommunicable Diseases 2012–2016, part of the European Food and Nutrition Action Plan 2015–2020, the "elimination of trans fats in food and their replacement with poly-unsaturated fats", is a priority (World Health Organization, 2012, 2014). Reducing trans-fats typically used in very processed foods has the potential benefit of reducing diet and therefore health inequalities. In the UK, reducing trans-fats in many product categories reduced trans-fats' consumption in the whole population but particularly in lower-income groups who had the highest intakes (Hutchinson et al., 2017).

Targets also include reducing the total and the saturated fat content of foods. Low-fat foods can be produced by reducing fat-based ingredients in the formulation, but this has the disadvantage of negatively affecting the physicochemical and sensory properties of the food. Fat replacement strategies applied by the food industry use fat substitutes which are materials with similar chemical and physical properties as fats

**TABLE 6.1**
**Reformulation Schemes for Salt, Sugar, and Fat in Different EU Countries**

| Country | Type of Reformulation | Start Date | Initiative | Industry Involved | Targets |
|---|---|---|---|---|---|
| Austria | Trans-fatty acids | 2009 | Federal Ministry for Health | Food processing industry | max 2 g TFAs/100 g total fat |
| | Salt | 2010 | | Bakery industry | 15% reduction |
| Bulgaria | Salt, sugar, and fat | 2009 | Ministry for Health | Requirements of schoolchildren healthy diet with less salt, sugar and fat in buffets and canteens | Regulation No 37 |
| France | Salt | 2002 | French Agency for Food Safety | Consumers | 20% reduction in consumption over 5 years, i.e. to 6–8 g a day on average |
| | | 2010 | Ministry of Feeding, Agriculture and Fishery | Food processing industry | - |
| Finland | Fat and salt | 2000 | Finnish Heart Association (Suomen Sydänliitto) | Food processing industry<br>Labelling | "Heart label" or "A Better Choice" label (Sydänmerkki, Parempi valinta–merkki) |
| Germany | Trans-fatty acids<br>Salt | 2008 | Federal Ministry for Food, Agriculture and Consumer Protection ((BMELV)<br>Federal Institute for Risk Assessment (BfR) | Food processing industry | - |
| Hungary | Salt | 2012 | Ministry of Health | Bakery industry | - |

(*Continued*)

**TABLE 6.1 (*Continued*)**
**Reformulation Schemes for Salt, Sugar, and Fat in Different EU Countries**

| Country | Type of Reformulation | Start Date | Initiative | Industry Involved | Targets |
|---|---|---|---|---|---|
| Italy Sardinia | Salt | 2007 | Gruppo Inter-societario di Intervento sul Consumo di Sale in Italia – GIRCSI Ministry of Health | Bakery products and soups | 10% reduction by 2011 |
| | | 2009 | Ministry of Health and National Associations of Bakers | Bakery and pasta industry | 10% reduction |
| | | 2008 | Local authorities | Campaign to consumers | 16% reduction in consumption |
| Romania | Salt | 2011 | Ministry of Health Romalimenta (Food Industries Federation) | Food processing industry | - |
| Spain | Salt | 2008 | Spanish Confederation of Bakery Organizations (CEOPAN) | Bakery products | 20% reduction (2005–2008) |
| | | 2010 | Ministry of Health and Social Policy | Food processing industry and HoReCa industry | 20% reduction |
| UK | Salt | 2006 | Department of Health and Social Care, Food Standards Agency | Food processing industry | Voluntary 15% reduction although different reduction percentages, depending on the food product, see reference (PHE, 2020): Salt reduction targets for 2024 |

*Source:* A European network to follow-up the reformulation of food. Identification and exchange of good practices for SMEs and consumers (SALUX), GA No: 20101210100865.

and oils and which can replace fat on a weight-to-weight basis. These materials can be obtained by enzyme-modified oils and fats and can also be synthesized chemically. Some contain energy, while others are low in calories or are calorie-free. The three main categories of fat substitutes are: fat, carbohydrate, and protein-based.

**Fat-based fat substitutes**, with more fatty acids than triglycerides, are too large to be digested, and therefore do not contribute to dietary fat or energy. However, large amounts may cause a loss of fat-soluble vitamins or gastrointestinal side effects. Fat-based fat substitutes are used in baked goods, chocolate, confectionary, snacks, and savoury products (Marcus, 2013).

Common fat-based fat substitutes are:

- *Caprenin* (caprocaprylobehenic triglyceride molecule; energy density: 5 kcal/g; functional properties: emulsify, stabilize, texturize, lubricate, flavour carrier; application: candy, confectionary, a cocoa butter substitute);
- *Olestra* (or *Olean*; sucrose polyester; energy density: 0 kcal/g; functional properties: texturize, lubricate, flavour carrier; application: reduced-fat snacks, potato chips; products containing olestra must be labelled correctly as olestra may cause abdominal cramping and loose stools and inhibit the absorption of some nutrients);
- *Salatrim* (acyl triglyceride molecule; energy density: 5 kcal/g; functional properties: emulsify, stabilize, texturize, lubricate, flavour carrier; application: cheese, dips, sauces, dairy desserts, confectionary) (O'Sullivan, 2016).

**Carbohydrate-based fat substitutes** have some functional properties which help to add form and structure like fat: texturizer, water holding, thickening, gelling but a lower energy density: 4 kcal/g for starches and polysaccharide, 0 kcal/g for gums and cellulose. They cannot be used for cooking or frying.

Examples of carbohydrate-based fat substitutes include:

- starches (corn, potato, tapioca, rice, maize, waxy maize) used in processed meats, margarines, sauces, dressings, baked foods;
- gums: guar, locust bean, xanthan used in bakery goods; carrageenan used in processed meats, yogurts, salad dressings, desserts, ice cream, chocolate; pectin used in sauces; Arabic gum used in dressings;
- methylcellulose used in frozen desserts, powdered soups/sauces; microcrystalline cellulose used in dairy, salad dressing, sauces desserts;
- polysaccharide: maltodextrin used in processed meats, dairy spreads, salad dressings, baked foods, frozen desserts; polydextrose used in confectionary, spreads, salad dressings, baked foods, frozen desserts, sauces, toppings; β-glucan used in baked foods.

**Protein-based fat substitutes** such as egg white, milk, and whey are blended to trap water and create a creamy liquid that is similar to fat. They contribute less total fat and fewer calories (energy density: 4 kcal/g) than the fat they replace. Protein-based fat substitutes cannot be used for baking or frying, since heat causes a change in their structure – they gel and lose their creaminess. Protein-based fat substitutes are used to replace the fat in baked goods, butter, cheese, dairy products, ice cream, mayonnaise, salad dressings, and sour cream.

**TABLE 6.2**
**Examples of Typically High Fat Foods Available on the Market with Lower Fat Content**

| No. | Type of Food/ | Reformulation Type | Replacers for Fat | Country Origin | Labelling Nutritional Claims |
|---|---|---|---|---|---|
| 1 | Butter | Lowering fat content | Milk normalization | Romania/Hungary/ Slovak Republic/ | Low fat content |
| 2 | Cheese | Lowering fat content | - | Spain | 30% less fat |
| 3 | Pork pulp ham/chicken breast ham/Victoria turkey salami/turkey salami/chicken breast with pepper/beef hamburger/salami | Lowering fat content | - | Romania/Italy | 1,5% fat/ reducing fat up to 77%–92%/ low fat content |
| 4 | Biscuits | Lowering fat content | - | Italy | 30% less fat |

Common protein-based fat substitutes include:

- egg white protein; milk protein; whey protein concentrate; and whey protein.
- microparticulated protein (as *Simplesse* with role as stabilizer and texturizer, energy density: 4 kcal/g, used in cheese, yogurt, dips, mayo, dairy spreads, desserts);
- white egg protein and xanthan gum (*Trailblazer,* with role as stabilizer and texturizer, energy density: 4 kcal/g; used in: dairy, soups, sauces, baked foods).

Table 6.2 provides some European examples of high-fat foods where fat has been reduced.

### 6.2.3 Sugars

Sweetening of food is associated with increased palatability and increased consumption of beverages or nutrient-dense foods (Onaolapo et al., 2020) and sweetened baked products are one of the highest contributors to added sugars. Reformulation to reduce sugar in these products may be an effective method to reduce overall added sugar intake. If added sugar is replaced by low-calorie carbohydrates (prebiotic fibres) or non-nutritive sweeteners (NNS), further calorie reduction may be possible (Luo et al., 2019).

If more than 10% of sucrose is removed from a sweetened baked product, there will be obvious sensory and textural defects that will not be acceptable to the consumer. To further reduce sucrose, other low-calorie, carbohydrates such as oligosaccharides and polysaccharides can be used as bulking agents. Alternative sugars such as tagatose and isomaltulose are both refined like sucrose; however, tagatose has fewer calories and isomaltulose is slowly digested by the human body and thus elevates glycaemic response more mildly. Polydextrose is another sucrose alternative, one that is widely available and preferred by food manufacturers. It is a suitable bulk sugar replacement when used with NNS such as sucralose and stevia (Luo et al., 2019). Inuline, maltodextrin, and resistant maltodextrin can also be used to replace sucrose.

Sugar alcohols or polyols are widely used by the food industry to produce low-calorie foods and foods for patients with diabetes. They contribute sweetness, texture, and bulk to baked products and can replace sucrose on a one-to-one basis, yet, except for xylitol, they have a lower intensity of sweetness than sucrose and NNS are usually required. The major limit of polyols is their laxative effect when consumed in high quantities, and statements regarding this effect are required for polyol-containing foods. Xylitol is a suitable polyol sweetener in sucrose-free cakes; however, replacing all sucrose with xylitol significantly affects product acceptance due to its high hygroscopicity. Erythritol has an unfavourable low solubility though it can substitute up to 50% of sucrose in both cakes and biscuits with the same consumer acceptance. Sorbitol, isomalt, lactitol, and maltitol are all competent as complete sucrose replacers in non-yeast-raised baked products without significant adverse effects on quality.

NNS substitutes such as Stevia and its derivatives, including leaf extract, rebaudioside A, steviosides, and the commercial ingredient Stevianna®, have been widely studied and found to be suitable as alternative sweeteners in most products. Fifty percent sucrose replaced by Stevianna® (rebaudioside A 1%, erythritol 99%) in cocoa- and vanilla-flavoured muffins had no significant impact on quality based on both instrumental and sensory analyses, and successfully reduced sucrose content from 20% to 10%. Similarly, Vatankhah et al. (2017) showed that stevioside could replace up to 50% of sucrose in sweet bread and even achieved a higher overall acceptability than control (20% of sucrose).

Table 6.3 summarizes some of the reformulated products, lower in sugar, currently on the market. Both locally produced and international imported products are represented.

### 6.2.4 Salt

Salt (sodium chloride or NaCl) is a commonly used food ingredient or condiment, usually for enhancing taste and /or preservation. The effect of salt on food taste depends on the form: solid (sodium chloride crystals) or solution, with solutions being more intensely perceived. Reducing salt in food affects not only the "salty" flavour but also other organoleptic characteristics such as texture and hydration as sodium chloride allows proteins to bind with fats, thereby retaining water (Parniakov et al., 2020). At the EU level, it is estimated that 95% of sodium is consumed in the form of salt (European Commission 2012) and almost 75% of salt in the diet comes from prepared food/fast food where salt is added both for taste and preservation. A portion of pizza, for example, contains around 50% of the recommended daily consumption (Parniakov et al, 2020). According to the EU strategy for salt reduction, 12 food categories contributing to high salt intake have been identified

**TABLE 6.3**
**Examples of Typically High Sugar Foods Available on the Market with Lower or No Sugar Content**

| No. | Type of Food | Reformulation | Sugar Replacers | Country Origin | Labelling Nutritional Claim |
|---|---|---|---|---|---|
| 1 | Chocolate | Less sugar | Maltitol/coconut sugar/ maltodextrin/mannitol/ fibres (inulin) | France | Less 55% sugars/low glycemic index/less 96% sugars/low sugar/less 91% sugars |
| | | | Fibres and jam | Belgium | No added sugars |
| | | No sugars added | Eritritol/maltitol<br>Steviol glycosides<br>Inulin | Romania | No sugars added/19%–23% less calories compared with the ones containing sugar/rich in fibres |
| 2 | Biscuits | Low sugar content/no sugar/replacing sugar by sweeteners | Manitol/maltitol/brown cane sugar<br>Fructo-oligosaccharides fibres/eritriol/lactitol | France | Less 33–37–52–58–78–87–91% sugars/no added sugars |
| | | | | Hungary | Low sugar content |
| | | | | Spain | With sweeteners/no sugar/ low impact on glycemic index |
| 3 | Bars | Sugar replaced by sweeteners | Maltitol, steviol glycosides | Spain | No sugar added |
| | | Sugar replaced by sweeteners | Maltitol | Romania | No sugar added, with sweeteners |
| 4 | Wafers | Replacing sugar by sweeteners | Maltitol | Romania | No sugars added, with sweetener |
| 5 | Candies | Replacing sugar by sweeteners | Maltitol syrup<br>Acesulfam-K<br>Isomalt | Germany | No added sugars |
| 6 | Spreadable cream with cacao and hazelnut/ Halva | Replacing sugar by sweeteners | Steviol glycosides,<br>Eritriol, inulin/maltitol syrup<br>Sorbitol | Romania | No added sugars/with sweeteners, no added sugars |
| 7 | Muesli with cereals, seeds and fruits | No exogenous sugars added | - | France/ Romania | No added sugars |
| 8 | Jams and syrups | No sugar | Apple juice | Austria | No added sugars |
| | | No sugar, with sweeteners | Sodium cyclamate, acesulfam-K, sucralose, saccharin | | 0% sugar |
| | | No exogenous sugar added | Agave syrup | | No added sugar |

(bread, meat products, cheese, ready meals, soup, breakfast cereals, fish products, crisps and savoury snacks, catering meals, restaurant meals, sauces, condiments and spices, and potato products). Countries are advised to select at least five product types to target through their national nutrition action plans and strategies (World Health Organization, 2013).

Much research has been carried out to successfully reduce salt in high contributing foods. For example, in the UK, salt in bread and breakfast cereals has been substantially reduced (Parliamentary Office of Science and Technology (POST), 2021). However, a dramatic reduction of sodium in bread, for example, negatively affects yeast growth and the development of gluten networks, affecting the texture. Various studies show no differences among bread baked with 0.3% or 0.6% salt; however, the omission of salt changed crumb structure and caused sensory changes in texture and flavour during storage (Belz et al., 2012). In cheeses, a reduction of salt limits the initial microbial activity that favours the curing of these products.

Salt is inexpensive so any substitute will inevitably increase the price of the products. However, salt reduction can sometimes be achieved without using any additional ingredients. For example, in low-salt bread production, salt reduction can be replaced by modifying or introducing different technological phases, such as packing in a protective atmosphere, pasteurization of packaged bread, or irradiation (Belz et al., 2012).

The most commonly used salt replacers are (Institute of Medicine, 2010):

- inorganic salts: potassium chloride, potassium sulfate, calcium chloride, and magnesium sulfate which are used in many foods, including cheeses, breads, and meats;
- mixtures of inorganic salts with NaCl in up to a 50:50 ratio;
- salts with altered crystal structure (e.g., micronized salt): porous and star-shaped structures, created by manipulating the salt drying process, allow greater salty taste with smaller amounts of salt; particularly useful in applications where salt is used on the surface of food products;
- monosodium glutamate (MSG) and other glutamates are used in foods to replace some salt; other glutamate salts such as monopotassium glutamate or calcium diglutamate may further reduce sodium;
- yeast extracts and hydrolyzed vegetable protein – often contains MSG but is seen as a "natural" alternative to MSG use;
- nucleotides including inosine-5′-monophosphate (IMP) and guanosine-5′-monophosphate impart the taste of umami; found to act synergistically with glutamates to enhance salty tastes in some foods;
- amino acids, especially arginine and related compounds – L-arginine is reported to enhance the saltiness of foods with low to moderate levels of salt;
- dairy concentrates – reported to allow moderate sodium reductions in a variety of products;
- herbs and spices provide other flavouring characteristics and may, for some people, help alleviate blandness following salt removal;
- compounds that reduce bitterness including adenosine-5′-monophosphate, 2,4-dihydroxybenzoic acid (DHB), lactose, sodium gluconate, and mixtures

**TABLE 6.4**
**Examples of Typically High Salt Products Available on the Market with Lower Salt Content**

| No. | Type of Food | Reformulation Type | Replacers for Salt | Origin Country | Labelling Information |
|---|---|---|---|---|---|
| 1 | Meat products: Turkey rolls/ Mediterranean ham/ soft chicken liver pate/chicken frankfurters | Lowering salt content with 30% of the mean value existing on the market | - | Romania | Information available on the website (http://www.santivia.ro/) |
| 2 | Dairy products: smocked and unsalted pressed cheese/ naturally unsalted pressed cheese/goat telemea | Removing salt from the recipe | | | No salt |
| 3 | No salt bread | | | | |
| 4 | Corn snacks and crackers | | | | |
| 5 | Bread | Removing salt from the recipe | | UK | Traffic light labelling improved due to reduction in salt of up to 50% |
| 6 | Breakfast cereals | Removing salt from the recipe | | | Traffic light labelling improved due to reduction in salt of up to 50% |

for use in combination with potassium chloride – designed to mask bitterness of potassium chloride or reduce bitterness from other food components that are usually masked by salt; allow partial reduction of total sodium content;

- mixtures of NaCl substitutes and enhancers – proprietary mixtures are produced by many companies; mixtures consist of a number of ingredients such as non-sodium salts, yeast extracts, potassium chloride, sodium, and sodium gluconate.

Table 6.4 provides examples of low-salt products.

The most successful approach to salt reduction is the use of micronized salt. It is smaller in size (from 250–500 μm to 5–10 μm) and provides a salty taste more quickly and intensely since the microparticles come into solution faster and interact with taste receptors in the oral cavity through more connections. Micronized salt allows salt reduction in products such as pastries, pizzas, bread, and cheese by 30%. The SODA-LO Salt Microspheres base their effectiveness on this principle (Noort et al., 2010). Potassium chloride is perhaps the most frequently used solution for the reduction of sodium in the diet since its taste closely approximates that of chloride. However, salt intensity is perceived as 30% less and it has a slight metallic taste.

Protein hydrolysates of vegetable origins are the most common amino acids used. In addition to saltiness, they provide a "meaty" flavour to products, although appreciation of this depends on the consumer and are stable to heat (Parniakov et al., 2020). Sea plants can also be a good alternative for providing a salty taste. Dried extracts from plants of the genus *Salicornia* and *Eucheuma* are rich in potassium chloride and low in sodium. They also contain iodine, which makes them optimal substitutes for iodized salt, as well as vitamins and unsaturated fatty acids (Barreira et al., 2017).

Another salt reduction strategy is changing the processing method. The application of some treatments like pasteurization or ultra-pasteurization (ultra-high temperature); freezing and/or cooling; curing (e.g., cheeses); drying (e.g., sausages); fermentation; preservation at high pressures which destroys microorganisms, and adding salts that decrease the activity of microorganisms in water, such as potassium chloride (Parniakov et al., 2020), can be great options to minimize the salt content. A current approach to reduce sodium in processed foods and meat products is based on improving salt diffusion by employing novel processing technologies, such as high-pressure processing, pulsed electric fields (PEFs), and ultrasound (Inguglia et al., 2017). Ultrasound has reduced salt by 30% in processed meats such as ham (Barretto et al., 2018). High hydrostatic pressures (HPPs) have also emerged as an alternative technology to heat treatment for food preservation (Barba et al., 2012).

## 6.3 FOOD TRANSPORT AND DISTRIBUTION IN CITIES

Logistics for the food sector demand high levels of food safety and traceability, such as short-lead time and distinct handling procedures. For fresh, frozen and prepared food, temperature-controlled technology is required together with just-in-time deliveries and dedicated facilities and vehicles (Mahajan et al., 2017). In the last decade, the global food supply system has experienced critical disruptions, such as price surges and shortages, resulting from the financial crisis of 2007–2008 and extreme weather events. More recently, the COVID-19 pandemic has placed exceptional stresses on food supply chains, with issues related to transport and logistics, as well as considerable shifts in demand. The consequences of global food disruptions include reduced food access and food security (Morgan and Sonnino, 2011). Transport and logistics operations are a key element of sustainable food distribution systems that improve access to healthy and affordable food. Perishable foods need to be transported in refrigerated trucks, stored in refrigerated warehouses, and displayed in refrigerated cases. The added costs associated with fresh foods, that non-perishable processed products do not have to consider, directly affect the availability of fruit and vegetables in stores and ultimately food choice for the consumers.

### 6.3.1 The Last Mile for Food

Food logistics in an urban environment are an important yet problematic aspect of the supply chain, due to the high number of receivers (supermarkets and food outlets) and the resulting lack of efficiency in transport operations (Morganti & Gonzalez-Feliu, 2015).

The last mile deliveries from local warehouses, distribution centres, suppliers, and farmers to urban food outlets and consumers are often characterized by small volumes, high frequency, non-homogeneous transport units (pallets, parcels, boxes, etc.) and a wide range of commercial vehicles, such as vans, small trucks, and lorries (ibid 2015). The receivers, both businesses and households, set increasingly high-performance standards that must be met, including shorter time windows, no minimum order amount and higher frequency of deliveries. Empty runs and long dwell times at loading and unloading points are frequent and they can represent a significant waste of resources. Inefficient food transport operations generate a larger amount of waste in terms of food that is lost during the loading and unloading activities, transit, and delivery. Food losses are highest for fruits and vegetables where on average 4%–15% of production is lost along the distribution phase (Gustavsson et al., 2011), generating additional costs usually reflected in the price paid by consumers.

To reduce food losses during last mile deliveries, several factors need to be taken into account: temperature, humidity and water loss, atmospheric composition, physical injury and mixed load (Vigneault et al., 2009). Many trucks and vans deliver several types of produce in a single journey. Although last mile deliveries are usually short trips (from local warehouses to city outlets), the quality of the load can be compromised if, for example, produce is mixed with products with different storage requirements (ibid 2009). As a result, the fleet should be equipped with adequate temperature control and air circulation systems to ensure quality preservation of perishable goods. In more general terms, refrigerated vehicles have higher energy requirements than standard vehicles, increasing transport costs. From a socio-economic perspective, factors such as fluctuating fuel prices, shortage of skilled drivers forcing higher wages, and increased regulation governing driver hours (Rodrigue, 2020) also contribute to the complexity of last mile for food contributing to higher transport costs, differentiated by type of food and how perishable it is.

Other issues related to the last mile for food deal with urban environmental sustainability and the way food circulates in cities. Road transport, almost the sole mode for urban deliveries, is one of the most polluting per unit of distance travelled (Rodrigue, 2020) and it generates negative effects on traffic (Quak and Koster, 2009) and on air quality, especially refrigerated vans (Yang et al., 2021).

### 6.3.2 Fruit and Vegetable Distribution Issues

Besides constraints related to food transport, retailing management operations associated with perishable goods play an important role on defining the range of fresh products available in stores. Fresh foods have a short shelf-life, and their value declines as appearance declines (Shewfelt, 2017). Fresh foods are refrigerated as soon as possible to slow rotting, but refrigeration requires energy which increases costs both in transport and in the retail destination. Upon arrival at the retail destination, produce should be refrigerated; but since display cabinets in many retailers do not have the refrigeration capacity to cool produce, fruits and vegetables may not be at their optimum temperature before being stacked for display (Vigneault et al., 2009).

### 6.3.3 Preserving the Variety of Distribution Channels: Independent Retailers

Perishable goods deliveries for independent retailers and small food services in urban areas are characterized by small-scale distribution of goods. Shop keepers, hotel, and restaurants owners ask for high frequency and express deliveries of limited number of parcels, in a narrow time window. Food deliveries are usually informal logistics activities, most of them directly operated by food suppliers, producers, and shop owners, with limited delivery consolidation measures. Moreover food outlets are located in the whole urban area and their fragmentation represents a critical issue for efficient delivery planning (Morganti and Gonzalez-Feliu, 2015). Potential benefits resulting from improved deliveries systems in the urban food sector have been investigated with increasing interest; however, costs specifically associated with cold chain transport, as well as the scarcity of space available for logistics platforms and the limited availability of public finances, reduce the opportunity to implement consolidation measures. Scenarios describing fragmented, frequent, and small deliveries to urban food outlets have been described by different studies, for cities of various size, for example, Winchester, UK (Cherrett et al., 2009), and Melbourne, Australia (Aljohani & Thompson, 2018). In terms of vegetables, only 12% are now purchased from family run grocer shops in the UK and the majority, 72%, are sold in supermarkets where transport costs are cheaper due to bulk deliveries which is reflected in the cost to the consumer. However, there are down sides as smaller retailers are more likely to better connect producers with consumers and provide diverse foods for the local population. Furthermore, there are wider losses to society as small grocers are often centres of communities (Pretty, 2001; Hughes, 1996).

### 6.3.4 Food Hubs

The urban food distribution system includes a variety of stakeholders who oversee logistics operations: producers, wholesalers, retailers, shop and restaurant owners, and shippers who contribute in different ways to the local provisioning system and who assure connections at a regional and global level. Within this scenario, the wholesale produce market (WPM) offers an effective solution to reduce the fragmentation of urban food deliveries and the subsequent transport costs for fresh foods. When the market authority or the management body can provide transport and delivery services and consolidate in one vehicle deliveries to multiple receivers from different suppliers, the WPM is not only a marketplace but becomes also a logistic platform. In different European countries and in the US, wholesale markets started a renovation process based on the concept of a Food Hub (FH), as defined by Morley and Morgan (2009):

> partnership based arrangements that coordinate the distribution of a range of food products from producers of a uniform provenance to conventional or hybrid markets.

Three core components characterized the FH function on urban food supply system:

i. Aggregation, distribution, and wholesale

ii. Active coordination
iii. Permanent facilities together with additional logistics, marketing, and communication services.

The FH concept has been applied to the wholesale produce market and to different entities operating in the urban food distribution system, such as cooperatives of producers and associations of private wholesalers (Palacios-Argüello et al., 2017).

An example is in the city of Parma, Italy, where the WPM re-designed its functions around the concept of the FH (Morganti & Gonzalez-Feliu, 2015). The authority pursued three goals: reducing air pollution with low-carbon vans; improving the resources efficiency and cost-effectiveness of produce deliveries while incorporating external costs; and contributing to the access of healthy food in the community, assuring that it is available to small local businesses. Similar projects need a strong support and commitment from different local stakeholders, only achievable with long-lasting partnerships created during the early stages of the initiative.

## 6.4 CONCLUSIONS

The food industry is global, providing a wide range of foods of which 80% are processed to some degree. Many manufactured foods are too high in fats, sugars, and salt which has led to intakes of lower-than-optimal diets. As most consumers are now used to eating food that tastes sweeter, fattier, and saltier than is good for our health, the food industry has focused on a wide range of innovative solutions to produce healthier foods and non-alcoholic beverages. Due to the role of fats, sugars, and salt in food preservation and sensory attributes, a compromise is necessary to balance what consumers want to eat and what they should eat to maintain health. Nevertheless, progress has been made in the last two decades through reformulation; and the wide reach of reformulated products has the potential to reduce inequalities in diet and health. Consumption patterns vary by region, resulting in some countries prioritizing reductions of one nutrient over another. The process of food reformulation needs co-creation, multidisciplinary, and education-based activities involving all food producers and food businesses.

Food deliveries, particularly in urban environments, are the least efficient part of the supply chain, due to the high number of receivers and to their increasingly high requirements. In the case of fresh foods which are usually lowest in salt, sugar, and fat, distinct handling procedures and temperature-controlled transport represent additional constraints to these last mile deliveries. Inefficiencies in food logistics also have an impact on the competitiveness of food outlets which in turn influence the access to affordable healthy food. Food hubs in urban areas offer one solution but further last food mile schemes supported by public sector policies are needed to reduce the impact on local air pollution while improving availability of healthy foods.

In conclusion, consistent, fair, and enforced regulation, across different regions of the world, to compel food producers to produce and deliver healthy food is required to ensure a healthy food environment for all.

## REFERENCES

Albuquerque, T., G., Santos, J., Silva, M. A., Beatriz, M., Oliveir, P.P., & Costa, H. S. 2018. An update on processed foods: Relationship between salt, saturated and trans fatty acids contents. *Food Chemistry*, 267, pp. 75–82.

Aljohani, K., & Thompson, R. 2018. The impacts of relocating a logistics facility on last food miles–The case of Melbourne's fruit & vegetable wholesale market. *Case Studies on Transport Policy*, 6(2), 279–288.

Barba, F. J., Esteve, M. J., & Frígola, A. 2012. High pressure treatment effect on physicochemical and nutritional properties of fluid foods during storage: A review. *Comprehensive Reviews in Food Science and Food Safety*, 11, pp. 307–322.

Barreira, L., Resek, E., Rodrigues, M.J, Rocha, M.I., Pereira, H., Bandarra, N., Moreira da Silva, M., Varela, J., & Custódio, L. 2017. Halophytes: Gourmet food with nutritional health benefits? *Journal of Food Composition and Analysis*, 59, pp. 35–42.

Barretto, L.T., Rodrigues Pollonio, M.A., Telis-Romero, J., & da Silva Barretto, A.C. 2018. Improving sensory acceptance and physicochemical properties by ultrasound application to restructured cooked ham with salt (NaCl) reduction. *Meat Science*, 145, pp. 55–62.

Belc, N., Smeu, I., Macri, A., Vallauri, D., & Flynn, K. 2019. Reformulating foods to meet current scientific knowledge about salt, sugar and fats. *Trends in Food science & Technology*, 84, 25–28.

Belz, C.E.M., Ryan, A.M.L., & Arendt, E.K. 2012. The impact of salt reduction in bread: A review. *Critical Reviews in Food Science and Nutrition*, 52, 514–524.

Cherrett, T., McLeod, F., Maynard, S., Hickford, A., & Allen, J. 2009. Understanding retail supply chains to enable 'greener' logistics – A case study of 'delivery' and 'take-back' mechanisms in Winchester – Final Report. https://www.researchgate.net/publication/237760979_Understanding_retail_supply_chains_to_enable_'greener'_logistics_-_A_case_study_of_'delivery'_and_'take-back'_mechanisms_in_Winchester

DEFRA. 2020. Food statistics in your pocket: Process and expenditure. https://www.gov.uk/government/statistics/food-statistics-pocketbook/food-statistics-in-your-pocket-prices-and-expenditure.

Domenech-Asensi, G., Merola, N., Lopez-Fernandez, A., Ros-Berruezo, G., & Frontela-Saseta, C. 2016. Influence of the reformulation of ingredients in bakery products on healthy characteristics and acceptability of consumers. *International Journal of Food Sciences and Nutrition*, 67(1), 74–82.

EUFIC. 2010. The greatest thing since sliced bread? A review of the benefits of processed foods. http://www.eufic.org/en/food-production/article/the-greatestthing-since-sliced-bread-a-review-of-the-benefits-of-processed.

European Commission (EC). 2012. Survey on members states' implementation of the EU salt reduction framework. https://ec.europa.eu/health/sites/default/files/nutrition_physical_activity/docs/salt_report1_en.pdf

Gustavsson, J., Cederberg, C., Sonesson, U., Otterdijk, R.V., & Meybeck, A. 2011. Global food losses and food waste: Extent, causes and prevention. In *Interpack*. Rome, Italy: Food and Agriculture Organization of the United Nations.

Hughes, D. 1996. Dancing with an elephant: Building partnerships with multiples. Paper presented at *The Vegetable Challenge Conference*, London, May 21, The Guild of Food Writers.

Hutchinson, J., Rippin, H.L., Jewell, J., Breda, J.J., & Cade, J.E. 2017. Comparison of high and low trans-fatty acid consumers: Analyses of UK National Diet and Nutrition Surveys before and after product reformulation. *Public Health Nutrition*, 21(3), 465–479.

Inguglia, E. S., Zhang, Z., Tiwari, B.K., Kerry, J.P., & Burgess, C. M. 2017. Salt reduction strategies in processed meat products – A review. *Trends in Food Science & Technology*, 59, pp.70–78.

Institute of Medicine. 2010. *Strategies to Reduce Sodium Intake in the United States.* Washington, DC: The National Academies Press. doi: 10.17226/12818.

Luo, X., Arcot, J., Gill, T., Louie, J.K.Y., & Rangan, A. 2019. A review of food reformulation of baked products to reduce added sugar intake. *Trends in Food Science & Technology*, 86, pp. 412–425.

Mahajan, R., Garg, S., & Sharma, P. B. 2017. Processed food supply chain: A framework for literature review. *Journal of Advances in Management Research*, 14(1), 91–109. doi: 10.1108/JAMR-05-2016-0035.

Marcus, J.B. 2013. Chapter 6- Lipids basics: Fats and oils in foods and health: Healthy lipid choices, roles and applications in nutrition, food science and the culinary arts. In *Culinary Nutrition*, edited by Jacqueline B. Marcus. Cambridge, MA: Academic Press, pp. 231–277. ISBN 9780123918826, doi: 10.1016/B978-0-12-391882-6.00006-6.

Morgan, K., & Sonnino, R. 2011. The urban foodscape: World cities and the new food equation. *Cambridge Journal of Regions, Economy and Society*, 3(2), 209–224.

Morganti, E. 2019. Food and urban logistics. In: *Urban Logistics: Management, Policy and Innovation in a Rapidly Changing Environment*, edited by M. Browne & S. Behrends. London: Kogan Page Publishers, 196–208. https://www.koganpage.com/product/urban-logistics-9780749478711

Morganti, E., & Gonzalez-Feliu, J. 2015. City logistics for perishable products. The case of Parma's Food Hub. *Case Studies in Transport Policy*, 3 (2), 120–128.

Morley, A., & Morgan, S. (2009). Alternative food hubs: The missing middle in sustainable local food network? Report for the Welsh Assembly Government.

Noort, M. W.J., Bult, J. H.F, Stieger, M., & Hamer, R.J. 2010. Saltiness enhancement in bread by inhomogeneous spatial distribution of sodium chloride. *Journal of Cereal Science*, 52(3): 378–386.

O'Sullivan, M.G. 2016. Low-fat foods: Types and manufacture. In *Encyclopedia of Food and Health*, edited by Benjamin Caballero, Paul Finglas & Fidel Toldrá. Cambridge, MA: Academic Press, pp. 571–575.

Onaolapo, A.Y., Onaolapo, A.J., & Olowe, A. 2020. Chapter 9 - An overview of addiction to sugar. In *Dietary Sugar, Salt and Fat in Human Health*, edited by Harry G. Preuss & Debasis Bagchipp. Cambridge, MA: Academic Press, pp. 195–216.

Palacios-Argüello, P., Morganti, E., & Gonzalez-Feliu, J. 2017. Food hub: Una alternativa para alimentar las ciudades de manera sostenible. *Revista Transporte y Territorio*, 17:10–33

Parliamentary Office of Science and Technology (POST). 2021. Food and drink reformulation to reduce fat, sugar and salt. https://post.parliament.uk/research-briefings/post-pn-0638/.

Parniakov, O., Mikhrovska, M., Toepfl, S., Roselló-Soto, E., Pinto, C.A., Saraiva, J.A., & Barba, F.J. 2020. Current and future strategies to reduce salt consumption. In *Agri-Food Industry Strategies for Healthy Diets and Sustainability. New Challenges in Nutrition and Public Health*, edited by Francisco J. Barba, Predrag Putnik & Danijela Bursać Kovačević. Cambridge, MA: Academic Press, pp. 155–175.

Popkin, B.M. 2015. Nutrition transition and the global diabetes epidemic. *Current Diabetes Reports*, 15, 64.

Popkin, B.M., Adair, L.S., & Ng, S.W. 2012. Global nutrition transition and the pandemic of obesity in developing countries. *Nutrition Reviews*, 70(1), 3–21. doi: 10.1111/j.1753-4887.2011.00456.x. PMID: 22221213; PMCID: PMC3257829.

Pretty, J. 2001. Some benefits and drawbacks of local food systems. University of Essex, Briefing Note for TVU/Sustain AgriFood Network, November 2nd.

Public Health England (PHE). 2020. *Salt Reduction Targets for 2024.* London: PHE Publications. https://assets.publishing.service.gov.uk/government/uploads/system/uploads/attachment_data/file/915406/2024_salt_reduction_targets_070920-FINAL-1.pdf, accessed: 20.03.2021

Quak, H.J., & de Koster, M.B.M. 2009. Delivering goods in urban areas: How to deal with urban policy restrictions and the environment. *Transportation Science*, 43(2), 211–22.

Rodrigue, J. 2020. *The Geography of Transport Systems*. New York: Routledge, 456 pages. ISBN 978-0-367-36463-2.

Shewfelt, R.L. 2017. Why can't we find more locally produced and fresher food in our supermarkets and restaurants? In *Defense of Processed Food*, edited by Susan Safren. Cham: Copernicus. doi: 10.1007/978-3-319-45394-1_3.

The European Consumer Organisation. 2015. Informed food choice for healthier consumers, BEUC position on nutrition.

Turnera, C., Aggarwalb, A., Wallsc, H., Herforthd, A., Drewnowskie, A., Coatesf, J., Kalamatianoua, S., & Kadiyalaa, S. 2018. Concepts and critical perspectives for food environment research: A global framework with implications for action in low- and middle-income countries. *Global Food Security*, 18, 93–101.

Vatankhah, M., Garavand, F., Mohammadi, B. & Elhamirad, A.H. 2017. Quality attributes of reduced-sugar Iranian traditional sweet bread containing stevioside. Journal of Food Measurement and Characterization, 11, 1233–1239.

Vigneault, C., Thompson, J., We, S., Hui, C., & LeBlanc, D. 2009. Transportation of fresh horticultural produce. *Postharvest Technologies for Horticultural Crops*, edited by Noureddine Benkeblia. Vol. 2, Trivandrum: Research Signpost. pp. 1–24. ISBN: 978-81-308-0356-2.

World Health Organization. 2012. Action plan for implementation of the European strategy for the prevention and control of noncommunicable diseases 2012–2016. http://apps.who.int/medicinedocs/documents/s19752en/s19752en.pdf. Accessed 20.01.2017.

World Health Organization. 2013. Mapping salt reduction initiatives in the WHO European region. http://www.euro.who.int/__data/assets/pdf_file/0009/186462/Mapping-salt-reduction-initiatives-in-the-WHO-European-Region.pdf. Accessed 20.01.2017.

World Health Organization. 2014. European food and nutrition action plan 2015–2020. Denmark: Copenhagen. http://www.euro.who.int/_data/assets/pdf_file/0008/253727/64wd14e_FoodNutAP_140426.pdf.

World Health Organization. 2015a. Eliminating trans fats in Europe. A policy brief. Denmark: Copenhagen. http://www.euro.who.int/_data/assets/pdf_file/0010/288442/Eliminating-trans-fats-in-Europe-A-policy-brief.pdf?ua=1.

World Health Organization. 2015b. Guideline: Sugars intake for adults and children. https://www.who.int/publications/i/item/9789241549028. Accessed 10.01.2021.

World Health Organization. 2018. Healthy diet – Key facts. http://www.who.int/en/news-room/fact-sheets/detail/healthy-diet.

World Health Organization. 2019. Replace trans fat: An action package to eliminate industrially produced trans-fatty acids. https://www.who.int/docs/default-source/replace-transfat/1-replace-framework-updated-june-2019-ke.pdf. Accessed 10.01.2021.

Yang, Y., Davis, G.C., & You, W. 2019. Measuring food expenditure poverty in SNAP populations: Some extensions with an application to the American Recovery and Reinvestment Act. *Applied Economic Perspectives and Policy*, 41, 133–152. doi: 10.1093/aepp/ppy004.

Yang, Z, Tate, J.E., Morganti, E., & Shepherd, S.P. 2021. Real-world $CO_2$ and $NO_X$ emissions from refrigerated vans. *Science of the Total Environment*, 763, 142974. doi: 10.1016/j.scitotenv.2020.142974.

# 7 The Role of the Food Industry in Public Health Nutrition

*Simon Capewell and Ffion Lloyd-Williams*
University of Liverpool

## CONTENTS



## 7.1 INTRODUCTION

Our food environments are powerfully shaped by the food industry which naturally prioritises profits, over health. Total UK food supply chain company revenues annually exceed £120 billion, with sales of manufactured food and drink exceeding £75 billion, representing some 20% of total UK manufacturing (Food and Drink Federation 2021). The food industry is essential for food provision in every country; however, the manufacturing of ultra-processed foods high in saturated fats, sugars and

DOI: 10.1201/9781003043720-7 

salt raises major concerns for diet quality and health. These ultra-processed products (UPPs) are made from processed substances extracted or refined from whole foods for example, oils, hydrogenated oils and fats, flours and starches, variants of sugar, and cheaper parts or remnants of animal foods and additives – with little or no whole foods (Monteiro et al. 2018). UPPs include sugar-sweetened beverages (SSBs) – drinks with added sugar including non-diet soft drinks and sodas, flavoured juice drinks, sports drinks, energy drinks and sweetened teas.

Over 90% of UK food industry profits come from UPPs including SSBs with barely 5% of profits coming from fruit and vegetables (Statista 2020). Ultra-processing thus represents a simple and highly profitable business model. It "adds value" to basic materials; for instance, turning one bag of potatoes costing 50 p into ten bags of crisps sold for £2.50 or more. The multinational food corporations recently reported an average gross profit margin of 37%, three-fold higher than the 10%–15% profit for fruit and vegetables. Thus in 2019, estimated UK fruit and vegetable wholesalers' profits were just £1.5 billion (Statista 2020).

In this chapter, we will briefly consider the producing and marketing, by industry, of UPPs, SSBs and convenience food and snacks. All are high in energy, saturated fats, sugars or salt or all four. We will then examine the tactics industry uses to minimise regulation and taxation and thus maximise profits. We finish with lessons learnt from previous public health successes in tobacco and alcohol control. Many are directly applicable to achieving healthier food environments in the UK and beyond.

## 7.2 HEALTHY AND UNHEALTHY DIETS AND ULTRA-PROCESSED PRODUCTS

The key features of a healthy diet are well defined by WHO and country-specific organisations such as the American Heart Association (AHA) in the US and the Public Health England (PHE) Eatwell Guide in the UK (see Chapter 1). A healthy diet gives preference to fruits, vegetables and wholegrain foods as well as foods high in polyunsaturated fats (canola) or monounsaturated fats (olive oil), lean meats and meat alternatives such as beans or tofu, and avoiding industrial trans-fats. Unhealthy dietary patterns are also well defined, being high in saturated animal fats, salt and sugars (hence high-fat sugar salt or "HFSS").

Packaged foods are much more likely to be categorised as HFSS. There is no one universally agreed method to classify foods that are HFSS and ultra-processed but one increasingly popular method is the NOVA system. NOVA usefully describes the nature, extent and purpose of food processing, categorising all foods into four groups (Monteiro et al. 2018). UPPs typically include soft drinks; sweet and savoury packaged snacks; confectionery; mass-produced packaged breads, buns, biscuits and cakes; hot dogs, poultry and fish "nuggets"; reconstituted meat products; "instant" soups and noodles; industrialised desserts and industrially pre-prepared pizzas, pies and other dishes and meals (Monteiro et al. 2018).

Diets high in UPPs thus contain more energy, fats and sugars and salt and less fruits and vegetables (Monteiro et al. 2018). UPPs now dominate the food supplies in high-income countries and are rapidly increasing in low- and middle-income countries.

In a recent UK study, ultra-processed foods accounted for 57% of total energy intake, with most adults and children exceeding the recommended limit of 10% of energy from free sugars. Conversely, eliminating ultra-processed foods could potentially halve free sugar intake (Monteiro et al. 2018). However, intakes of UPPs are much lower in some countries such as Portugal, demonstrating that it is possible even for wealthy countries to consume less processed diets.

## 7.3 MARKETING OF ULTRA-PROCESSED PRODUCTS

UPPs are designed to be hyper-palatable, attractive and consumable anywhere, at any time. Their formulation, presentation and marketing thus promote overconsumption, and their long shelf-life further increases their profitability. Marketing of UPPs is covered in more detail in Chapter 14; the reliance of fast food businesses and supermarkets (where most food is purchased) on what is nationally available from food companies is highlighted in Chapters 8 and 5, respectively.

The UK food industry expenditure to promote "unhealthy" foods for purchase in retail settings exceeded £250 million in 2014 (Public Health England 2015) and has continued to rise since then. Furthermore, the companies producing the top 18 UK brands annually spent over £140 million advertising their products, mainly crisps, confectionery and sugary drinks (Obesity Health Alliance, 2017). This spend was 28 times the £5 million UK government budget for their flagship healthy eating campaign Change4Life, run by PHE in the same year (O'Dowd 2017).

UPP marketing often also includes sponsorship. Large expensive events rely on funding from industry, notably from UPP companies. Thus in 2012, McDonalds and Coca-Cola, the official London Olympics sponsors, repeatedly exaggerated the benefits of physical activity to address the obesity epidemic, as opposed to reducing the consumption of HFSS foods and sugary drinks.

## 7.4 THE "BIG 10" UPP FOOD AND BEVERAGE COMPANIES

Globally, most processed food consumed each day is produced by one of just ten multinational corporations. Hence, the striking infographic (Figure 7.1) in the 2013 Oxfam's report "Behind the Brands: Food justice and the "Big 10" food and beverage companies". These ten huge multinational corporations are Associated British Foods (ABF), Coca-Cola, Danone, General Mills, Kelloggs, Mars, Mondelez International (previously known as Kraft), Nestlé, PepsiCo and Unilever (Figure 7.1). They together create the narrow stem of an "hour-glass" between producers and consumers – a small number of purchasing desks which can powerfully influence contemporary food markets. Furthermore, these giant food multinationals hide behind a profusion of labels (Figure 7.1), concealing their substantial industrial power and market control. In 2019, the most valuable food brands worldwide ranked Nestlé first, with a global brand value of roughly US$20 billion, and Danone ranked second being valued at some US$8 billion (Statista 2020). The obligation to maximise profit for shareholders ensures that UPP production and promotion is prioritised over healthier options (Capewell & Lloyd-Williams 2018).

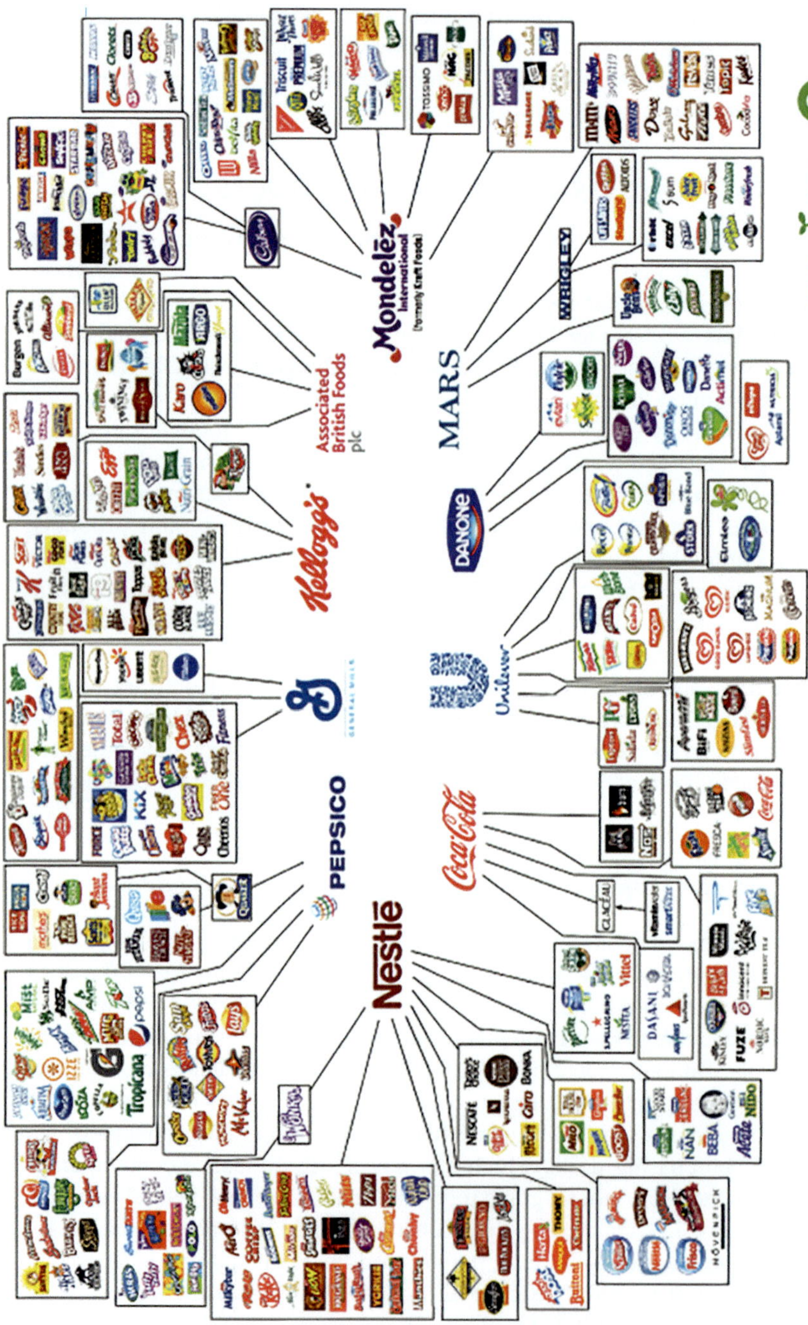


**FIGURE 7.1** Behind the brands: Food Justice and the "Big 10" food and beverage companies. (Reprinted with permission from Joki Gauthier at Oxfam, 2012. Available at http://www.behindthebrands/take-action/.org.)

## 7.5 IMPACT OF FOOD INDUSTRY PRACTICE ON SOCIO-ECONOMIC INEQUALITIES IN DIET

Ultra-processed food and SSBs are generally cheaper and thus more affordable for lower-income households (Backholer et al. 2016). In the UK, local authority areas with a higher deprivation score have five times more fast food outlets compared with more affluent areas (Public Health England 2018). Recent UK and US studies have therefore described these neighbourhoods as "food swamps" – areas with a high density of establishments selling high-calorie fast food and junk food (Cooksey-Stowers, Schwartz, Brownell 2017). The *presence* of "food swamps" (however defined) was a stronger predictor of obesity rates than the *absence* of full-service grocery stores ("food deserts"). Furthermore, the food swamp effect was even stronger in countries with greater income inequality and less mobility of residents.

In order to reduce inequalities in diet, it is necessary for policies and programmes to have more impact in lower-income populations. Backholer et al. (2016) reviewed studies within high-income countries to examine the effects of an SSB price increase on beverage purchases or consumption. Tax on SSB was effective, and sometimes delivered even greater benefits for lower socio-economic groups, for instance in Mexico (Colchero 2016).

The double burden of malnutrition (DBM) also demonstrates dramatic inequalities. DBM, defined as the simultaneous manifestation of both undernutrition and overweight and obesity, affects most low-income and middle-income countries (LMICs). This can make food policy decision-making particularly complex. Popkin, Corvalan and Grummer-Strawn (2020) describe the dynamics of the DBM in LMICs and how it differs markedly by socio-economic level. DBM has increased in the poorest LMICs, mainly due to increases in overweight and obesity. Indonesia is the largest country with a severe DBM, but numerous other Asian and sub-Saharan African countries also face this problem. The increases in overweight mainly reflect very rapid changes in the food system, particularly the availability of cheap ultra-processed food and beverages in LMICs, and major reductions in physical activity at work, transportation, home and leisure due to introductions of activity-saving technologies. Increased understanding then helps to identify crucial drivers and possible options for addressing the DBM at all levels. Double-duty actions (DDAs) aim to simultaneously tackle both undernutrition and problems of overweight, obesity and diet-related non-communicable diseases (DR-NCDs) in a more holistic way. Hawkes et al. (2020) identify ten DDAs to potentially reduce the risk of both undernutrition, obesity and DR-NCDs. Tackling this double burden is unlikely to get easier. The world trade in highly processed food products is growing fast, with middle-income countries becoming the major commodity suppliers to world markets (Food and Drink Federation 2021). UK food exports in 2020 totalled some £10 billion, of which highly processed foods accounted for almost £6 billion.

## 7.6 UK PUBLIC HEALTH ACTIONS TO PREVENT CHILDHOOD OBESITY

Obesity has been on the policy agenda for almost two decades in the UK, particularly since the *Foresight Report* in 2007. However, a coherent strategy has been lacking.

Obesity only really started to gain traction as a policy issue when the estimated societal cost of obesity in the UK reached £27 billion per year, with NHS costs then exceeding £5 billion (both probably underestimates) (Public Health England 2017). Obesity initiatives then multiplied, particularly in the last decade as the link to the steep rise in type 2 diabetes was increasingly recognised. Unfortunately, most of the initial policy initiatives emphasised politically unchallenging approaches such as information, education and "personal choice". All these individual-focused interventions are weak or ineffective and have, thus, actually been supported by the industry (Royal College of Paediatrics and Child Health 2015). However, after increasingly acknowledging the failure of these past strategies to reduce obesity, the UK is now identifying more population-wide effective interventions.

### 7.6.1 UK Parliamentary Health Select Committee and the WHO

The Parliamentary Health Select Committee, chaired by Sarah Wollaston MP, a public health advocate, examined the evidence base for preventing childhood obesity in the UK in 2015 and again in 2017 (House of Commons Health Committee 2015). They advocated "bold action" and produced important recommendations (Table 7.1). Crucially, they highlighted the importance of the obesogenic environment and recognised that it represents a large and complex problem. It would thus require a comprehensive, multifactorial and multilevel approach, because any single intervention in isolation would likely have minimal impact on this complex system.

Internationally, the Commission on Ending Childhood Obesity (ECHO), 2016, likewise stated in its Final Report that governments had a moral responsibility to act on behalf of children (World Health Organisation 2016). The extensive harms of food marketing targeting children were then further emphasised in 2018 by the WHO Committee on the Rights of the Child (World Health Organisation 2018). They concluded that countries had an obligation to protect the rights of children by adopting comprehensive measures to reduce the impact of HFSS marketing on children.

**TABLE 7.1**
**Health Select Committee (UK) Recommendations: A Comprehensive Prevention Strategy Comprising 12 Evidence-Based Interventions**

↓↓ Restrictions on advertising to children
↑↑ Reformulation
↑↑ 20% tax on full sugar soft drinks
↓↓ Price promotions
↓↓ Placement of food and drink in retail environment
↑↑ Labelling
↓↓ Portion sizes and caps
↑↑ Nutrition standards in ALL schools
↑↑ Support local authorities and wider public sector
↑↑ Early interventions
↓↓ Calorie reduction (not just sugar)
↑ Physical activity

### 7.6.2 UK Government Policies

Subsequent UK progress has been patchy thus far. A Soft Drinks Industry Levy (SDIL) or "sugar-tax" on sugary drinks was announced in 2016 and implemented in April 2018 (Gov.uk 2018). Further restrictions on advertising to children were implemented in 2016 and legislated in 2021. Voluntary industry reformulation of diverse food groups was subsequently supervised by PHE. The intention was to follow the same path successfully achieved by salt reduction in the last decade (Hyseni et al. 2017a, HM Government 2018), but progress has been minimal thus far.

Progress slowed even more in March 2020 with the onset of the coronavirus pandemic, then accelerated after the UK Prime Minister personally highlighted the increased importance of obesity prevention policies to reduce coronavirus risk. But will industry support this potentially important initiative?

Unless the rise in childhood obesity is arrested and then reversed, particularly the recent increase in inequalities in childhood obesity, millions of people will face a life shortened by obesity, type 2 diabetes and other chronic diseases. And both the NHS budget and UK economy will be further challenged.

## 7.7 UPP INDUSTRY DENIALISM TACTICS

The harms generated by the tobacco, alcohol, agro-chemical, fossil fuel, gambling, Big Tech, UPP and beverage corporations (the "Unhealthy Commodity Industries" or UCIs) are now increasingly recognised.

UPP and UCI corporations are legally obliged to preserve profits. Unfortunately, that inevitably results in undermining the most effective public health interventions – taxation and regulation. The role of corporate political activity (CPA) in undermining public health regulation has long been recognised in tobacco control circles (Chapman 2008). However, it was only in 2009 that Brownell and Warner published a seminal review entitled "Big tobacco played dirty and millions died, how similar is big food?" (Brownell & Warner 2009).

The last decade has witnessed a large increase in research in UCIs. Thus, Freudenberg described the prevailing ideology of the "the corporate consumption complex", and the resulting "hyper-consumption" across modern society; while Gilmore described UCI multinational corporations as "vectors of disease" (Gilmore et al., 2011). Hastings and Stuckler have separately detailed the powerful harmful influences that sophisticated UCI marketing campaigns are having on health (Capewell & Lloyd-Williams 2018). In 2010, UPP industry "denialism" tactics were further highlighted by McKee and Diethelm (2010), and the commonalities and links between the "Big Tobacco", "Big Alcohol" and "Big Food" corporations were then detailed in a *PLOS Medicine* series (Stuckler & Nestle 2012), and an extensively referenced *Lancet* review memorably entitled "Profits and Pandemics" by Moodie et al. (2013). They recommended public regulation and market intervention as the best, evidence-based mechanisms to minimise industry harms. Also that UCIs should have no role in the formation of national or international NCD policy (Moodie et al. 2013).

### 7.7.1 The Merchants of Doubt

Why are UPP industry players so keen to market doubt? Doubt can paralyse the legislative process. Doubt potentially undermines the solid evidence generally needed to justify a new public health policy (Oreskes & Conway 2010). For instance, John Yudkin catalogued the health harms of sugar in 1972. But industry actors successfully maintained sufficient doubts to ensure policy paralysis for three more decades (Lustig 2014). Only then could public health activists such as Lustig, MacGregor, Malhotra and Capewell begin to build successful UK healthy alliances, raising public concern and thus energising politicians to develop effective policies (Capewell & Lloyd-Williams 2018).

To be effective, public health messages need to be simple and clear ("Sugar Is The New Tobacco", *is an example of this*). Thus, public health advocates pragmatically distil sufficient evidence to satisfy public and politicians. They use a "balance of probabilities" criterion and actively reject industry saboteurs attempting to reframe the debate using the "beyond all reasonable doubt" criterion. This perfectionist standard is admirable, but inappropriate. *For instance, consider the causal links between smoking and lung cancer, or human activity and global warming. Agreed by 99% scientists, but still contested by vested commercial interests.* Furthermore, this pragmatism can create a tension with research colleagues who traditionally value "uncertainty" (i.e. doubt) as a fundamental component of the scientific process.

### 7.7.2 The HARMS Denialism Tactics Used by Tobacco and UPP Industry Actors

Mialon and colleagues have usefully identified, described and comprehensively categorised UCI denialism tactics as part of corporate political activity (CPA). UPP industry actors use multiple CPA strategies, particularly "information and messaging" and "constituency building" strategies. These deny, discredit, delay and dilute the effective interventions which might threaten profits, notably regulation and taxation (Mialon & da Silva Gomes 2019).

How best to communicate these and detailed comprehensive models of UPP industry tactics to the wider public is of interest. Building on existing research (Mialon & Gomes F da 2019), we offer *HARMS* as a mnemonic. Although this is new and not yet universally accepted; in our opinion, it is a useful framework. H A R M S stands for Heaps of money; Attack; Recruiting allies; Misinformation; and Substitution of ineffective policies (Table 7.2):

1. **Heaps of money**, hospitality and gifts. For instance, funding journalists, scientists (see below), political parties and politicians to delay legislation and weaken regulation. Around two thirds of US Congress representatives declare food industry funding (Nestlé 2013).
2. **Attack**. The UCI actors will target individuals, organisations and even countries (for example, the 2016 Philip Morris legal onslaught on Uruguay's tobacco control measures). Industry will use both actual litigation and also the simple threat which itself can achieve "regulatory chill".

**TABLE 7.2**
**HARMS Tactics Used by Tobacco & UPP Food Industries to Deny, Discredit, Delay and Dilute Effective Interventions**

| HARMS: Tactics Used by Tobacco and Food Industries to Block Market Regulation |
|---|
| *H Heap money on politicians, journalist & scientists* |
| *A Attack* |
| Neutralise, discredit, fragment and destabilise opponents: "Nanny State, Anti-business" |
| Litigation, challenge policies in courts, threaten legal action or "job losses" |
| *R Recruit* |
| Build *internal* constituencies, alliance and trade association. *External* constituencies, other sectors; policy makers; media; unions; civil society, consumers, employee, public; Astroturf (*fake grassroots organisations*) |
| *M Misinform* |
| Reshaping evidence; lobbying (direct or via third parties); increase doubt; procrastinate |
| *S Substitute ineffective interventions* |
| Voluntary, self-regulation, public–private partnerships, education, individual choice |

*Source:* Inspired by data from Savell et al. (2014).

UPP industries often use front organisations to fight on their behalf. In the UK, for instance, these include "free-market" think tanks like Institute of Economic Affairs (IEA) and Tax-Payers Association (TPA) and associated "libertarians". International co-ordination is then provided by the less-than-transparent Atlas Network (University of Bath 2020). These industry actors might mount *ad-hominem* attacks on public health advocates or accuse them of being "nanny state" or "anti-business", claiming that "this regulation will hurt jobs and the economy" (which it rarely does).

3. **Recruiting** allies and building up internal constituencies and trade associations to create political opposition coalitions. UPP actors also energetically recruit policy makers, media, civil society and consumer groups. For example, the American Beverage Association recently mobilised opposition to sugary drinks taxes by financing hostile media adverts, providing "charitable" funding to local community groups, and "astroturfing" – creating fake grassroots opposition organisations (De Lacy-Vawdon & Livingstone 2020).
4. **Misinformation** via blunt propaganda and more subtle biasing of the evidence. UCI corporations annually spend millions on "research" studies to undermine the basic evidence of harm. For instance, the Global Energy Balance Network (GEBN) attempted to blame children's obesity entirely on physical inactivity (Barlow et al. 2018). Industry can then hire "independent experts" or "independent think tanks" to lobby policy makers, or use "front groups" to misinform the media and public, generate doubt and therefore delay proposed regulation. Thus leading to politicians using the perceived "lack of scientific consensus" to justify policy inaction,

for instance, UPP industry propaganda framing using the term "Balanced Diet". Scientifically undefined, it implies that a bit of everything is ok, including ultra-processed foods and SSBs. "Balanced diet" is thus a shibboleth identifying industry-friendly framing (Chapter 12 provides more detail on misinformation and propagandists).

5. **Substituting** ineffective or weak interventions such as education, "individual choice" tropes, public–private partnerships, self-regulation or voluntary agreements. Anything other than regulation or taxation represents a good distraction (Knai et al. 2015a,b) (Table 7.2).

## 7.8 EFFECTIVE STRATEGIES TO CONTROL CONSUMPTION OF HARMFUL COMMODITIES

The understanding of corporate denial tactics has progressively disseminated across the wider policy arena and is now recognised by WHO (Chan 2013, WHO 2018) and the UN Special Rapporteurs on the Right to Food (2011) and on the Right to Health (2016).

### 7.8.1 Lessons from Tobacco Control and Alcohol Control

Effective tobacco control, painfully achieved over six decades, has generated valuable lessons. Crucially the need for comprehensive strategies which address each of the "3 As" – Affordability, Acceptability and Availability (Capewell & Lloyd-Williams 2018). Affordability includes increasing prices and taxes on all tobacco products. Acceptability includes advertising bans, smoke-free laws and plain packaging. Availability includes the elimination of previously ubiquitous vending machines, age checks in retail outlets and licensing of retailers. These comprehensive tobacco control strategies succeed by decreasing smoking initiation, reducing consumption and increasing quitting (Capewell & Lloyd-Williams 2018).

The UK, Ireland, Australia and USA can now boast some of the best tobacco control policies in the world. Trend analyses of smoking prevalence consistently demonstrate the successive impact of wave after wave of effective interventions taken from the "3A's" portfolio.

Public health alliances are thus continuing to battle and win against CPA. The tobacco industry is increasingly constrained by regulation and taxation, particularly in high-income countries. Progressive control globally has been powerfully assisted by the legally binding Framework Convention on Tobacco Control (FCTC), now adopted in some 180 countries (World Health Organisation 2005). Furthermore, the learning from the public health triumphs over Big Tobacco, and many other health threats over the last two centuries offer valuable lessons for the future. These lessons can be summarised using the SUPPORT framework (described below), and then applied across a wide range of issues.

### 7.8.2 The SUPPORT Pathway to Policy Success

Notable public health triumphs include clean water, sanitation, pollution control, slavery abolition, immunisation, seat belts and smoke-free interventions. The pathways for each of these can be usefully summarised by the mnemonic SUPPORT (Table 7.3).

**TABLE 7.3**
**SUPPORT Pathway Summarising Past and Future Public Health Triumphs**

| |
|---|
| ***S*CIENTIFIC evidence** emerges |
| ***U*NDERSTANDING** spreads |
| ***P*ROFESSIONALS accept** the scientific paradigm |
| ***P*UBLIC & POLITICIANS** become aware of the evidence, then supportive of remedies |
| ***O*PPOSITION from vested interests** is anticipate, then progressively **OVERCOME**, then |
| ***R*EGULATION is introduced**, often strengthened by |
| ***T*AXATION to reinforce regulations** |

UK tobacco control offers an excellent illustration of SUPPORT in action. Scientific evidence that tobacco causes heart disease and lung cancer became irrefutable in the 1950s and 1960s. A wider Understanding then spread across the scientific community, then more widely. Professionals such as doctors initially challenged it, but then progressively accepted the concept. The growing evidence about tobacco harms, was then diffused through the population, increasing Public understanding and awareness. Often amplified by committed advocates, that dissemination then progressively shifted opinion, first the general public, followed by Politicians. These policy makers then had little choice but to accept the will of the electorate and, crucially, resist intense industry lobbying. Because, as always, these proposals faced predictable Opposition from commercial vested interests and industry-funded pro-smoking lobbying groups. However, that opposition was then progressively Overcome to pave the way for Regulation. Recent successes include progressive marketing restrictions, reinforced in 2007, by smoke-free legislation banning smoking in enclosed public spaces (a major blow to smoking Acceptability). England subsequently increased the age at which tobacco products can be purchased, introduced picture warnings on packaging, banned vending machines and rolled out standardised packaging for tobacco products (Centre for Public Impact 2019). All reinforced by progressive rises in Taxation. Always popular with governments, taxes raise revenues which can potentially be fed back into public health schemes, fruit and vegetable subsidies or school breakfast clubs (as with the recent UK sweetened drinks industry levy (SDIL) (Gov.uk 2018)).

SUPPORT may thus offer a potentially useful framework to apply to public health successes, both historical and more recent ones such as UPP reformulation and sugary drinks taxation (Table 7.3).

### 7.8.3 The Public Health Effectiveness Hierarchy

These lessons from Tobacco Control have been successfully applied across a wider range of issues, demonstrating a phenomenon we have described as the "effectiveness hierarchy" of public health interventions (Capewell & Capewell 2018). Thus "downstream" preventive activities targeting individuals (such as primary prevention medications or 1:1 health education advice or leaflets to exercise or stop smoking) consistently achieve much smaller net health benefits than comprehensive, population-wide, policy interventions aimed further "upstream" (for instance, smoke-free legislation, tobacco taxes, alcohol minimum pricing or trans-fats elimination from foods). These are all "structural", improving the overall food environment, rather than depending on "agentic" and time-limited individual behaviour responses. Our team has demonstrated a clear effectiveness hierarchy in healthy diet strategies to reduce salt (Hyseni et al. 2017a) and trans-fats (Hyseni et al. 2017b). Our salt systematic review found that multi-component strategies (involving both upstream and downstream interventions) generally achieved the biggest reductions in salt consumption across an entire population (−4 g/day in Finland and Japan, −3 g/day in Turkey and −1.3 g/day in the UK). Mandatory reformulation alone might achieve −1.5 g/day, much more than voluntary reformulation (−0.8 g/day), school interventions (−0.7 g/day), short-term dietary advice (−0.6 g/day), nutrition labelling (−0.4 g/day), tax- and community-based counselling (−0.3 g/day) or health education media campaigns (−0.1 g/day) (Hyseni et al. 2017a).

Likewise industrial trans-fat intake still exceeds WHO targets in most countries. We systematically reviewed interventions to reduce trans-fat consumption. Multi-component interventions which included a legislative ban to eliminate trans-fats from food products were the most effective strategy. Reformulation and other multi-component interventions can also achieve useful reductions. However, "downstream" interventions consistently achieve smaller reductions (Hyseni et al. 2017b, c)).

Upstream structural policies are not just powerful, they also tend to be more cost-effective and equitable (Masters et al. 2017, Capewell & Capewell 2018). This is very apparent when broadly considering interventions to promote healthy eating. McGill et al. (2015) categorised healthy eating interventions using a "5P's" framework (Price, Place, Product, Promotion and Person). We found differential effects on healthy eating outcomes by socio-economic position. "Upstream" interventions categorised as "Price" (fiscal measures) generally decreased health inequalities and were more effective in lower socio-economic groups. All interventions that combined taxes and subsidies consistently decreased health inequalities. Conversely, "downstream" "Person" interventions (individual-based information, education and dietary counselling) had a smaller impact and also tended to widen health inequalities (McGill et al. 2015).

### 7.8.4 Successes in Controlling Industrial Trans-Fats and Salt

Building on a decade of progressive restrictions, Denmark was the first country to implement a national regulatory policy to eliminate industrially produced trans-fatty acids (ITFAs) in 2003. This defined a mandatory national limit (industrially produced TFA <2/100 g total oils and fats in all foods).

Regulation in Denmark then prompted the UK Food Standards Agency (now Public Health England) to encourage voluntary industry reformulation in 2008.

In the US, New York City regulation on ITFA content (<0.5% energy content) prompted major manufacturers to simplify their production chains by voluntarily implementing that standard nation wide. ITFA blood levels rapidly halved thereafter (Dietz & Scanlon 2012). It was then politically easy to transform this voluntary approach to mandatory in 2015 using a "no longer generally recognized as safe" (GRAS) ruling (United States Food and Drug Administration 2015).

As discussed above, the biggest reductions in salt consumption across entire populations have likewise mostly been achieved by multi-component strategies always including upstream policy interventions. Exemplars include Finland and Japan, Turkey and the UK (Laverty et al. 2019).

## 7.9 IMPLICATIONS FOR FUTURE RESEARCH AND POLICY

The focus of nutrition research has moved in one century from food safety to adequate supply and then to diet quality. The healthy diet consensus now emphasises fruit and vegetables, nuts and pulses, fish and olive oil, as in the DASH and Mediterranean Diets, and demonises UPPs and SSBs (see Chapter 3 on school food environments). Meanwhile, multinational corporations are energetically expanding their markets into middle-income countries using HARMS denial tactics (Capewell & Lloyd-Williams 2018). Fortunately, global research targeting the UCI and UPP industries has recently increased exponentially, supported by the *INFORMAS* collaboration (involving 22 countries as of May 2020) (INFORMAS 2020) and the GECI Network (2018).

Monteiro and colleagues suggest that the extinction of both the tobacco and UPP industries would benefit everyone (Monteiro et al. 2018). However, food policy progress represents a more complex challenge than tobacco control – the UPP corporations claim privileged status by currently feeding "billions" of people every day. Yet, every food multinational is haunted by the spectre of the tobacco industry – their arrogance and aggression provoked major regulation and taxation. The UPP industry is thus keen to avoid making the same mistake; especially now when facing increasing pressure from health professionals, public and politicians. The industry will therefore need to evolve by radical product reformulation, reducing potential harms and increasing health benefits while preserving profits. That strategy could win public support, and thus avoid political regulation.

The majority of great tobacco and food policy successes have been achieved by healthy alliances, often led by independent non-government organisations such as *El Poder del Consumidor* in Mexico, *CASH, Action on Sugar, Childrens' Food Campaign, & Consumers Association* in the UK, *the European Heart Network, the Center for Science in the Public Interest (CSPI)* in the US and *the Centre for Health Science and Law* in Canada. Important encouragement and support has come from the global network of activists and advocates in the World Public Health Nutrition Association (WPHNA) and GEC-PH (2018). Building public support has usually been crucial. For instance, in Mexico, *El Poder del Consumidor* overcame major obstacles from industry wealth and government inertia. They used Bloomberg funding to conduct a text-book three-phase messaging campaign – Expose the Human Drama (highlighting numerous diabetes and obesity deaths); Culprit Identification (exposing the industries producing SSBs) and then Present Solutions (Tax SSBs and spend the revenue on safe drinking water in schools, previously lacking).

## 7.10 CONCLUSIONS

Ultra-processed foods and SSBs mass-produced by the UPP food industry are energy-dense and high in salt, sugars and saturated fats. Poor diet generates some 40% of preventable NCDs (more than tobacco, alcohol and inactivity combined). But tackling dietary-related NCDs is difficult. These transnational UPP corporations aim to maximise profit and avoid regulation using HARMS denialism tactics, much like the tobacco industry in past decades. However, major lessons can be learnt from previous successes in tobacco (and alcohol) control, by employing a comprehensive strategy which includes the "3As" of Affordability, Acceptability and Availability (Capewell & Lloyd-Williams 2018). "Upstream", population-wide regulatory and fiscal approaches are much more effective than "downstream" behavioural interventions. Advocacy, activism and public engagement are all essential to travel successfully along the entire SUPPORT path, from the initial scientific evidence to finally achieving effective regulation and taxation. Only then can we ensure that scientific evidence is translated into effective policies delivering healthier food environments for everyone.

## ACKNOWLEDGEMENTS

We thank Ann Capewell and Paul Jameson for their perennial support and encouragement. We thank Prof Sian Griffiths, BMB Editor, for publishing our earlier exploration of these fascinating issues (Capewell & Lloyd-Williams 2018).

## REFERENCES

Backholer K, Sarink D, Beauchamp A, Keating C, Loh V, Ball K, Martin J, Peeters A. (2016) The impact of a tax on sugar-sweetened beverages according to socio-economic position: a systematic review of the evidence. *Public Health Nutrition* 19(17): 3070–3084.

Barlow P, Serôdio P, Ruskin G, et al. (2018) Science organisations and Coca-Cola's 'war' with the public health community: insights from an internal industry document. *Journal of Epidemiology Community Health* 72: 761–763.

Brownell KD, Warner KE. (2009) The perils of ignoring history: Big Tobacco played dirty and millions died. How similar is Big Food? *Milbank Quarterly* 87: 259–294. doi:10.1111/j.1468-0009.2009.00555.

Capewell S, Capewell A. (2018) An effectiveness hierarchy of preventive interventions: neglected paradigm or self-evident truth? *Journal of Public Health (Oxford)* 40(2): 350–358. doi:10.1093/pubmed/fdx055.

Capewell S, Lloyd-Williams F. (2018) The role of the food industry in health: lessons from tobacco? *British Medical Bulletin* 125(1): 131–143. doi:10.1093/bmb/ldy002.

Centre for Public Impact. (2019) Smoking ban in the United Kingdom, 2 September 2019. https://www.centreforpublicimpact.org/case-study/smoking-ban-united-kingdom/ (last accessed 9/11/2021).

Chan M. (2013) Director-general of the World Health Organization WHO director-general addresses health promotion conference opening. *Eighth Global Conference on Health Promotion Helsinki*, Finland, 10 June 2013.

Chapman S. (2008) *Public Health Advocacy and Tobacco Control: Making Smoking History.* Oxford, UK: Wiley-Blackwell. ISBN: 978-0-470-69163-2.

Colchero, MA, Popkin, BM, Rivera, JA, Ng, SW. (2016). Beverage purchases from stores in Mexico under the excise tax on sugar sweetened beverages: Observational study. *BMJ*: 352 doi:10.1136/bmj.h6704 (Published 6 January 2016).

Cooksey-Stowers K, Schwartz MB, Brownell KD. (2017) Food swamps predict obesity rates better than food deserts in the United States. *International Journal of Environmental Research and Public Health* 14(11): E1366. doi:10.3390/ijerph14111366.

de Lacy-Vawdon C, Livingstone C. (2020) Defining the commercial determinants of health: a systematic review. *BMC Public Health* 20: 1022. doi:10.1186/s12889-020-09126-1.

Dietz WH, Scanlon KS. (2012) Eliminating the use of partially hydrogenated oil in food production and preparation. *Journal of American Medical Association* 308(2): 143–144. doi:10.1001/jama.2012.7379.

Food and Drink Federation. (2021) Economic contribution and growth opportunities. https://www.fdf.org.uk/economic-contribution.aspx (last accessed 06.07.2021).

GECI Network (Governance, Ethics, and Conflicts of Interest in Public Health). (2018) GECI – PH Beirut – Network. https://www.wphna.org/blog/governance-ethics-and-conflicts-interest-public-health-geci-ph-beirut-network (last accessed 9/11/2021).

Gilmore AB, Savell E, Collin J. (2011) Public health, corporations and the new responsibility deal: promoting partnerships with vectors of disease? *Journal of Public Health* 33: 2–4. doi:10.1093/pubmed/fdr008.

Gov.uk (2018) Soft drinks industry levy comes into effect. https://www.gov.uk/government/news/soft-drinks-industry-levy-comes-into-effect (last accessed 9/11/2021).

Hawkes C, Ruel MT, Salm L, Sinclair B, Branca F. (2020) Double-duty actions: seizing programme and policy opportunities to address malnutrition in all its forms [published correction appears in *Lancet* 395(10221): 338]. *Lancet* 395(10218): 142–155. doi:10.1016/S0140-6736(19)32506-1.

HM Government. (2018) Childhood obesity: a plan for action Chapter 2, June 2018. https://assets.publishing.service.gov.uk/government/uploads/system/uploads/attachment_data/file/718903/childhood-obesity-a-plan-for-action-chapter-2.pdf (last accessed 9/11/2021).

House of Commons Health Committee. (2015) Childhood obesity—brave and bold action. First report of session 2015–16. https://publications.parliament.uk/pa/cm201516/cmselect/cmhealth/465/465.pdf (last accessed 26.05.2020).

Hyseni L, Elliot-Green A, Lloyd-Williams F, et al. (2017a) Systematic review of dietary salt reduction policies: evidence for an effectiveness hierarchy? *PLoS One* 12:e0177535. doi:10.1371/journal.pone.0177535.

Hyseni L, Bromley H, Kypridemos C, O'Flaherty M, Lloyd-Williams F, Guzman-Castillo M, Pearson-Stuttard J, Capewell S. (2017b) Systematic review of dietary trans-fat reduction policies: evidence for an effectiveness hierarchy? *WHO Bulletin* 95(12): 821–830. doi:10.2471/BLT.16.189795.

Hyseni L, Atkinson M, Bromley H, et al. (2017c) The effects of policy actions to improve population dietary patterns and prevent diet-related non-communicable diseases: scoping review. *European Journal of Clinical Nutrition* 71(6): 694–711. doi:10.1038/ejcn.2016.234.

INFORMAS. (2020) Benchmarking food environments. https://www.informas.org/ (last accessed 9/11/2021 ).

Knai C, Petticrew M, Durand MA, Scott C, James L, Mehrotra A, Eastmure E, Mays N. (2015a) Has a public–private partnership resulted in action on healthier diets in England? An analysis of the Public Health Responsibility Deal food pledges. *Food Policy* 54. doi:10.1016/j.foodpol.2015.04.002.

Knai C, Petticrew M, Durand MA, Scott C, James L, Mehrotra A, Eastmure E, Mays N. (2015b) The Public Health Responsibility Deal: has a public-private partnership brought about action on alcohol reduction? *Addiction* 110(8): 1217–1225. doi:10.1111/add.12892.

Laverty AA, Kypridemos C, Seferidi P, et al. (2019) Quantifying the impact of the Public Health Responsibility Deal on salt intake, cardiovascular disease and gastric cancer burdens: interrupted time series and microsimulation study. *Journal of Epidemiology & Community Health* 73: 881–887.

Lustig R. (2014) *Fat Chance: The Hidden Truth about Sugar, Obesity and Disease.* New York: Harper Collins.

Masters R, Anwar E, Collins B, Cookson R, Capewell S. (2017) The return on investment of public health interventions: a systematic review. *Journal of Epidemiology & Community Health* 71(8): 827–834. doi:10.1136/jech-2016-208141, https://jech.bmj.com/content/71/8/827.full.

McGill R, Anwar E, Orton L, et al. (2015) Are interventions to promote healthy eating equally effective for all? Systematic review of socioeconomic inequalities in impact. *BMC Public Health* 15: 457. doi:10.1186/s12889-015-1781-7.
McKee M, Diethelm P. (2010) How the growth of denialism undermines public health. *British Medical Journal* 341: c6950. doi:10.1136/bmj.c6950.
Mialon M, da Silva Gomes F. (2019) Public health and the ultra-processed food and drink products industry: corporate political activity of major transnationals in Latin America and the Caribbean. *Public Health Nutrition* 22(10): 1898–1908.
Monteiro C, Moubarac J, Levy R, Canella D, Louzada M, Cannon G. (2018). Household availability of ultra-processed foods and obesity in nineteen European countries. *Public Health Nutrition* 21(1), 18–26. doi:10.1017/S1368980017001379.
Moodie R, Stuckler D, Monteiro C, et al. (2013) On behalf of The Lancet NCD Action Group. Profits and pandemics: prevention of harmful effects of tobacco, alcohol, and ultra-processed food and drink industries. *Lancet* 381: 670–679 doi:10.1016/S0140-6736(12)62089-3.
Nestle M. (2013) *Food Politics: How the Food Industry Influences Nutrition and Health.* Oakland, CA: University of California Press.
O'Dowd A. (2017) Spending on junk food advertising is nearly 30 times what government spends on promoting healthy eating. *British Medical Journal* 359: j4677. doi:10.1136/bmj.j4677.
Obesity Health Alliance. (2017) A "Watershed" moment: Why it's prime time to protect children from junk food adverts. http://obesityhealthalliance.org.uk/wp-content/uploads/2017/11/A-Watershed-Moment-report.pdf (last accessed 26.05.2020).
Oreskes N, Conway EM (2010). *Merchants of Doubt: How a Handful of Scientists Obscured the Truth on Issues from Tobacco Smoke to Global Warming.* New York: Bloomsbury Press. ISBN: 10-1596916109.
OXFAM. (2013) Briefing paper no. 166 26 February 2013. Behind the brands: Food justice and the 'Big 10' food and beverage companies. https://www.behindthebrands.org/images/media/Download-files/bp166-behind-brands-260213-en.pdf (last accessed 9/11/2021).
Popkin BM, Corvalan C, Grummer-Strawn LM. (2020) Dynamics of the double burden of malnutrition and the changing nutrition reality. *Lancet.* 395(10217): 65–74. doi:10.1016/S0140-6736(19)32497-3.
Public Health England. (2015) Sugar reduction: from evidence into action, 22 October 2015. https://www.gov.uk/government/publications/sugar-reduction-from-evidence-into-action (last accessed 9/11/2021).
Public Health England. (2017) Guidance health matters: obesity and the food environment, 31st March 2017. https://www.gov.uk/government/publications/health-matters-obesity-and-the-food-environment/health-matters-obesity-and-the-food-environment--2 (last accessed 9/11/2021).
Public Health England. (2018) Fast food outlets: density by local authority in England, 29th June 2018. https://www.gov.uk/government/publications/fast-food-outlets-density-by-local-authority-in-england (last accessed 9/11/2021 ).
Royal College of Paediatrics and Child Health. (2015). Tackling England's childhood obesity crisis. A report to inform the development of the UK Government's childhood obesity strategy.
Savell E, Gilmore AB, Fooks G. (2014) How does the tobacco industry attempt to influence marketing regulations? A systematic review. *PLoS One* 9: e87389. doi:10.1371/journal.pone.0087389.
Statista. (2020) Prices and access. Food and nutrition. https://www.statista.com/markets/415/topic/468/food-nutrition/#overview (last accessed 06.07.2021).
Stuckler D, Nestle M. (2012) Big food, food systems, and global health. *PLoS Medicine* 9: e1001242. doi:10.1371/journal.pmed.1001242.

United States Food and Drug Administration. (2015) Final determination regarding partially hydrogenated oils. Docket no. FDA-2013-N-1317. Federal Register 80(116). Washington DC: U.S. Government Publishing Office. Available from: https://www.gpo.gov/fdsys/pkg/FR-2015-06-17/pdf/2015-14883.pdf (last accessed 17.05.2020).

University of Bath. (2020) Tobacco tactics website. https://tobaccotactics.org/wiki/atlas-network/ (last accessed 26.05.2020).

WHO (2005) (Conference of the parties to the WHO FCTC). Framework convention on tobacco control, 27 February 2005. http://www.who.int/fctc/text_download/en/ (last accessed 26.05.2020).

WHO Commission on Ending Childhood Obesity (ECHO). (2016) Ending childhood obesity final report, 25 January 2016. https://www.who.int/end-childhood-obesity/final-report/en (last accessed 26.05.2020).

WHO. (2018) Evaluating implementation of the WHO set of recommendations on the marketing of foods and non-alcoholic beverages to children. Progress, challenges and guidance for next steps in the WHO European Region. http://oro.open.ac.uk/57150/ (last accessed 9/11/2021 26.05.2020).

# 8 Fast Food and Out-of-Home Food Environments

*Charlotte E.L. Evans*
University of Leeds

*Ayyoub K. Taher*
Kuwait Institute for Scientific Research

*Cath Rycroft*
University of Leeds

*Pablo Monsivais*
Washington State University

## CONTENTS



## 8.1 INTRODUCTION

Fast food is categorised as food that is obtained from outlets where the main purpose is to buy food to take away. Although many fast food chains enable customers to eat in, the food is typically packaged to enable the food to be consumed off the premises, is paid for before eating, and does not involve table service (Burgoine et al., 2016).

DOI: 10.1201/9781003043720-8

The out-of-home food environment on the other hand is broader, including "sit-down" restaurants and cafes where table service is common and food is consumed on the premises. With the emergence of online ordering through platforms such as Uber Eats, customers may not visit the food outlet at all but instead order online and have the food delivered (Keeble et al., 2020). Restaurants that traditionally offered only eating in as an option have now signed up to delivery platforms in large numbers to widen their customer base, particularly as a result of the COVID-19 epidemic (Poelman et al., 2021). Eating out in many countries is very common and is a growing market. Over the last few decades, fast food consumption has increased dramatically in many countries across the world (Jia et al., 2021). In the UK, for example, 56% of adults reported they had bought food outside the home in the last month (in 2019) and 33% had purchased food from a fast food outlet, either directly or through an online platform (Food Standards Agency (FSA), 2019). Adolescents, young adults and lower-income families are more likely to regularly consume fast food and takeaways which may be due to easy access and lower prices as well as taste preferences and marketing (Jia et al., 2021). For adults, it is likely that higher exposure to fast food at home or at work or while commuting between the two is important in terms of risk of higher intakes and poor health (Burgoine et al., 2014).

Historically, fast food has tended to be higher in fats, particularly unhealthy fats such as trans- and saturated fats, higher in sugars and salt and lower in fruits and vegetables than home-cooked foods, resulting in adults and children with diets high in fast foods having lower-quality diets overall (Moore et al., 2009). Despite improvements in the quality of foods purchased from supermarkets (see Chapter 5) and schools (see Chapter 3), in many countries including the UK and the US, progress has been much slower in the improvement in quality of offerings in fast food outlets over the last two decades. This is a particular issue given that fast food is popular with young people who are disproportionally affected by poor diet in childhood, exacerbated by the fact that much of the marketing of fast food is aimed at children and adolescents (discussed further in Chapter 14 on food advertising). Furthermore, fast food outlets are more common in areas of deprivation in the UK and elsewhere resulting in increasing inequalities in diet (Public Health England, 2017). This chapter reviews the available evidence about the relationships between fast food and out-of-home eating on diet quality and health outcomes and identifies where action has been taken to improve this key food environment, particularly in terms of reducing diet inequalities.

## 8.2 FAST FOOD AND DIET QUALITY

There is an established body of research suggesting that fast food consumption is associated with lower-quality diets for adults and children (Jaworowska et al., 2013). Some studies have reported on links between fast food consumption and intakes of individual foods and drinks such as sugar-sweetened beverages, fried foods and fruits and vegetables in the diet. A UK study using national data reported that adults and children who consumed fast food weekly or more often consumed more calories

(Goffe et al., 2017) and the greater energy intake was larger for those from less affluent households. Two US studies of children and adolescents, investigating the relationship of fast food (Bowman et al., 2004) and the relationship of fried foods away from home (Taveras et al., 2005) with diet quality, reported that regular consumption of either was positively associated with energy intake, fats and added sugars/sugary drinks, and negatively associated with the intake of fruit and non-starchy vegetables. Portion sizes of takeaway meals were also found to be high (see Chapter 15 for more information on portion sizes).

Other studies have measured the links between fast food consumption and overall diet quality. Analysis of adolescents aged 11–18 years in the UK National Diet and Nutrition Survey (NDNS) used the food-based validated diet quality tool DQI-A measuring quality, diversity and equilibrium; and reported a lower quality score for adolescents frequently consuming takeaways at least once per week (Taher et al., 2019). Moreover, a Canadian study involving school-aged adolescents (11–14 years) found that consumption of takeaway meals was negatively associated with the Healthy Eating Index as an assessment of their overall diet quality (Woodruff & Hanning, 2009). In terms of nutrients, analysis of US data from the National Health, Nutrition and Exercise survey reported that consuming fast food on a given day increased energy intake by 190 kcal, saturated fat intake by 3.5 g and sugars intake by 4 g; and reduced fibre intake by 0.4 g as well as some vitamins and minerals (An, 2016).

## 8.3 FAST FOOD, OBESITY AND HEALTH

Despite substantial evidence on the negative relationships of fast food with diet quality, research into the relationships of fast food intake and obesity produces a mixed picture. Studies examining the links between fast food, diet and health outcomes have generally taken one of two approaches. Some have used traditional dietary assessment instruments to identify fast foods in the diet, linking the consumption of these foods with diet quality, weight and health outcomes, either cross-sectionally (Schroder et al., 2007) or prospectively (Pereira et al., 2005). Alternatively, geographic approaches have linked measures of proximity or density of fast food outlets around residential, school or workplace addresses or post codes to measures of diet, weight and health outcomes (Jeffery et al., 2006). The preponderance of research in this area is cross-sectional in design, limiting causal inference between dietary behaviour and health outcomes (see Chapter 19 for more information on different types of evaluation). A systematic review published in 2019 identified 16 longitudinal studies (a stronger study design) as well as many cross-sectional studies, reporting on the relationship between fast food and obesity in children and adolescents up to age 18 years in different countries (Jia et al., 2021). The review reported that higher fast food restaurant access (measured by number, density or presence of fast food outlets) was associated with higher fast food consumption, although there were no strong or consistently positive associations with obesity. Approximately half of the longitudinal studies which were based in the US (8), UK (4), Canada (2) and Sweden (1) reported that higher access to fast food was associated with rising body mass index (BMI) or obesity rates but half did not indicate any relationship. A longitudinal UK study found inconsistent associations between access to fast food outlets and adolescent weight status (Green et al., 2018). In this study, although a positive association was found between BMI and number of fast food outlets along travel routes, exposure to fast food outlets was not systematically associated with changes in BMI or waist circumference over time.

For adults, there are no recent reviews investigating the longitudinal relationships of fast food and obesity, and individual studies again indicate mixed results. In Sweden, a longitudinal study with 11-year follow-up of over a million adults reported that there were no consistent associations between fast food outlets and obesity (Okuyama et al., 2020), and in Victoria, Australia, a longitudinal study of women living in disadvantaged neighbourhoods did not detect a relationship between availability of major chain fast food outlet availability and BMI (Lamb et al., 2017). In the US, a longitudinal study also found no significant associations between weight status of adults living in rural or urban areas and density of fast food outlets (Gibson, 2011). Another US study including adults with 7-year follow-up stated that there was no relationship between number of fast food outlets and obesity (Rummo et al., 2017).

Given the nutritional risks associated with fast food intake, research has also examined cardiometabolic outcomes. In Tehran, Iran, higher consumption of fast food was associated with a higher risk of metabolic syndrome (Bahadoran et al., 2013) in a large cohort of adults. This was more pronounced in younger adults under 30 years, overweight adults and those consuming lower intakes of fruits, vegetables and fibre. This has implications for risk of type 2 diabetes. A review of studies measuring triglycerides concluded that high intakes of fast food increase the risk of type 2 diabetes (Bahadoran et al., 2015). In the US, the Cardia study which has 25 years of follow-up measured access to fast food and convenience stores. The study reported increased risk of coronary artery calcification between follow-up years 15 and 25 with increased access to convenience stores but no relationships with fast food access (Kelman et al., 2019). In Canada, 5-year follow-up of more than 7,000 participants revealed that participants under 65 years living in areas with high exposure to fast food were nearly twice as likely to develop type 2 diabetes, but there was no relationship when adjustment was made for BMI (Polsky et al., 2016).

## 8.4 IMPACT OF FAST FOOD EXPOSURE ON DIET AND HEALTH INEQUALITIES

The exposure to fast food and other unhealthy food outlets such as convenience stores may vary across local areas and tend to be higher in disadvantaged areas in many countries such as the UK (Maguire et al., 2015). In addition to higher exposure, the relationships between fast food and diet quality and health may be different for individuals living in areas with more deprivation. Cross-sectional analysis of a large dataset of adults aged 38–72 years in Greater London, UK, reported independent associations of exposure to fast food and income and relationships with BMI and prevalence of obesity (Burgoine et al., 2018). In total, 18% of food outlets were classified as fast food but for the quarter of participants in the highest exposure category 24%–45% of food vendors were fast food outlets. Those with the highest exposure to fast food had 1.5 (95% CI 1.5–1.6) greater odds of being obese compared with those in the lowest exposure category; for those on the lowest incomes, this risk increased to 2.4 (95% CI 2.1–2.8) greater odds of being obese. Previous analysis elsewhere in the UK also highlighted a stronger association between fast food outlet exposure and obesity for individuals with lowest levels of education (Burgoine et al., 2016). Another study based in the Netherlands reported that households experiencing food insecurity consumed poorer quality diets, and this relationship was stronger with higher exposure to fast food outlets (van der Velde et al., 2020). These findings highlight the importance of specifically focussing on populations experiencing the double burden of lower socio-economic placement and an unhealthy food environment to reduce inequalities in diet and health.

## 8.5 ONLINE FAST FOOD DELIVERY

During the past 20 years, due to economic growth and wider reach of the internet, e-commerce including online food delivery has expanded worldwide. The growth of online food delivery has led to the situation where access to food can no longer be measured by a physical distance from the consumer to the food outlet but alternatively by the number of outlets willing to deliver to a specific location, particularly in cities where most of the online deliveries take place. With online food delivery, the variety of food service can extend out to 10 km and potentially much further (Maimaiti et al., 2018) increasing the availability and accessibility of fast food, far beyond the 1.6 km or 20-minute walk buffer typically used by researchers to define neighbourhood food environments (Wilkins et al., 2017) (REF).

The whole process of ordering food online is set up to make ordering easy, assisted by the use of applications or "apps". Food delivery app service providers can be classified into the food retailer itself (e.g., KFC, Dominos or McDonalds), and intermediaries such as Uber Eats, Just Eats and Deliveroo. With intermediaries, customers order food via an app and the order is passed to the food outlet that prepares the food. The outlet then hands the order over to a courier (either working for the food outlet or the delivery service) who then delivers it to the customer, usually within 20 or 30 minutes. The cost of delivery is in the region of £2–3 per delivery.

The number of customers ordering food online is growing and is set to increase further. The market share of delivered food is increasing, and Compound Annual Growth Rate (CAGR) report that the expected annual growth revenues stand at 9.6%, which in turn are predicted to generate a global market volume of US$137.6 billion by 2023 (Kung & Guan-Yu, 2017). In Australia, for example, online deliveries have grown by more than 70% over the last 5 years (Bates et al., 2020). Analysis of 2018 data from five countries found that overall, 15% of the population had used online food delivery in the last 7 days, a much lower rate than had visited a food outlet in person (63%) (Keeble et al., 2020).

Online food delivery is more popular with adolescents and young adults as well as households with children (Keeble et al., 2020). This is a worry as young people also typically consume diets higher in free sugars and lower in vegetables than population averages (Taher et al., 2019). This review also found that identifying as being from an ethnic minority and being more highly educated (in all countries except the UK) was linked to heavier use of online deliveries. Young people in large countries such as China, the US, India and Brazil have led this global trend (Li et al., 2020) which is also increasing elsewhere. Rates currently vary by country, and in some countries such as Greece, there are much lower rates of usage of online food delivery (Kamenidou et al., 2019). The COVID-19 pandemic and the associated closure of restaurants to indoor dining has likely accelerated the rise in usage in many age groups (Poelman et al., 2021).

Online delivery increases access to fast food and potentially encourages an even more sedentary lifestyle as well as potentially reducing cooking skills. Hence, there are clear public health challenges faced by the rising trend in food delivery. There is little regulation of these online delivery sites (Bates et al., 2020), and little is reported on the nutritional quality of food sold on these platforms. As with all takeaway foods, there are issues around portion size, energy density, lack of vegetables and promotion of food waste by continually offering online promotions. One study in Brazil looked at marketing of food during the COVID-19 pandemic and found that unhealthy foods high in fats, sugars and salt were regularly advertised or provided with cheaper rates or delivery options (Horta et al., 2020).

The fast food industry has been further impacted during COVID-19 including a potentially permanent shift to more digital food purchasing (Cummins et al., 2020). In order to make sure that this sector develops in a sustainable way which serves the wellbeing of all stakeholders involved, interventions and regulation are needed to improve nutritional quality without reducing food choices.

## 8.6 OUT-OF-HOME EATING AND DIET

Less research has been published on relationships between diet quality and health and consumption of out-of-home eating at sit-down food outlets such as cafes and restaurants. In the UK, analysis of national data reported that energy intakes were higher for adults who ate out of the home weekly or more (Goffe et al., 2017), but the same relationship was not seen for children. A separate study of the same data found that more frequent out-of-home eating was associated with lower dietary quality overall, as well as higher odds of obesity in adults. When examining the types of outlets included in out-of-home dining, the authors found that the association was driven by utilisation of fast food outlets (Penney et al., 2017). Analysis of British adolescents revealed that eating out-of-home did significantly impact diet quality score in the UK, but this impact was smaller compared to eating takeaways (Taher et al., 2019). Adolescents typically consume high levels of non-core foods and drinks such as sugary drinks, confectionery, crisps, pizza and fried foods (Toumpakari et al., 2016) and eating occasions outside the home are higher in non-core foods than eating at home in this age group (Toumpakari et al., 2019).

Out-of-home eating was associated with poor quality diet in children (Ziauddeen et al., 2018), perhaps because children's menus are often high in fats, sugars and salt (Hobin et al., 2014).

An Irish study involving children showed that a small but statistically significant decline in nutrient intakes was observed among high consumers of foods outside the home. The greatest contribution to energy intake came from products that were consumed out of the home such as chips, processed meats, sauces and beverages (Burke et al., 2007).

## 8.7 INTERVENTIONS AND PROGRAMMES

### 8.7.1 Interventions to Improve Fast Food Environments

Despite a large number of studies identifying fast food as an important factor in terms of diet quality and health outcomes, there are fewer published evaluations of interventions that have successfully reduced fast food access or improved offerings from fast food outlets compared with interventions in the retail and school food environments. An assessment of nutritional quality of fast food in the US over 14 years from 1997/1998 to 2009/2010 found that there were only slight improvements in offerings over this time frame, mainly small reductions in fats and sugars, and a modest increase in the overall healthiness of menu offerings, based on the Healthy Eating Index, indicating interventions are needed in this food environment.

Interventions to reduce the dietary and health risks from fast food have taken one of three approaches. First, the use of menu labelling in food outlets gained popularity in the late 2000s and early 2010s in the USA with the passage of the Affordable Care Act, which included public health-oriented provisions, with menu labelling in chain restaurants, including major fast food chains. Although presumed to be an enabling intervention, the theory of this approach essentially shifts the burden to consumer, requiring them to recognise and interpret posted nutrition information and make prudent choices accordingly. Evidence on the effectiveness of menu labelling has been equivocal at best (see Chapter 13).

A second approach goes beyond posting nutrition information to change menu offerings within restaurants to improve their nutritional profile. Examples include the introduction of healthier alternatives and reformulation of recipes to reduce the content of key ingredients, such as salt and saturated and trans-fats to a limit. Compared to menu labelling interventions, there have been fewer evaluations of reformulation interventions, and evidence is uneven. For example, some states in the US such as New York have brought in regulations to restrict the use of artificial trans-fats in fast food, including French fries (Angell et al., 2012) and published some initial evaluation of this new regulation. Trans-fats reduced by 2.4 g (95% CI 2.0–2.8 g) per purchase, which is likely to have a significant impact on health although this wasn't assessed (Angell et al., 2012).

Training of chefs working in fast food outlets through a 3-hour masterclass with the goal of improving meal quality has been tested in England. Aims of the training included reducing fats, sugars and salt and increasing fibre and fruit and vegetables as well as reducing portion sizes. Different methods were suggested such as changing the placement of salt cellars and replacing sauces with low sugar/salt versions. Changes were made in all of the 18 food outlets involved although less than half of the planned changes were made (Hillier-Brown et al., 2019).

A slightly different approach is to ask customers whether they would like to down-size their portion of starchy food rather than the more common suggestion in fast food restaurants to supersize the customer's portion. One study did just this in Chinese fast food restaurants and found that 14%–33% of customers chose the down-size option, reducing their energy intake by about 200 kcal (Schwartz et al., 2012). It did not make a difference whether customers were offered a modest monetary discount or not. Information on a similar programme in Japan to increase vegetables in fast food outlets by offering a nominal monetary discount is provided in Chapter 16 on nudging.

A third intervention approach is at the neighbourhood or community level, where local authorities use planning or "zoning" policy to stem proliferation of fast-food "takeaways" in neighbourhoods, towns, and cities. Zoning or planning approaches are one structural response to the dramatic rise in the number of fast food outlets in communities and predicated on the notion that reducing the relative concentration of fast food outlets (while increasing the availability of healthier food retailing) will reduce consumer tendencies to patronise these restaurants. However, this approach can be controversial, with businesses and developers contesting any restrictions on their ability to develop and operate restaurants freely. In the UK, the use of planning controls to limit fast food outlets was flagged as promising as part of "whole-system" approaches to obesity prevention (see Chapter 20). There are some local authorities where this has had some measurable impact on reshaping the food environment, but there have been few studies of the impact of such policies on diet and health.

One notable exception has been the evaluation of the so-called "fast food ban" in California. In 2008, the Los Angeles City Council introduced an ordinance to prevent the opening or expansion of new fast food outlets in south Los Angeles, where it was perceived that a high density of these restaurants was contributing to "food deserts" and excess rates of overweight and obesity. In a pair of reports (Sturm & Cohen, 2009; Sturm & Hattori, 2015), evaluating the impact of the ban on the environment, diet, and weight, 1 and 4 years after the introduction of the ban, no discernible impacts were found on the food environment with minimal impacts on population diet, primarily on intakes of sugar-sweetened beverages. Paradoxically, overweight and obesity increased to a greater extent in the ban area than in other areas of Los Angeles.

Recent efforts to introduce policies at a regional level may be more likely to target reducing the density of fast food outlets near schools (Keeble et al., 2019), thereby focussing on improving children's diets.

### 8.7.2 Interventions to Improve Eating Out-Of-Home Other Than Fast Food

There are fewer intervention studies evaluating out-of-home eating than fast food although policies on labelling are becoming more common. For example in the UK, from April 2022, menus of food outlets are required to display energy values of meals (Deparment of Health and Social Care, 2021) (see Chapter 13 for more information on menu labelling). A systematic review of US community-based food outlets identified a range of different strategies to improve healthy choices (Gittelsohn et al., 2013). Most included signage and labelling to identify healthier choices, but a minority reduced portion sizes or improved healthiness of offerings which generally resulted in higher frequency in purchasing of healthier options. Results from a randomised control trial study show that education-based interventions on how to make wise food-related decisions showed some improvement on adolescents' snack food choices (the healthier option) (Ochoa-Aviles et al., 2017). Although daily fruit and vegetable intake decreased in both intervention and control groups, the intake of unhealthy snacks and added sugar decreased significantly in the intervention group at the end of the trial. More research is needed in this area.

## 8.8 CONCLUSIONS AND NEXT STEPS

The global fast food market is growing, particularly in middle- and high-income countries and is associated with lower diet quality in terms of vegetables, sugars, fats and salt. However the relationship with health outcomes such as obesity and type 2 diabetes is not consistent in adults or children. Access to fast food appears to mediate the relationship between deprivation and health and therefore high density of fast food in deprived areas is of particular concern. Online fast food delivery platforms have exacerbated the impact of fast food on diet quality, and therefore, interventions to improve the fast food environment must incorporate both in-person and online purchasing. Policies to reduce access around schools and other localities where children tend to group have the potential to partly improve food environments for young people. However, programmes to improve the quality of food available in fast food outlets are also required. Research in low-income countries is sparse and more is needed, particularly for countries transitioning from a traditional diet to a more globally influenced diet.

## ACKNOWLEDGEMENTS

The authors are grateful to Nastasia Belc for her references on online fast food.

## REFERENCES

An, R. 2016. Fast-food and full-service restaurant consumption and daily energy and nutrient intakes in US adults. *Eur J Clin Nutr,* 70, 97–103.

Angell, S. Y., Cobb, L. K., Curtis, C. J., Konty, K. J. & Silver, L. D. 2012. Change in trans fatty acid content of fast-food purchases associated with New York City's restaurant regulation: a pre-post study. *Ann Intern Med,* 157, 81–86.

Bahadoran, Z., Mirmiran, P., Hosseini-Esfahani, F. & Azizi, F. 2013. Fast food consumption and the risk of metabolic syndrome after 3-years of follow-up: tehran lipid and glucose study. *Eur J Clin Nutr,* 67, 1303–1309.

Bahadoran, Z., Mirmiran, P. & Azizi, F. 2015. Fast food pattern and cardiometabolic disorders: A review of current studies. *Health Promot Perspect,* 5, 231–240.

Bates, S., Reeve, B. & Trevena, H. 2020. A narrative review of online food delivery in Australia: challenges and opportunities for public health nutrition policy. *Public Health Nutr,* 1–11. https://doi.org/10.1017/S1368980020000701

Bowman, S. A., Gortmaker, S. L., Ebbeling, C. B., Pereira, M. A. & Ludwig, D. S. 2004. Effects of fast-food consumption on energy intake and diet quality among children in a national household survey. *Pediatrics,* 113, 112–118.

Burgoine, T., Forouhi, N. G., Griffin, S. J., Wareham, N. J. & Monsivais, P. 2014. Associations between exposure to takeaway food outlets, takeaway food consumption, and body weight in Cambridgeshire, UK: population based, cross sectional study. *BMJ,* 348, g1464.

Burgoine, T., Forouhi, N. G., Griffin, S. J., Brage, S., Wareham, N. J. & Monsivais, P. 2016. Does neighborhood fast-food outlet exposure amplify inequalities in diet and obesity? A cross-sectional study. *Am J Clin Nutr,* 103, 1540–1547.

Burgoine, T., Sarkar, C., Webster, C. J. & Monsivais, P. 2018. Examining the interaction of fast-food outlet exposure and income on diet and obesity: evidence from 51,361 UK Biobank participants. *Int J Behav Nutr Phys Act,* 15, 71.

Burke, S. J., Mccarthy, S. N., O'Neill, J. L., Hannon, E. M., Kiely, M., Flynn, A. & Gibney, M. J. 2007. An examination of the influence of eating location on the diets of Irish children. *Public Health Nutr,* 10, 599–607.

Cummins, S., Berger, N., Cornelsen, L., Eling, J., Er, V., Greener, R., Kalbus, A., Karapici, A., Law, C., Ndlovu, D. & Yau, A. 2020. COVID-19: impact on the urban food retail system and dietary inequalities in the UK. *Cities & Health*, 1–4.

Deparment of Health and Social Care. 2021. News story: Calorie labelling on menus to be introduced in cafes, restaurants and takeaways.

Food Standards Agency (FSA). 2019. The food and you survey.

Gibson, D. M. 2011. The neighborhood food environment and adult weight status: estimates from longitudinal data. *Am J Public Health,* 101, 71–78.

Gittelsohn, J., Lee-Kwan, S. H. & Batorsky, B. 2013. Community-based interventions in prepared-food sources: a systematic review. *Prev Chronic Dis,* 10, E180.

Goffe, L., Rushton, S., White, M., Adamson, A. & Adams, J. 2017. Relationship between mean daily energy intake and frequency of consumption of out-of-home meals in the UK National Diet and Nutrition Survey. *Int J Behav Nutr Phys Act,* 14, 131.

Green, M. A., Radley, D., Lomax, N., Morris, M. A. & Griffiths, C. 2018. Is adolescent body mass index and waist circumference associated with the food environments surrounding schools and homes? A longitudinal analysis. *BMC Public Health,* 18, 482.

Hillier-Brown, F., Lloyd, S., Muhammad, L., Summerbell, C., Goffe, L., Hildred, N., Adams, J., Penn, L., Wrieden, W., White, M., Lake, A., Moore, H., Abraham, C., Adamson, A. & Araujo-Soares, V. 2019. Feasibility and acceptability of a Takeaway Masterclass aimed at encouraging healthier cooking practices and menu options in takeaway food outlets. *Public Health Nutr,* 22, 2268–2278.

Hobin, E., White, C., Li, Y., Chiu, M., O'Brien, M. F. & Hammond, D. 2014. Nutritional quality of food items on fast-food 'kids' menus': comparisons across countries and companies. *Public Health Nutr,* 17, 2263–2269.

Horta, P. M., Matos, J. P. & Mendes, L. L. 2020. Digital food environment during the coronavirus disease 2019 (COVID-19) pandemic in Brazil: an analysis of food advertising in an online food delivery platform. *Br J Nutr,* 1–6.

Jaworowska, A., Blackham, T., Davies, I. G. & Stevenson, L. 2013. Nutritional challenges and health implications of takeaway and fast food. *Nutr Rev*, 71(5), 310–318.

Jeffery, R. W., Baxter, J., Mcguire, M. & Linde, J. 2006. Are fast food restaurants an environmental risk factor for obesity? *Int J Behav Nutr Phys Act,* 3, 2.

Jia, P., Luo, M., Li, Y., Zheng, J. S., Xiao, Q. & Luo, J. 2021. Fast-food restaurant, unhealthy eating, and childhood obesity: a systematic review and meta-analysis. *Obes Rev*, 22 Suppl 1, e12944.

Kamenidou, I. C., Mamalis, S. A., Pavlidis, S., Bara, E. Z. G. 2019. Segmenting the generation Z Cohort University students based on sustainable food consumption behavior: a preliminary study. *Sustainability,* 11, 837.

Keeble, M., Burgoine, T., White, M., Summerbell, C., Cummins, S. & Adams, J. 2019. How does local government use the planning system to regulate hot food takeaway outlets? A census of current practice in England using document review. *Health Place,* 57, 171–178.

Keeble, M., Adams, J., Sacks, G., Vanderlee, L., White, C. M., Hammond, D. & Burgoine, T. 2020. Use of online food delivery services to order food prepared away-from-home and associated sociodemographic characteristics: A cross-sectional, multi-country analysis. *Int J Environ Res Public Health,* 17(14), 5190.

Kelman, J., Pool, L. R., Gordon-Larsen, P., Carr, J. J., Terry, J. G., Rana, J. S. & Kershaw, K. N. 2019. Associations of unhealthy food environment with the development of coronary artery calcification: the CARDIA study. *J Am Heart Assoc,* 8, e010586.

Kung, L.-C. & Guan-Yu, Z. 2017. The optimal pricing strategy for two-sided platform delivery in the sharing economy. *Trans Res,* 101, 1–12.

Lamb, K. E., Thornton, L. E., Olstad, D. L., Cerin, E. & Ball, K. 2017. Associations between major chain fast-food outlet availability and change in body mass index: a longitudinal observational study of women from Victoria, Australia. *BMJ Open,* 7, e016594.

Li, C., Mirosa, M. And Bremer, P. 2020. Review of online food delivery platforms and their impacts on sustainability. *Sustainability,* 12, 5528.

Maguire, E. R., Burgoine, T. & Monsivais, P. 2015. Area deprivation and the food environment over time: a repeated cross-sectional study on takeaway outlet density and supermarket presence in Norfolk, UK, 1990–2008. *Health Place*, 33, 142–147.

Maimaiti, M., Zhao, X., Jia, M., Ru, Y. & Zhu, S. 2018. How we eat determines what we become: opportunities and challenges brought by food delivery industry in a changing world in China. *Eur J Clin Nutr,* 72, 1282–1286.

Moore, L. V., Diez Roux, A. V., Nettleton, J. A., Jacobs, D. R. & Franco, M. 2009. Fast-food consumption, diet quality, and neighborhood exposure to fast food: the multi-ethnic study of atherosclerosis. *Am J Epidemiol,* 170, 29–36.

Ochoa-Aviles, A., Verstraeten, R., Huybregts, L., Andrade, S., Van Camp, J., Donoso, S., Ramirez, P. L., Lachat, C., Maes, L. & Kolsteren, P. 2017. A school-based intervention improved dietary intake outcomes and reduced waist circumference in adolescents: a cluster randomized controlled trial. *Nutr J,* 16, 79.

Okuyama, K., Li, X., Abe, T., Hamano, T., Franks, P. W., Nabika, T. & Sundquist, K. 2020. Fast food outlets, physical activity facilities, and obesity among adults: a nationwide longitudinal study from Sweden. *Int J Obes (Lond),* 44, 1703–1711.

Penney, T. L., Jones, N. R. V., Adams, J., Maguire, E. R., Burgoine, T. & Monsivais, P. 2017. Utilization of away-from-home food establishments, dietary approaches to stop hypertension dietary pattern, and obesity. *Am J Prev Med,* 53, e155–e163.

Pereira, M. A., Kartashov, A. I., Ebbeling, C. B., Van Horn, L., Slattery, M. L., Jacobs, D. R., Jr. & Ludwig, D. S. 2005. Fast-food habits, weight gain, and insulin resistance (the Cardia study): 15-year prospective analysis. *Lancet,* 365, 36–42.

Poelman, M. P., Gillebaart, M., Schlinkert, C., Dijkstra, S. C., Derksen, E., Mensink, F., Hermans, R. C. J., Aardening, P., De Ridder, D. & De Vet, E. 2021. Eating behavior and food purchases during the COVID-19 lockdown: a cross-sectional study among adults in the Netherlands. *Appetite,* 157, 105002.

Polsky, J. Y., Moineddin, R., Glazier, R. H., Dunn, J. R. & Booth, G. L. 2016. Relative and absolute availability of fast-food restaurants in relation to the development of diabetes: a population-based cohort study. *Can J Public Health,* 107, 5312.

Public Health England. 2017. Health matters: obesity and the food environment.

Rummo, P. E., Guilkey, D. K., Ng, S. W., Meyer, K. A., Popkin, B. M., Reis, J. P., Shikany, J. M. & Gordon-Larsen, P. 2017. Does unmeasured confounding influence associations between the retail food environment and body mass index over time? The Coronary Artery Risk Development in Young Adults (CARDIA) study. *Int J Epidemiol,* 46, 1456–1464.

Schroder, H., Fito, M., Covas, M. I. & Investigators, R. 2007. Association of fast food consumption with energy intake, diet quality, body mass index and the risk of obesity in a representative mediterranean population. *Br J Nutr,* 98, 1274–1280.

Schwartz, J., Riis, J., Elbel, B. & Ariely, D. 2012. Inviting consumers to downsize fast-food portions significantly reduces calorie consumption. *Health Aff (Millwood),* 31, 399–407.

Sturm, R. & Cohen, D. A. 2009. Zoning for health? The year-old ban on new fast-food restaurants in South La. *Health Aff (Millwood),* 28, w1088–w1097.

Sturm, R. & Hattori, A. 2015. Diet and obesity in Los Angeles County 2007–2012: is there a measurable effect of the 2008 "Fast-Food Ban"? *Soc Sci Med,* 133, 205–211.

Taher, A. K., Evans, N. & Evans, C. E. 2019. The cross-sectional relationships between consumption of takeaway food, eating meals outside the home and diet quality in British adolescents. *Public Health Nutr,* 22, 63–73.

Taveras, E. M., Berkey, C. S., Rifas-Shiman, S. L., Ludwig, D. S., Rockett, H. R., Field, A. E., Colditz, G. A. & Gillman, M. W. 2005. Association of consumption of fried food away from home with body mass index and diet quality in older children and adolescents. *Pediatrics,* 116, e518–24.

Toumpakari, Z., Haase, A. M. & Johnson, L. 2016. Adolescents' non-core food intake: a description of what, where and with whom adolescents consume non-core foods. *Public Health Nutr,* 19, 1645–1653.

Toumpakari, Z., Tilling, K., Haase, A. M. & Johnson, L. 2019. High-risk environments for eating foods surplus to requirements: a multilevel analysis of adolescents' non-core food intake in the National Diet and Nutrition Survey (NDNS). *Public Health Nutr,* 22, 74–84.

Van Der Velde, L. A., Zitman, F. M. P., Mackenbach, J. D., Numans, M. E. & Kiefte-De Jong, J. C. 2020. The interplay between fast-food outlet exposure, household food insecurity, and diet quality in disadvantaged districts. *Public Health Nutr,* 1–20.

Wilkins, E. L., Morris, M. A., Radley, D. & Griffiths, C. 2017. Using geographic information systems to measure retail food environments: discussion of methodological considerations and a proposed reporting checklist (Geo-FERN). *Health Place,* 44, 110–117.

Woodruff, S. J. & Hanning, R. M. 2009. Effect of meal environment on diet quality rating. *Can J Diet Pract Res,* 70, 118–124.

Ziauddeen, N., Page, P., Penney, T. L., Nicholson, S., Kirk, S. F. & Almiron-Roig, E. 2018. Eating at food outlets and leisure places and "on the go" is associated with less-healthy food choices than eating at home and in school in children: cross-sectional data from the UK National Diet and Nutrition Survey Rolling Program (2008–2014). *Am J Clin Nutr,* 107, 992–1003.

# 9 Community Food Environments

*M. Susan Caswell*
University of Waterloo

*Margaret A. Allman-Farinelli*
University of Sydney

*Dana L. Olstad*
University of Calgary

*Patti-Jean Naylor*
University of Victoria

**CONTENTS**



DOI: 10.1201/9781003043720-9

## 9.1 INTRODUCTION

The socioecological model highlights the breadth of the potential uses of the term 'community'. For the purposes of this chapter, the term community is used to refer to specific geographically defined locations and the settings within them that are governed by regional, state and local government decision-making bodies and policies. Schools, workplaces, restaurants and homes are all organizational settings within geographic communities that are sources of food or influences on nutrition that are dealt with elsewhere in this text. There are, however, other community settings where food is served or sold, two of which are addressed herein: transportation hubs (e.g. train and bus stations) and public and private recreation and sports facilities. We first provide an overview of what is known about the food environment in these two community settings to illustrate the size and scope of the issues to be addressed if we want to improve their food environments and their impact on the purchasing and consumption patterns of individuals. Second, we highlight potential interventions that may help to improve these food environments by reviewing the evidence pertaining to strategies to improve the food environment in one community setting: publicly or privately funded recreation and sport facilities (typically called leisure or health centres or sports clubs in European countries and Australia). Primarily we present evidence about the effectiveness of both regional- and community/setting-level policy and capacity-building in effecting sustainable change to the quality of these food environments. We also address the potential for interventions in these settings to narrow dietary inequities in order to provide researchers and practitioners with ideas they can implement in community settings to improve diet and health (de Leeuw, 2017).

## 9.2 FOOD AND BEVERAGE AVAILABILITY IN COMMUNITY AND PUBLIC SPACES

An adapted comprehensive whole of setting model (Naylor et al., 2010) developed for the recreation and sport environment provides a broad view of opportunities to promote healthful eating patterns in community spaces (see Figure 9.1) that is underpinned by policy and includes education about healthy eating (e.g. cooking classes, health promotion message boards, newsletters), staff and volunteers working in the setting (e.g. guidelines or policy around healthy food choices at meetings, lunch room environments), fundraising (e.g. intermittent selling of food to raise money for charity or sport), public events (e.g. community celebrations of national holidays held at the facility), the marketing environment and food security (e.g. providing locations for community gardens).

With respect to food availability within most community spaces, the two main ways for the public to access food are via cafes/restaurants/concessions and vending machines. Both cafes and concessions are staffed and have specific opening hours, but cafes typically have seating areas and more comprehensive cooking facilities and food options while concessions or snack bars typically have limited or no seating areas and cooking equipment (hereafter referred to as either cafes or concessions). Vending machines provide ready access to a selection of foods and drinks at any time of the day without the need for staff. Vending is a billion-dollar industry globally

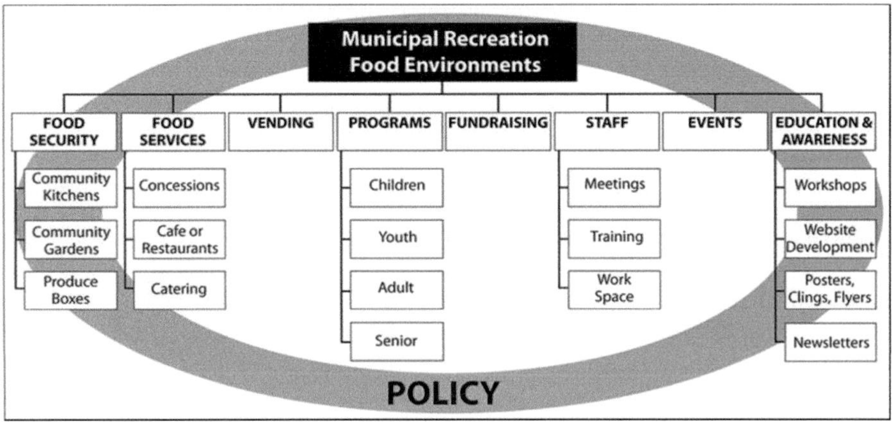


**FIGURE 9.1** Food environment framework. (Adapted from Naylor et al. (2010), figure 1. Reproduced under CC 3.0, http://creativecommons.org/licenses/by/3.0/.)

(Euromonitor International, 2019) and has a significant influence on dietary patterns. For example, a secondary analysis of data from the National Nutrition and Health Examination Survey (NHANES 2005–2014) in the United States (US) showed that 3.9% of adults consumed food from vending machines on the day of recall in a variety of settings (Onufrak et al., 2019) and included primarily sugar-sweetened beverages, salty grain snacks, candies and potato chips. Indeed, it has been well documented that vending machines have a negative impact on food purchasing and eating practices in many settings including schools, tertiary institutions and workplaces (Grech & Allman-Farinelli, 2015).

## 9.3 COMMUNITY TRANSPORTATION HUBS

Each working day millions of adults and children around the world travel to work and study using public transportation. To provide some context for the public health importance of these settings, one in four people use public transport for travel to and from work and study in Sydney, Australia (Australian Bureau of Statistics, 2018), and in some European jurisdictions such as London, it is closer to three in four (Department for Transport, 2019). During this commute, they will encounter vending machines, concessions, cafes and other outlets offering foods and beverages and be exposed to numerous advertisments for foods around or within transportation hubs, trains and buses (Signal et al., 2017).

### 9.3.1 Vending Food and Beverages

Similar to other community settings, vending machines provide food and beverages for commuters and travellers at any time of the day or night. Two different studies conducted in Australia and the US have assessed the contents of vending machines at railway stations and highway rest areas, respectively. A 2012 cross-sectional study audited vending machine offerings in the Greater Sydney area at railway stations (Kelly et al., 2012). The sample ($n = 100$) consisted of 30% of all railway stations and included 40%, 39% and 21% from low, medium and high socioeconomic status (SES) areas, respectively. Fifty-nine percent of stations housed at least one vending machine with the average being 2.1 machines in low SES, 2.3 in medium SES and 1.5 in high SES community locations. Of the more than 5,168 machine slots, 40% were for cold beverages, 59% for snack foods and 1% for hot beverages. Most drinks and beverages were classified as 'unhealthy'. Sugar-sweetened beverages comprised 65% of all drink slots and unhealthy snacks comprised 97% of all food slots. Healthy beverages, mostly bottled waters, were less expensive than unhealthy beverages but healthy snacks cost more. Passengers waiting on a train platform (where most machines were located, see Figure 9.2) are a captive audience for purchasing these 'unhealthy' products.

Similar to public transportation settings, each year millions of drivers and their passengers purchase food and beverages from vending machines at more than 1,800 public or private rest areas across the US (McGuirt et al., 2019). Research conducted in 2018 in North Carolina in the US found that among the 30 rest stops studied, cold beverage vending machines (average 4.1 per rest area) were most common followed by snack machines (average 2.9 per rest area) (McGuirt et al., 2019). Less common were hot beverage machines (average 0.6 per rest area), combination machines (0.2 per rest area) and ice cream machines (0.1 per rest area). The distribution of healthy and unhealthy products in the 241 vending machines, perhaps unsurprisingly, was weighted towards 'unhealthy' foods and beverages (89% of snack items, 62% of cold beverages and 70% of hot beverages were classified as unhealthy). While this section has summarized existing research on vending in transport hubs, there is less

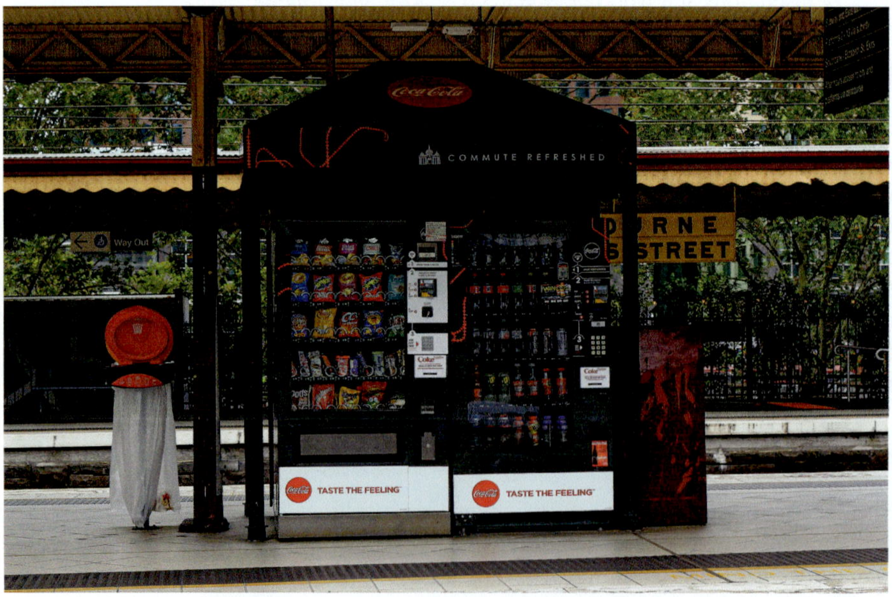


**FIGURE 9.2** Vending machine on Melbourne train station. https://www.shutterstock.com/image-photo/melbourne-victoria-australia-jan-26-2017-1773350366.)

information on cafes and concessions. There is however published research on food marketing in these community spaces.

### 9.3.2 Food and Beverage Marketing

Audits of 558 public transit stops, including train stations, bus and tram stops with a shelter across 20 areas in Melbourne, Australia (Settle et al., 2014), found that one in three displayed advertisments for food or beverages, with cold drinks advertised the most frequently. Those shelters in lower SES areas advertised more fast food, flavoured milk and fruit juice while those in higher SES locations featured more diet beverages.

Sainsbury et al. (2017) audited 178 train stations in the Sydney Metropolitan area in both summer and winter. They collected information on products, brands and the location and format of all advertising. Nearly 30% of all advertisements promoted food and beverages; 54% of those were on the train platform or visible from the train platform with just over 50% of ads on vending machines themselves. Of greater concern was that 84% of food and beverage advertisements were for discretionary (i.e. unhealthy) foods. Thus, vending machines not only provided access to unhealthy foods for patrons but also served as a non-broadcast source of out-of-home advertising.

### 9.3.3 Interventions in Transportation Hubs

It is clear that transport hubs, trains and buses are an important intervention setting to improve both the accessibility and marketing of healthy food choices. When planning interventions in transport hubs, the complexity of this environment needs to be taken into account. For instance, ownership of rail systems varies by country. In the UK, ownership of rail networks is currently privatized (Haywood, 2005), whereas rail networks in Australia are government owned (Australian Government, 2020). Station development also engages local urban planning (Haywood, 2005). Strategies to scale-up initiatives to change these food environments will need to be adapted to a variety of different contexts and organizational structures. Planning and implementation of interventions may be influenced by the number of stakeholders or different processes that influence the food provided. Interventions could also target not only the hubs and stops but the journey itself on buses or trains. While there is a paucity of information about interventions in transportation hubs and other settings, lessons from initiatives in community recreation and sports facilities, described later in this chapter, may be relevant and transferable.

## 9.4 RECREATION AND SPORT FACILITIES

Recreational physical activity and sports facilities including non-elite community sports clubs have a wide reach (McFadyen et al., 2018) and are an integral part of even the most isolated communities. Public accessibility and the fact that children and youth represent a substantive portion of their user base (Naylor et al., 2015) make recreation and sport facilities an important setting in which to promote healthy behaviours (Meganck et al., 2015).

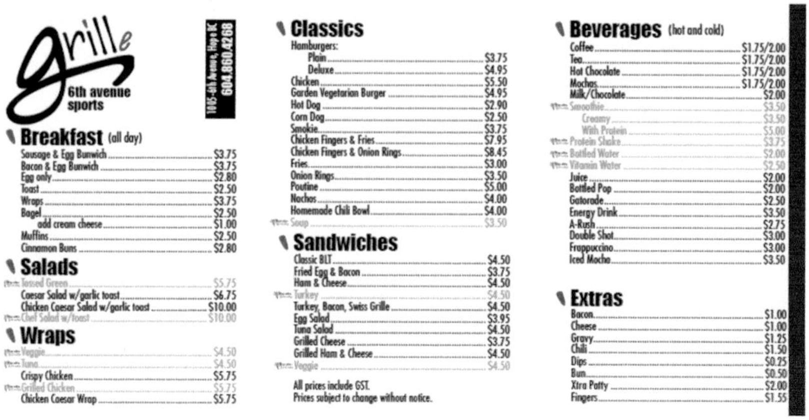
Grille
6th avenue sports
1005-6th Avenue, Hope BC
604.860.4268

**Breakfast** (all day)

| | |
|---|---|
| Sausage & Egg Bunwich | $3.75 |
| Bacon & Egg Bunwich | $3.75 |
| Egg only | $2.80 |
| Toast | $2.50 |
| Wraps | $3.75 |
| Bagel | $2.50 |
| add cream cheese | $1.00 |
| Muffins | $2.50 |
| Cinnamon Buns | $2.80 |

**Salads**

| | |
|---|---|
| Tossed Green | $5.75 |
| Caesar Salad w/garlic toast | $6.75 |
| Chicken Caesar Salad w/garlic toast | $10.00 |
| Chef Salad w/toast | $10.00 |

**Wraps**

| | |
|---|---|
| Veggie | $4.50 |
| Tuna | $4.50 |
| Crispy Chicken | $5.75 |
| Grilled Chicken | $5.75 |
| Chicken Caesar Wrap | $5.75 |

**Classics**

| | |
|---|---|
| Hamburgers: | |
| Plain | $3.75 |
| Deluxe | $4.95 |
| Chicken | $5.50 |
| Garden Vegetarian Burger | $4.95 |
| Hot Dog | $2.90 |
| Corn Dog | $2.50 |
| Smokie | $3.75 |
| Chicken Fingers & Fries | $7.95 |
| Chicken Fingers & Onion Rings | $8.45 |
| Fries | $3.00 |
| Onion Rings | $3.50 |
| Poutine | $5.00 |
| Nachos | $4.00 |
| Homemade Chili Bowl | $4.00 |
| Soup | $3.50 |

**Sandwiches**

| | |
|---|---|
| Classic BLT | $4.50 |
| Fried Egg & Bacon | $3.75 |
| Ham & Cheese | $4.50 |
| Turkey | $4.50 |
| Turkey, Bacon, Swiss Grille | $4.50 |
| Egg Salad | $3.95 |
| Tuna Salad | $4.50 |
| Grilled Cheese | $3.75 |
| Grilled Ham & Cheese | $4.50 |
| Veggie | $4.50 |

All prices include GST.
Prices subject to change without notice.

**Beverages** (hot and cold)

| | |
|---|---|
| Coffee | $1.75/2.00 |
| Tea | $1.75/2.00 |
| Hot Chocolate | $1.75/2.00 |
| Mochas | $1.75/2.00 |
| Milk/Chocolate | $2.00 |
| Smoothie | $3.50 |
| Creamy | $3.50 |
| With Protein | $5.00 |
| Protein Shake | $3.75 |
| Bottled Water | $2.00 |
| Vitamin Water | $2.50 |
| Juice | $2.00 |
| Bottled Pop | $2.00 |
| Gatorade | $2.50 |
| Energy Drink | $3.50 |
| A-Rush | $2.75 |
| Double Shot | $3.00 |
| Frappuccino | $3.00 |
| Iced Mocha | $3.50 |

**Extras**

| | |
|---|---|
| Bacon | $1.00 |
| Cheese | $1.00 |
| Gravy | $1.25 |
| Chili | $1.50 |
| Dips | $0.25 |
| Bun | $0.50 |
| Xtra Patty | $2.00 |
| Fingers | $1.55 |

**FIGURE 9.3** Concession menu at a sports centre in Canada.

As well as a healthy environment for physical activities, community recreation and sport facilities or clubs are ideally positioned to exemplify a healthy food environment (Meganck et al., 2015) across a range of food services that are often present. Vending machines are the most common food source in this setting. In one study of recreation facilities in British Columbia, Canada (Naylor et al., 2010), facilities ($n = 101$) had an average of 3.6 (range: 0–19 machines) beverage machines and 1.9 (range: 0–12) snack machines. Large urban facilities generally had more vending machines than small urban or rural facilities. Sixty-one percent of facilities surveyed also had a cafe or concession (see Figure 9.3) open during peak times, 32% provided food during facility-based childcare and on average 2.5 food-related sport team fundraisers were held onsite each year (Naylor et al., 2010). In the UK, research evaluating the food environment in both public and private leisure centres and health clubs found that in public venues, the average number of vending machines was 2.8 (SD = 1.6) and 35% had a cafe or restaurant, whereas private facilities had significantly fewer machines at 1.5 (SD = 0.9) (Nowak et al., 2012).

### 9.4.1 Vending Food and Beverages

The food in vending machines situated in recreation and sport facilities has not typically been health promoting. For instance, the percentage of unhealthy beverages and snacks (high in salt, saturated fat and/or sugar) available in vending machines in Canadian facilities in three provinces ranged from 65% to over 90% of items (Olstad et al., 2020). These disappointing proportions resemble those in other jurisdictions such as Australia (Boelsen-Robinson et al., 2020) and the UK (Nowak et al., 2012). In one UK study, vending machine food offerings were categorized using the School Food Trust criteria and only 0.4% of vending snack offerings and 14% of beverages were classified as 'permitted for sale' (Nowak et al., 2012). Vending machines, however, are not the only source of unhealthy foods in recreation and sport facilities.

### 9.4.2 Concessions and Cafes

Evidence also indicates that the healthfulness of venue concession offerings resembles the pattern found in vending machines. A New Zealand study involving stakeholder interviews and an assessment of venue food offerings found that more than 62% of foods sold were unhealthy (Carter et al., 2019). Data from the Eat, Play, Live trial in Canada compared concession food offerings of facilities located in provinces with voluntary nutrition guidelines for recreation and sport facilities to those located in provinces without such guidelines. Facilities in provinces with voluntary nutrition guidelines had a reduced Nutrition Environment Measures Survey for Restaurants (rNEMS-R; Saelens et al., 2007) score of 37% of the ideal, and 80% of packaged snacks and 73% of beverages for sale were categorized based on the guidelines as 'Do Not Sell' (non-nutritious, energy-dense foods). In facilities with no provincial guidelines, the rNEMS-R score was 24% of the ideal score and 94% of packaged snacks and 80% of beverages were categorized as 'Do Not Sell' (Olstad et al., 2020). The proportion of facilities with unhealthy foods (e.g. French fries, potato chips/crisps, high fat main dishes like hot dogs) on their menus was also high (Olstad et al., 2020). Thus, the foods available in concessions and vending machines may support less healthful dietary practices.

### 9.4.3 Food and Beverage Marketing

There is emerging evidence that extensive food and beverage sponsorship and marketing occurs in recreation and sport facilities (Westberg et al., 2021). More than half of all marketing in facilities in the Canadian based Eat, Play, Live trial was for the 'Least Healthy' products with another fifth from a 'Less Healthy' category (Prowse et al., 2018). To further exacerbate this, research in two Canadian provinces investigated vendor-supported healthfulness labelling and found 21.5% of products were labelled as healthier than their nutrient content supported (Prowse et al., 2019). This labelling approach is only one of many marketing tools used by distributors to encourage food purchasing in recreation and sport settings.

Food marketing in the recreation and sport environment consists of marketing exposures in the form of signage, branding, pricing promotions and product placement (Prowse et al., 2018) and also sponsorship of sports and physical activity events that utilize the facilities through naming rights (e.g., hockey or football league names), logos on uniforms, branded participant products (e.g., water bottles) and product vouchers (Westberg et al., 2021). Sponsorship has been shown to influence brand preferences and loyalty, attitudes and food preferences and consumption (Caswell & Hanning, 2018). Thus, food-related sponsorship of teams, leagues and events in a facility can act as a unique influence on that food environment. A survey of recreation and sport facilities in British Columbia, Canada, showed almost one fifth of facility respondents reported receiving financial and corporate incentives and about one quarter reported sponsorship from companies associated with unhealthy food products (Naylor et al., 2010). This study did not ask specifically about sponsorship of teams, leagues and events that rented or used the facilities. Two studies conducted in Australian community sport clubs showed that 17% and 26%, respectively

(Westberg et al., 2021), had sponsorship and, similar to studies elsewhere (Westberg et al., 2021), half of that sponsorship came from companies associated with unhealthy food products. Interestingly, the most common sponsorship arrangement was a brand or logo on children's uniforms (Kelly et al., 2010a).

## 9.5 INTERVENING IN COMMUNITY ENVIRONMENTS: THE EXAMPLE OF RECREATION AND SPORT FACILITIES

Two intervention approaches have been explored extensively in recreation and sport facilities, namely policy interventions (regional/state or facility level) and capacity-building (Naylor et al., 2015; Olstad et al., 2019), which can also be described as implementation support strategies (McFadyen et al., 2018). Implementation support is typically used to enhance policy implementation but can target practice and environmental changes as well. We highlight what is known about these two strategies and how they interact.

### 9.5.1 The Use of Policy to Change Recreation and Sport Facility Food Environments

Several policy areas and options have been identified as opportunities to positively influence food environments and individuals' eating practices within recreation and sport facilities (Olstad & Raine, 2013). Policy action can be taken at many levels across the socioecological framework (see Chapter 1), but the most obvious at the macro level is government-level policy. However, policy action at the meso level, within a community/municipality (applying to one or more sport or recreation facilities within the geographic boundary) or organizational (applying to a single recreation facility) setting, is also common. Both policy levels have the potential to alter societal norms and values and to thereby positively affect dietary practices.

Some prior evidence suggested local government and facility managers perceived that food policy in community recreation facilities and sport clubs was outside their mandate and not relevant to them (Allender et al., 2011). However, policy for promoting healthy food/eating environments has become a priority in some jurisdictions. For example, research in Australia surveying health promotion, nutrition, physical activity and sports management found healthy food availability at canteens and reducing sponsorship by companies selling primarily unhealthy food and beverages ranked second only to alcohol practices as a health priority (Kelly et al., 2014).

### 9.5.2 Government (Regional/State) Level Policy – Nutrient Profiling Standards or Guidelines

The government-level policy approach we know most about is nutrient profiling standards or guidelines, which can be mandatory or voluntary. For instance, the policy approach taken in many Canadian jurisdictions to address the health profile of food and beverages sold in recreation and sport facilities has been voluntary provincial nutrition guidelines (Olstad et al., 2020). Nutrient profiling guidelines have been applied to food and beverages sold in vending machines and in concessions/cafes (Olstad et al., 2020). These guidelines both define what constitutes a healthy or an unhealthy food option and establish standards for their availability (Kelly et al., 2014). In most cases, expert-derived nutrition guidelines categorize products on a scale of healthfulness (e.g. in British Columbia, Canada, these categories are ‘Do Not Sell’, ‘Sell Sometimes’ and ‘Sell Most’) using detailed nutrient content and portion size criteria (British Columbia Ministry of Health, 2014).

Voluntary guidelines in sports facilities may have a positive but limited impact on the healthfulness of foods offered. Assessment of the impact of voluntary nutrition guidelines in Alberta, Canada, highlighted that awareness, adoption and implementation of the guidelines remained low 1 year following their release (Olstad et al., 2011). More recently, the Canadian Eat, Play, Live trial results demonstrated that facilities in provinces with voluntary nutrition guidelines had healthier food environments than those in provinces without guidelines, and that those with guidelines that also received an 18-month capacity-building intervention significantly improved the quality of their food environments (Olstad et al., 2019). Nevertheless, the overall quality of their food environments remained relatively poor.

A study in four US cities (Green et al., 2020) demonstrated that city-level policies around vending machines in venues where children spend time (including recreation centres) could be effective but were not always fully implemented. The cities in the study each committed to different percentages of healthy snack offerings and implemented a compliance monitoring mechanism indicating that the policies were not voluntary. When a selection of vending machines in each city were audited for policy compliance, the proportion of healthy snacks was lower than the goal in three of the cities, but goal compliance for beverages was higher overall. There was higher compliance to beverage guidelines in US cities with regulated guidelines compared to in the Canadian Eat, Play, Live study where guidelines were voluntary (Olstad et al., 2019). However, in terms of snacks, for the facilities in the Canadian study that received both guidelines and a capacity-building intervention, compliance levels (i.e. percentage of snacks meeting or not meeting the guideline standard) were similar to the US study (Green et al., 2020). This likely reflects the lack of availability of healthy and palatable snack options compared to less healthy (Naylor et al., 2015; Westberg et al., 2021).

In addition, the Eat, Play, Live trial showed a potential ‘health halo’ effect from provincial voluntary nutrient guideline implementation, as despite the fact that marketing was not addressed in the guidelines, the proportion of marketing exposures promoting ‘Least Healthy’ products was lower in guideline provinces compared to non-guideline provinces (48% versus 74%) (Prowse et al., 2018). Child-targeted and sports-related marketing techniques promoting ‘Least Healthy’ products were also less common in guideline province facilities compared to non-guideline province sites. Thus, a provincial nutrition profiling standard potentially served as a catalyst for, or represented more global changes in, the socio-cultural food environment.

The studies described above highlight the need for interventions to improve the implementation of healthy food and beverage policies in recreation and sport centres.

In the case of voluntary policies, additional capacity-building interventions and monitoring of standards are needed (Green et al., 2020; Olstad et al., 2019).

### 9.5.3 Facility-Level Policy – The Case of Contracts

Beyond government-level policy, cities or municipalities and even individual facilities are often in a position to enact localized policy approaches including vending and concession contracts (Lane et al., 2019). Many facilities participating in the Stay Active Eat Healthy initiative in British Columbia, Canada, reported developing facility-level policy statements as a step in changing their food environments (Naylor et al., 2015) although their specific content and impact was not examined. The Eat, Play, Live study assessed vending contracts and found that facilities that included a health stipulation in their contract had a lower proportion of 'Do Not Sell' beverages and snacks than those facilities that had no health stipulations (Lane et al., 2019). However, few contracts identified specific standards for food and beverages which may be important to meeting provincial standards (Lane et al., 2019). Furthermore, events such as fundraising are often excluded from contracts but are important in maintaining a healthy food culture (Kelly et al., 2010b). Mandatory food procurement policies which align with healthier vending contract standards have been identified as a potential policy approach to improve food environments in recreational settings (Raine et al., 2018) but, similar to policies addressing marketing to children in this setting, have not yet been studied. These more localized policy tools appear important to enhancing the food environment either in the context of higher-level policies or not.

### 9.5.4 Building Capacity for Action

Related to the issue of food policy implementation and other strategies to improve the healthfulness of food environments is that of capacity-building or the provision of implementation support strategies (see Table 9.1). Emerging evidence from Canada and Australia has highlighted the importance of providing implementation support to achieving changes in the healthfulness of food provided in recreation and sport facilities. A 2018 systematic review identified three controlled interventions that evaluated the effectiveness of strategies to enhance healthy food and beverage policy implementation in non-elite sport clubs or recreation facilities' policies, practices and environments (McFadyen et al., 2018). These included 'quality improvement initiatives, education and training, performance feedback, prompts and reminders, implementation resources, financial incentives, penalties, communication and social marketing strategies, professional networking, the use of opinion leaders, an implementation consensus process or a combination of strategies' (McFadyen et al., 2018). These types of strategies have often been referred to as capacity-building in the health promotion literature (Hawe et al., 2009) and in some of the recreation and sport facility food environment literature (Naylor et al., 2015) but are otherwise described in implementation science literature as implementation support strategies (Leeman et al., 2017a). Since this review, one further randomized trial was conducted in Canada (Olstad et al., 2019) which also used capacity-building (Leeman et al., 2017b)

**TABLE 9.1**
**Key Implementation Support Strategies**

| Key Implementation Support Strategies Identified in the Literature as Important to Implementation of Food Environment Change Initiatives |
|---|
| • A project coordinator/knowledge broker/support officer who provided technical support to organizational representatives or champions<br>• Audits of food and/or beverages and a feedback report to organizational representatives<br>• Training (online or in-person)<br>• Small grants for implementation cost recovery (e.g. to hire a nutritionist to review concession menus or to purchase vending products for patron taste-testing or to reduce the cost of healthy items) or incentives (e.g. recognition, accreditation)<br>• Educational materials (online or printed resources, newsletters and powerpoint presentations for decision makers/opinion leaders and staff to enhance buy-in)<br>• Cross-facility sharing and professional networking |

and linking systems theory (Orlandi et al., 1990). The Canadian study (Olstad et al. 2019) included many of the strategies previously described and also provided public-facing marketing materials focused on healthy choices (e.g., clings for doors and machines), facilitated cross-facility sharing and used the whole of setting model previously described (Figure 9.1). All four studies demonstrated that implementation support strategies enhanced implementation of at least one organizational policy or practice related to improving the food environment.

### 9.5.5 Implementation: A Critical Issue

With government- and local-level policy and capacity-building emerging as efficacious options for improving community food environments, there is also an ever-increasing body of evidence documenting perceived barriers to implementation within these environments. These include competing priorities, financial constraints and fears, social/cultural norms, stakeholder buy-in, lack of an advocate or champion and the absence of community support (Kirk et al., 2021; Westberg et al., 2021). Capacity-specific barriers identified included lack of expertise, lack of government support and lack of time (Meganck et al., 2017). In regions with significant commitment to facility-level policy action, additional barriers identified included limited availability of products that met guideline standards, complexity of nutrition guidelines, lack of training and insufficient resources to implement nutrition guidelines (Olstad et al., 2013; Westberg et al., 2021).

Strongly entrenched norms include the sale of non-nutritious energy-dense snack foods (Carter et al., 2019; McIsaac et al., 2018) in these community environments. Carter et al. (2019) suggested that the high level of exposure has succeeded in normalizing these foods within these settings. Social norms clearly dictate expectations to stakeholders of the types of foods and beverages that should be available and underscore the fear of objections from patrons (McIsaac et al., 2018). Importantly, other primary barriers can be closely linked to this overarching barrier. For instance, social/cultural norms link directly to the fears of customer or revenue loss to competitive food options and the increased cost and spoilage of healthier food options (Vander Wekken et al., 2012; Westberg et al., 2021). Industry stakeholders also have financial concerns centred on consumer preferences and their unwillingness to pay higher prices associated with healthier foods and the increased operational costs associated with greater perishability (Vander Wekken et al., 2012). However, a growing body of evidence challenges the perception that offering healthier food and beverages results in financial losses (Boelsen-Robinson et al., 2017). Overcoming negative perceptions and allaying fears about reduced profitability may therefore be a key target for intervention.

Engaging stakeholders (e.g., public health officials, sport organizations, recreation facilitiy staff and food manufacturers and distributors) at all levels and establishing partnerships between sectors is critical to building and supporting a healthy food environment (Kirk et al., 2021). However, the capacity and willingness of sport organizations to engage and take action may be more limited due to a reliance on volunteers rather than paid staff. Furthermore, the idea that adopting a health-oriented approach to food offerings is important may not be shared by industry partners, whose primary responsibility is to generate a profit (Olstad et al., 2013) but a regulatory approach, that 'creates a level playing field' for purveyors of food and beverages has been identified as helpful (Olstad et al., 2013). Engaging champions (individuals who enthusiastically support and are knowledgeable about change strategies) to support local efforts can also facilitate healthy food initiatives and support implementation of mandatory regulations and voluntary guidelines (Kirk et al., 2021). All of the above can also be classified as implementation support strategies (see Table 9.2).

**TABLE 9.2**
**Areas of Potential Food Environment Action, Designed by the Authors**

| Areas of Potential Food Environment Action in Community Settings Distilled from the Literature |
|---|
| • Facility-level written food policy based on a whole of setting approach and encompassing concessions, vending, programming, events, fundraising, marketing and food security, and the environment for staff and volunteers<br>• Vending and concession contracts with specifically defined nutrient standards (healthy food provisions) and accountability mechanisms<br>• Reducing availability and promotion of unhealthy food and beverages in recreation and sport facilities, including in fundraising and in children's programming (e.g. summer sports camps)<br>• Restructuring corporate sponsorship arrangements to reduce/eliminate exposure to unhealthy food and beverages and their marketing<br>• Reducing/eliminating exposure to unhealthy food and beverage marketing and promotion<br>• Identifying facility staff with responsibility for facilitating a 'healthy food environment' by working with stakeholders, developing initiatives like consumer 'taste-testing' and monitoring policy and contract compliance |

## 9.6 VULNERABLE POPULATIONS

Policies and healthy nutrition environments and practices in community recreation and sport facilities have the potential to reduce dietary inequities as the broad reach of recreation and sport means that many vulnerable children and families are engaged in sport or recreation settings. In Australia, almost two thirds of children participate in sport (Kelly et al., 2014), and among those aged 15 years and older, sports participation is even higher at 87% (McFadyen et al., 2018). Where efforts are taken to create a healthy and welcoming environment (Allender et al., 2011)) and culturally tailored programming for different ethnic groups, there are increases in participation (Po'e et al., 2012). Many recreation facilities in Canada provide subsidies and free physical activity and sport programming for at-risk adults, children and youth. Outreach programming (i.e. programs delivered in community settings outside of the facility like a school or family resource centre) is also common (Canadian Parks and Recreation Association (CPRA), 2015). One of the goals of the Framework for Recreation in Canada (CPRA, 2015) is to ensure access to healthy food for those with constraints to sports participation. Similar efforts in Australia include sport clubs' provision of a healthy meal to disadvantaged and Indigenous youth (Kelly et al., 2010b). Although recreation and sport facilities may support equitable access to healthy food, if indeed healthy food is offered, it is important to note that in general, families with lower incomes typically have fewer opportunities for recreational and sport experiences due to the cost and resources needed for registrations, transportation and equipment (CPRA, 2015) meaning that the benefit of a healthy food environment in this setting is not necessarily equitable. Bowen et al. (2015) noted that 'obesogenic' nutrition environments may also be more pervasive in lower socioeconomic public areas. Further exacerbating the social divide, a qualitative investigation of guideline adoption in Alberta (Olstad et al., 2013) led to the suggestion that more advantaged regions with more connections to partners, initiatives and resources could be more likely to implement voluntary healthy eating policies while those in the most dire need due to neighbourhood socioeconomic conditions may be left without any policy benefits. Allender et al. (2011) argue that socioeconomic inequities are more likely to improve with a strong regulatory approach supporting multi-faceted intervention(s), suggesting that equitable change may only occur if implementation of nutrition policies in recreation and sport facility policies is mandatory rather than voluntary.

## 9.7 CONCLUSIONS

The food environment in community settings including within transportation hubs and recreation and sport facilities remains largely 'unhealthy' and thus fails to support healthy dietary practices and patterns among the populations using these facilities. It is clear from the literature that policy in the form of guidelines or standards for food sold in community settings is an important step in positively influencing their food environments, but in isolation their impact is limited. Multi-sectoral engagement and comprehensive capacity-building/implementation supports are required to support policy implementation. Although the research is limited, it appears that mandated policy with embedded accountability mechanisms may facilitate more meaningful improvements in community food environments compared to voluntary guidelines and should therefore be encouraged. Although providing a healthy food environment in community recreation and sport facilities holds promise for enhancing equitable access to healthy food, this remains largely unexamined in the research literature. Measuring the impact of food environment interventions on dietary practices and patterns is an important priority of future research, with a specific focus on their effectiveness within socioeconomically disadvantaged populations.

## REFERENCES

Allender, S. et al., 2011. Policy change to create supportive environments for physical activity and healthy eating: which options are the most realistic for local government? *Health Promotion International,* 27(2), pp. 261–274.

Australian Bureau of Statistics, 2018. Census of population and housing: commuting to work - more stories from the census, 2016. [Online] Available at: https://www.abs.gov.au/ausstats/abs@.nsf/Lookup/by%20Subject/2071.0.55.001~2016~Main%20Features~Feature%20Article:%20Journey%20to%20Work%20in%20Australia~40 [Accessed July 2020].

Australian Government, 2020. Background - organization of Australia's Railways. [Online] Available at: www.infrastructure.gov.au/rail/background.aspx [Accessed 2020].

Boelsen-Robinson, T. et al., 2017. The effect of a change to healthy vending in a major Australian health service on sales of healthy and unhealthy food and beverages. *Appetite*, 114, pp. 73–81.

Boelsen-Robinson, T. et al., 2020. Change in drink purchases in 16 Australian recreation centres following a sugar-sweetened beverage reduction initiative: an observational study. *BMJ Open,* 10:e029492. doi:10.1136/bmjopen-2019-029492

Bowen, D. J., Barrington, W. E. & Beresford, S. A., 2015. Identifying the effects of environmental and policy change interventions on healthy eating. *Annual Review of Public Health*, 36, pp. 289–306.

British Columbia Ministry of Health, 2014. Healthier choices in vending machines in B.C. public buildings policy. [Online] Available at: https://www2.gov.bc.ca/assets/gov/health/managing-your-health/healthy-eating/vending-policy-2014.pdf, [Accessed 2020].

Canadian Parks and Recreation Association (CPRA), 2015. Framework for recreation in Canada. [Online] Available at: www.cpra.ca/about-the-framework [Accessed 2020].

Carter, M.-A., Signal, L. N., Edwards, R. & Hoek, J., 2019. Competing teammates: food in New Zealand sports settings. *Health Promotion International*, 34, pp. 803–810.

Caswell, M. S. & Hanning, R. M., 2018. Adolescent perspectives of the recreational ice hockey environment and influences on eating behaviour revealed through photovoice. *Public Health Nutrition,* 21(7), pp. 1255–1265.

de Leeuw, E., 2017. Engagement of sectors other than health in integrated health governance, policy, and action. *Annual Review of Public Health*, 38, pp. 329–349.

Department for Transport, 2019. Transport Statistics Great Britain 2019 Moving Britain Ahead. [Online] Available at: assets.publishing.service.gov.uk [Accessed 2020].

Euromonitor International, 2019. Retailing 2019. [Online] Available at: www.euromonitor.com/passport [Accessed July 2020].

Grech, A. & Allman-Farinelli, M., 2015. A systematic literature review of nutrition interventions in vending machines that encourages consumers to make healthier choices. *Obesity Reviews*, 16, pp. 1030–1041.

Green, S., Glanz, K. & Bromberg, J., 2020. Facilitators and barriers to developing, implementing, and evaluating healthy vending policies in four cities. *Health Promotion Practice*, 22(5), pp. 670–675.

Hawe, P., Shiell, A. & Riley, T., 2009. Theorising interventions as events in systems. *American Journal of Community Psychology*, 43, pp. 267–276.

Haywood, R., 2005. Co-ordinating urban development, stations and railway services as a component of urban sustainability: an achievable planning goal in Britain? *Planning Theory & Practice,* 6(1), pp. 71–97.

Kelly, B. et al., 2014. Identifying important and feasible policies and actions for health at community sports clubs: a consensus-generating approach. *Journal of Science and Medicine in Sport*, 17, pp. 61–66.

Kelly, B. et al., 2010a. Food and drink sponsorship of children's sport in Australia: who pays? *Health Promotion International,* 26(2), pp. 188–195.

Kelly, B., Baur, L. A., Bauman, A. E. & King, L., 2010b. Examining opportunities for promotion of healthy eating at children's sports clubs. *Australian and New Zealand Journal of Public Health,* 34(6), pp. 583–588.

Kelly, B., Flood, V. M., Bicego, C. & Yeatman, H., 2012. Derailing healthy choices: an audit of vending machines at train stations in NSW. *Health Promotion Journal of Australia,* 23(1), pp. 73–75.

Kirk, S. et al., 2021. Appetite for change? Facilitators and barriers to nutrition guideline implementation in Canadian recreation facilities. *Health Promotion International*, pp. 1–11. doi:10.1093/heapro/daab017.

Lane, C. et al., 2019. Healthy vending contracts: so localized policy approaches improve the nutrition environment in publicly funded recreation and sport facilitities?. *Preventive Medicine Reports,* 16, pp. 1–7. doi:10.1016/j.pmedr.2019.100967

Leeman, J. et al., 2017a. Beyond "implementation strategies": classifying the full range of strategies used in implementation science and practice. *Implementation Science*, 12:125, pp. 1–9. doi: 10.1186/s13012-017-0657-x.

Leeman, J. et al., 2017b. Developing theory to guide building practitioners' capacity to implement evidence-based interventions. *Health Education & Behavior,* 44(1), pp. 59–69.

McFadyen, T. et al., 2018. Strategies to improve the implementation of policies, practices or programmes in sporting organizations targeting poor diet, physical inactivity, obesity, risky alcohol use or tobacco use: a systematic review. *BMJ Open,* 8: e019151. doi:10.1136/bmjopen-2017-019151

McGuirt, J. T., Heubner, G., Ward, R. & Jilcott Pitts, S. B., 2019. Food and beverage options at highway rest areas in North Carolina: a mixed-methods audit and geospatial approach. *Preventing Chronic Disease,* 17(16), p. E142.

McIsaac, J.-L. D., Jarvis, S., Spencer, R. & Kirk, S., 2018. "A tough sell": findings from a qualitative analysis on the provision of healthy foods in recreation and sport settings. *Health Promotion and Chronic Disease Prevention in Canada,* 38(1), pp. 18–22.

Meganck, J., Scheerder, J., Thibaut, E. & Seghers, J., 2015. Youth sports clubs' potential as health-promoting settings: profiles, motives and barriers. *Health Education Journal,* 74(5), pp. 531–543.

Meganck, J., Seghers, J. & Scheerder, J., 2017. Exploring strategies to improve the health promotion orientation of Flemish sports clubs. *Health Promotion International,* 32(4), pp. 681–690.

Naylor, P.-J. et al., 2010. Publicly funded recreation facilities: obesogenic environments for children and families? *International Journal of Environmental Research and Public Health*, 7, pp. 2208–2221.

Naylor, P.-J., Olstad, D. L. & Therrien, S., 2015. An intervention to enhance the food environment in public recreation and sport settings: a natural experiment in British Columbia, Canada. *Childhood Obesity,* 11(4), pp. 364–374.

Nowak, M., Jeanes, Y. & Reeves, S., 2012. The food environment in leisure centres and health clubs: how appropriate is it for children? *Nutrition & Food Science,* 42(5), pp. 307–314.

Olstad, D. L. & Raine, K. D., 2013. Profit versus public health: the need to improve the food environment in recreation facilities. *Canadian Journal of Public Health,* 104(2), pp. e167–e169.

Olstad, D. L. et al., 2011. Improving children's nutrition environments: a survey of adoption and implementation of nutrition guidelines in recreation facilities. *BMC Public Health,* 11:423, pp. 1–12. doi:10.1186/1471-2458-11-423

Olstad, D. L., Raine, K. D. & McCarger, L. J., 2013. Adopting and implementing nutrition guidelines in recreational facilities: tensions between public health and corporate profitability. *Public Health Nutrition,* 16(5), pp. 815–823.

Olstad, D. L. et al., 2019. Eat, Play, Live: a randomized controlled trial within a natural experiment examining the role of nutrition policy and capacity building in improving food environments in recreation and sport facilities. *International Journal of Behavioral Nutrition and Physical Activity,* 16:51, pp. 1–16. doi:10.1186/s12966-019-0811-8

Olstad, D. L. et al., 2020. Baseline results from the Eat, Play, Live trial: a randomized controlled trial within a natural experiement examining the role of nutrition policy and capacity building in improving food environments in recreation and sport facilities. *Food Policy,* 92, pp. 1–8. doi:10.10.16/j.foodpol.2020.101870

Onufrak, S. J. et al., 2019. Foods consumed by United States adults from non-school cafeterias and vending machines: NHANES 2005–2014. *American Journal of Health Promotion,* 33(5), pp. 666–674.

Orlandi, M. A., Landers, C., Weston, R. & Haley, N., 1990. Diffussion of health promotion innovations. In: K. Glanz, F. M. Lewis & B. K. Rimer, eds. *Health Behavior and Health Education: Theory, Rsearch, and Practice.* Washington, DC: Jossey-Bass/Wiley, pp. 288–313.

Po'e, E. K. et al., 2012. Systematic exposure to recreation centres increases use by Latino families with young children. *Childhood Obesity,* 8(2), pp. 116–123.

Prowse, R. J. et al., 2018. Food marketing in recreational sport settings in Canada: a cross-sectional audit in different policy environments using the Food and beverage Marketing Assessmen Tool for Settings (FoodMATS). *International Journal of Behavioral Nutrition and Physical Activity,* 15:39, pp. 1–11. doi:10.1186/s12966-018-0673-5

Prowse, R. J., Tomlin, D. L., Naylor, P.-J. & Raine, K. D., 2019. Exploring nutrition labelling of food and beverage vending machines in Canadian recreational sport settings. *Canadian Journal of Dietetic Practice and Research*, 80, pp. 55–62.

Raine, K. D. et al., 2018. Healthy food procurement and nutrition standards in public facilities: evidence synthesis and consensus policy recommendations. *Health Promotion and Chronic Disease Prevention in Canada,* 38(1), pp. 6–17.

Saelens, B. E., Glanz, K., Sallis, J. F. & Frank, L. D., 2007. Nutrition environment measures study in restaurants (NEMS-R): development and evaluation. *American Journal of Preventive Medicine*, 32(4), pp. 273–281.

Sainsbury, E., Colagiuri, S. & Magnusson, R., 2017. An audit of food and beverage advertising on the Sydney metropolitan train network: regulatory and policy implications. *BMC Public Health,* 17, p. 490. doi:10.1186/s12889-017-4433-2

Settle, P. J., Cameron, A. J. & Thornton, L. E., 2014. Socioeconomic differences in outdoor food advertising at public transit stops across Melbourne suburbs. *Austalian and New Zealand Journal of Public Health*, 38(5), pp. 414–418.

Signal, L. N. et al., 2017. Children's everyday exposure to food marketing: an objective analysis using wearable cameras. *International Journal of Behavorial Nutrition and Physical Activity*, 14, p. 137.

Vander Wekken, S., Sorensen, S., Meldrum, J. & Naylor, P.-J., 2012. Exploring industry perspectives on implementation of a provincial policy for food and beverage sales in publicly funded recreation facilities. *Health Policy*, 104, pp. 279–287.

Westberg, K. et al., 2021. Promoting healthy eating in the community sport setting: a scoping review. *Health Promotion International.* doi:10.1093/heapro/daab030

# 10 The Role of Places of Worship in the Food Environment

*Emma Tomalin*
University of Leeds

## CONTENTS



## 10.1 INTRODUCTION

Since the 1980s, there has been a shift towards considering the broader social ecosystem that shapes people's health and ought to therefore influence the selection of relevant sites for public health interventions. Despite this, the role of places of worship (PW) as public health settings in both high-income countries (HIC) and low- and middle-income countries (LMICs) has received patchy attention (Tomalin et al. 2019). While faith-based affiliations, ideas, actors and organisations can play negative as well as positive roles in health promotion and well-being, consideration of this has been weakly reflected in mainstream public health research and strategy globally. Within research on the food environment, some studies focus on the role that people's attitudes and culture play in shaping their choice of and access to certain foods, yet the specific role of religion and PWs is yet to be seriously considered (Turner et al. 2018).

There are a variety of types of PW across faith traditions and global regions, of varied use and significance. Across all religious traditions, playing a role in looking after a PW or donating money for its running costs and development is a religious duty. When forced or economic migrants move to new locations, setting up a space for worship is often a priority, to provide a 'home from home', meeting first in people's dwellings, sometimes using a room in a building intended for other purposes, before having the

DOI: 10.1201/9781003043720-10 

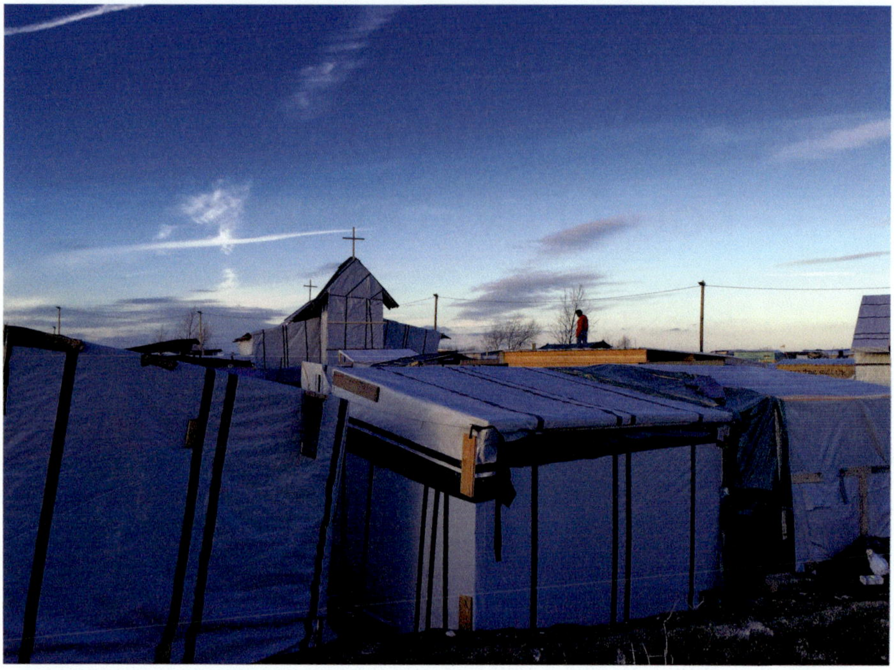

**FIGURE 10.1** St Michaels Church Calais Jungle seen from the South side. (Photo by Liam Stoopdice available at https://commons.wikimedia.org/wiki/File:St_Michaels_Church_Calais_Jungle.jpg. Reprinted with permission under license CC BY-SA 4.0, https://creativecommons.org/licenses/by-sa/4.0/deed.en.)

capacity to establish a dedicated space for worship or to purpose build a PW (Tomalin and Starkey 2017; see Figure 10.1). PWs are not ordinary spaces but through the activities that occur there and/or the presence of deities, they are sacred and transformative spaces that can deliver devotees into a so-called 'liminal' or 'threshold' state (Turner 1969). Usually there are some areas within PWs that are more sacred than others and where only trained and sanctified religious specialists can perform rituals, mediating between the people and the divine. However, many PWs also have non-sacred spaces, rooms or nearby buildings to carry out wider community activities.

For the communities who use them, PWs have a wider function that may not be obvious at first sight. They are spaces for bringing a faith community together, often involving the consumption of food reflecting regional cuisines and special diets (e.g. halal and kosher food, within Islam and Judaism; vegetarianism, within Hinduism, Jainism and Sikhism; periods of fasting, such as in Ramadan and during some Christian festivals) and rituals involving food (e.g. the blessing of food donations by the gods in Hindu temples, *prasad*, that are then received back by devotees; see Figure 10.2). They are also sites for pastoral care and psycho-social counselling, provided by trusted religious specialists; and locations where the beliefs and teachings of faith traditions are reinforced to maintain a community of believers. Beyond these functions, PWs also provide practical services including childcare and education, both in the tenets of the faith and wider schooling; they are locations where those in need can

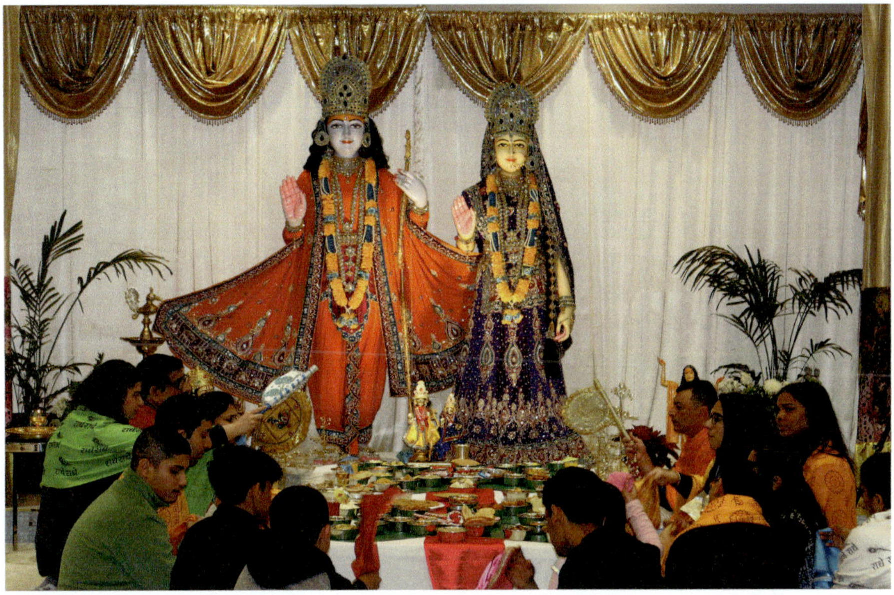

**FIGURE 10.2** A Chappan Bhog food offering in which 56 varieties of food are cooked by Hindu devotees. The food is then placed before the altar of the Hindu Deity, in this case, Shri Sita-Rama. Devotees partake by chanting a devotional song and fanning the Deity. The food is then distributed to guests and consumed as a Prasad, or devotional grace. (Photo by Bizmadhav1 available at https://commons.wikimedia.org/w/index.php?sort=relevance&search=prasad+offering+filetype%3Abitmap&title=Special:Search&profile=advanced&fulltext=1&advancedSearch-current=%7B%22fields%22%3A%7B%22filetype%22%3A%22bitmap%22%7D%7D&ns0=1&ns6=1&ns12=1&ns14=1&ns100=1&ns106=1#/media/File:Devotional_offering_of_food_to_Hindu_Deity_Shri_Sita-Rama.jpg. Reprinted with permission under licence CC BY-SA 4.0, https://creativecommons.org/licenses/by-sa/4.0/deed.en.)

receive charitable donations of food and other items (also see Chapter 11 for more information on food insecurity) and places where hospitals and clinics have been set up to treat those who have no access to healthcare. Therefore, PWs also play a role within the wider community in both HICs and LMICs. While many PWs are welcoming to everyone in their locality, this is not always the case, and they can be places that exclude certain groups (e.g. members of low caste groups in the case of some Hindu temples, women in the case of some mosques and LGBTIQ+ individuals in some Evangelical Christian places of worship). Therefore, it is important not to romanticise the role that PWs play in people's health and well-being as only being positive.

Both positive and negative, this account establishes that PWs are an important part of the wider social ecosystem emphasised in the Ottawa Charter that plays a role in shaping people's health and well-being, including diet and food choices (WHO 1986). Indeed, PWs have so many direct links to health and diet, suggesting that for communities with high levels of religious adherence, these spaces are important for public health actors to understand and to engage with. Turner et al. identify 'two key domains within the wider food environment construct' (2018: 95) where:

> The external domain relates to the world of opportunities and constraints that are 'out there' within a given context, and includes dimensions such as food availability, prices, vendor and product properties, and marketing and regulation. The personal domain includes a set of individual level dimensions, including food accessibility, affordability, convenience and desirability.
>
> *Turner et al. (2018: 95)*

They argue that research has focussed on the external food environment, and the personal food environment, which is most relevant to PWs, remains neglected. There is limited research on the existing and potential relevance of PWs as public health settings generally, and for the food environment specifically, in HICs and LMICs. The reasons for this neglect of faith in public health research and practice are complex but stem from a combination of lack of knowledge about how to engage with faith actors, and a distrust of approaches to health and healing that often differ from the biomedical model, where 'many communities attach a religious meaning to illness, in terms of an emic [insider] understanding of its causes, and hence the appropriate cures needed to treat it (e.g. a punishment from God that requires prayers; or a curse that requires ritual intervention)' (Tomalin et al. 2019: 59). Moreover, for national and global public health bodies, there is discomfort in partnering with faith actors and their PWs for fear of risking their perceived secular and neutral stance. This has been particularly challenging for humanitarian organisations, where despite the significant role that faith-based organisations play in humanitarian relief, including food aid, there is 'suspicion about the capacity of faith-motivated institutions to contribute to humanitarian objectives… practitioners and theorists alike have expressed concern with regards to their ability to adhere to humanitarian principles, particularly that of impartiality' (Kraft 2015: 396–397).

Nonetheless, there is a growing body of scholarship, currently at the margins of mainstream public health research, that 'recognises the strengths of a faith-inspired approach, where the support provided in faith-based settings and the trust that people place in religious leaders, as well as the tangible resources that religious settings have, can be a great asset in the pursuit of better global health outcomes' (Tomalin et al. 2019: 59). In the remainder of this chapter, I will examine some of this literature, drawing out examples of best practice, and identifying gaps for future research. I start by looking at PWs as 'healthy settings' in HICs, with a focus on research undertaken in Bradford in the UK. In the following section, I then explore the potential for food environment research within PWs in LMICs through the example of a recent initiative (2016) of the World Food Programme (WFP) to engage with faith actors and their communities.

## 10.2 PLACES OF WORSHIP AS HEALTHY SETTINGS AND THE FOOD ENVIRONMENT IN HIGH-INCOME COUNTRIES

The World Health Organisation's (WHO) 'healthy settings' initiative is an example of a holistic or ecosystem approach to health promotion. While research on healthy settings has been undertaken within schools, workplaces, hospitals, prisons and universities (Dooris 2005) (many of which are covered in other chapters in this book), there is virtually no research that examines PWs as healthy settings. This is despite the fact that as Corcoran et al. (2013) argue 'religious organisations and faith groups have often been able to engage in important roles in health … and thus have potential as a health promotion setting… [allowing]…access to some populations that traditional health promotion efforts may not reach, including specific ethnic groups and older people who may be traditionally low users of health care' (2013: 121–122). In HICs, research on faith, health and PWs tends to focus on improving health outcomes amongst 'seldom heard' groups, including individuals from 'Black, Asian and Minority Ethnic' (BAME) communities, due to their high levels of self-reported religious identification (Tomalin et al. 2019; November, 2014). Existing research that is relevant to the role of PWs as healthy settings, although not situated within the healthy settings literature, mainly comes from the USA and concerns interventions in Black churches (e.g. Newlin et al. 2012; Buta et al. 2011). There is a smaller literature from the UK focussing on South Asians (e.g. Maynard et al. 2017; Rao et al. 2012).

With respect to diet and food, as Turner et al. note, 'Food environment research to date has primarily been undertaken in response to the rapid rise of obesity and associated diet-related NCDs in HICs' (2018: 94). In the UK, this is reflected in the literature that takes religion into account where PWs are viewed as sites where public health interventions can take place, including relating to diet-related health and exercise (Maynard et al. 2009, 2017; Ghouri 2005; Rao et al. 2012; Boltri et al. 2008). However, alongside external collaboration, participation in religious activities at PWs, such as prayer or meditation, can have a positive impact on wellbeing and mental health (Nooney and Woodrum 2002) and religious leaders sometimes integrate health messages into their sermons or prayers (Tomalin et al. 2015). However, PWs not only play a role in shaping how people interact with food environments but are also food environments themselves. Some PWs provide food for the community as part of their religious service, such as the Sikh Langar (see Figure 10.3). Many PWs also step in during times of austerity and increased poverty, providing soup kitchens and foodbanks (Cloke et al. 2017; Joint Public Issues Team 2014; Singh 2015; Salonen 2016; Power 2017).

### 10.2.1 Case Study 1: Bradford, West Yorkshire, UK

Bradford has the largest proportion of people of Pakistani ethnic origin (20.4%) out of cities in the UK, and the fourth highest proportion of Muslims in England, with nearly one quarter of the population identifying as Muslim (City of Bradford Metropolitan District Council 2012). BAME communities in Bradford experience unequal outcomes with regard to several health conditions including obesity, depression, type 2 diabetes and smoking-related illness, as well as conditions linked to ethnic groups such as sickle cell anaemia, more prevalent in Asian, African or Caribbean populations (NHS 2012). People of South Asian, African and Caribbean heritage are also at greater risk for developing type 2 diabetes (Department of Health 2001). In a number of Bradford's neighbourhoods, high BAME occupancy rates correlate with some of the highest national levels of childhood obesity (NHS 2012). The prevalence of these health conditions cannot be linked to ethnicity alone and reflects structural factors such as poverty and deprivation, compounded by the fact that members of BAME

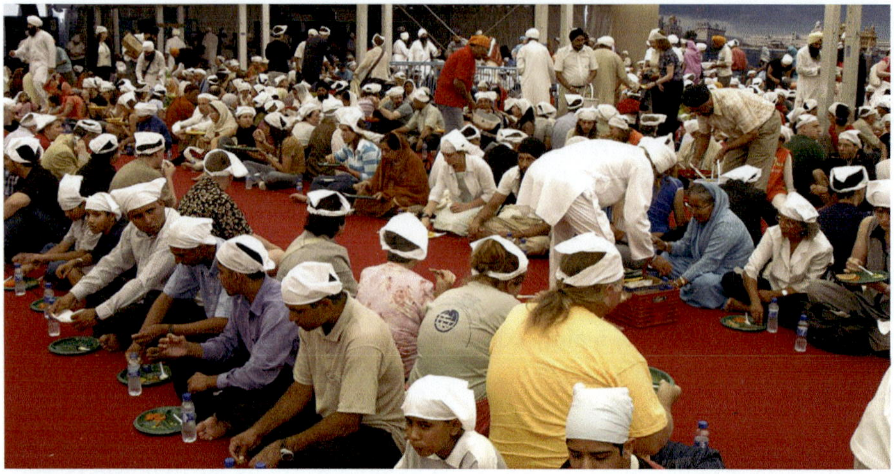

**FIGURE 10.3** A Sikh Langar. (Photo by Hari Singh available at https://en.wikipedia.org/wiki/Langar_(Sikhism)#/media/File:Langar.jpg. Reprinted with permission under licence CC BY-SA 3.0, https://creativecommons.org/licenses/by-sa/3.0/deed.en.)

communities are not always reached by mainstream health services and education and the inability of the mainstream health services to always recognise and respond to the specific needs of diverse communities.

In 2014, I led a small pilot project in Bradford, among the objectives of which were to:

- identify the health concerns prevalent within certain religious and/or ethnic groups, to understand how PWs could play a role in dealing with those issues.
- discover the attitudes of local 'religious leaders' (RLs), 'congregations' and public health (PH) actors in Bradford regarding PH practice in PWs.

We carried out one focus group with Muslim women and ten interviews (three with third sector organisations, two with public sector actors, one with an academic and four with representatives of PWs).[1] The issue of food poverty, diet and exercise emerged as a key theme. As a dietician told us, 'we've got a great food poverty/child poverty issue so a lot of faltering growth, where we might not see that elsewhere' which can lead to obesity, type 2 diabetes and high blood pressure and that 'even in children we're seeing that being diagnosed now'. While some put this down to the upsurge in cheap fast food, others drew attention to the normal lower birth weight of South Asian babies compared to White British, which can lead to early weaning. Coupled with lower-than-average breastfeeding rates in the Pakistani community in Bradford, this is a 'precursor for obesity'.

[1] Ethical permission for this research was granted by The University of Leeds Research Ethics Committee.

So, what role can PWs play? While one interviewee suggested that 'we could use faith organisations' as a way of educating people about breastfeeding and children's diet, the gendered use of the mosque presents potential barriers to this, as women are less likely to attend than men. Another interviewee in the Muslim women's focus group drew attention to activities carried out in community centres that support Muslim women, which may sometimes be linked to the mosque, such as exercise classes and education on nutrition. While the mosques may not always cater to women's needs, one Anglican Church was running a 'scones and samosas' group, for Muslim women. As the vicar told me, this project.

> ...has grown from the church's vision to serve the local community in a way that fosters well-being, includes the marginalised and encourages cross cultural and cross-faith relationships. It started out [...] talking to mums outside the school and they wanted to learn how to cook traditional English food like lasagne and pasta...So that also helps their language skills because they didn't know about measurements and all those sorts of things...But the focus on that is healthy cooking...They get about 14–20 mums, mainly mums go to school first and then come here...They're mainly Mirpuri Pakistanis...

It is common for children to attend the mosque after school for language and religious instruction. An interviewee from Early Childhood Services told us that his agency had introduced activities for children after school to help reduce obesity, but those kids were attending the mosque rather than these play schemes. He explained that they were beginning to work with the mosques to include more activity for the children. Another response to this was a Church which has set up an afterschool club, with activities and a healthy snack, predominantly for Muslim children, who attend until 5 pm when they go to the mosque.

An important contribution of PWs is the provision of emergency food aid. Research by Power et al. (2017) in Bradford examined the profile of the city's 67 community food aid providers. They found that 48% of them described themselves as faith-based, with 36% as Christian and 12% as Muslim. This high proportion of faith-based food banks is not uncommon in the UK, and faith-based food aid benefits 'from the use of a religious building rent-free, often including free utilities and facilities...[and]...Religious institutions were also the primary source of full- and part-time staff and volunteers' (2017: 259). Although Muslims do use the Christian and non-faith-based food banks, with a preference for the latter, they are more likely to use the ones at mosques. Given that nearly 25% of the city identifies as Muslim, these findings raise 'concerns about how well food aid in Bradford reflects the local demographic' (2017: 256). This is an important finding, because as the state increasingly relies on food banks, it cannot be assumed that they are necessarily reaching those most in need. The study found that the Christian food banks were more explicitly religious than the Muslim-run ones, including options to pray and join religious services, which could act as a barrier to Muslims accessing them. Muslims may also be deterred by the fear that the food will not be halal. However, Power et al. (2017) also suggest that 'The low use of food aid by Pakistani-Muslims in Bradford may...be attributable to the existence of alternative, hidden forms of food assistance among the Pakistani-Muslim community surrounding mosques' (2017).

## 10.3 PLACES OF WORSHIP AND THE FOOD ENVIRONMENT IN LOW- AND MIDDLE-INCOME COUNTRIES

Turner et al. note that food environment research had tended to focus on obesity and diet in HICs and that it 'needs to broaden its scope to also consider malnutrition' in LMICs, where food environment research is in its infancy (2018: 94). They draw attention to the fact that in both HICs and LMICs, most research has focussed on the external food environment, and that we know less about the personal food environment that involves 'people's individual preferences, acceptability, tastes, desires, attitudes, culture, knowledge and skills to shape the desirability of food vendors and products' (2019: 93). In LMICs, more so than HICs, the role of PWs on the personal food environment is important, given the high levels of religious adherence. In LMICs, a literature on faith and health developed earlier than in HICs, having its roots in the role that faith and PWs played in the HIV/AIDS crisis in Sub-Saharan African (Gunderson and Cochrane 2012). Prior to this, many hospitals in the 18th and 19th centuries in Africa and Asia developed as part of the Christian missionary enterprise continue to comprise a dominant proportion of national health systems. Nevertheless, the role that PWs and faith-based organisations play in the provision of food aid in humanitarian settings is under-researched as is the role that religion plays in shaping food choices and access to food in LMICs (see Figure 10.4).

Turner et al. (2020) carried out a systematic review of food environment research in LMICs. They found 70 articles that mentioned both food environment, its key

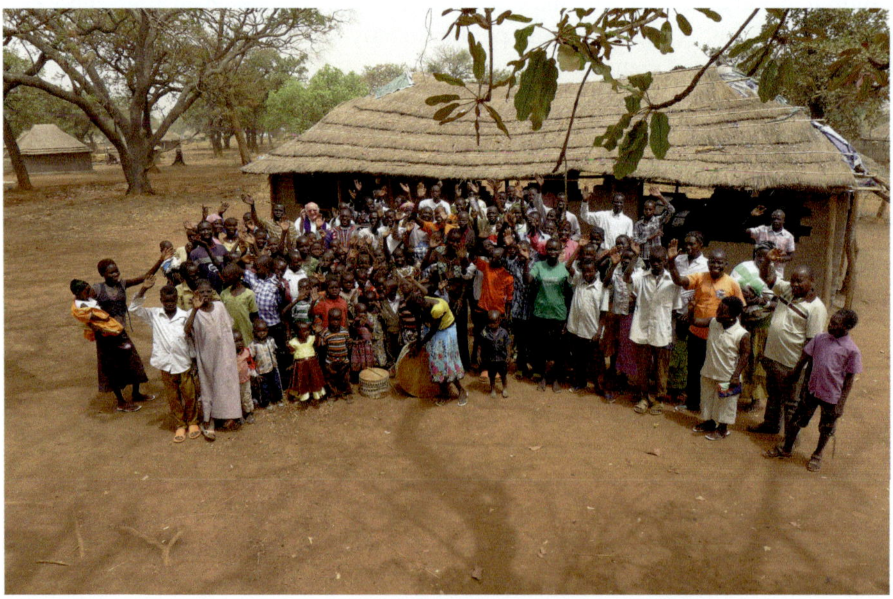

**FIGURE 10.4** Christians after Sunday Mass in South Sudan. (Photo by Earnst Ulz available at https://commons.wikimedia.org/wiki/File:P1050306_semilarge.jpg. Reprinted with permission under licence CC BY-SA 3.0, https://creativecommons.org/licenses/by-sa/3.0/deed.en.)

concepts and included reference to one or more LMICs. The studies included 22 LMICs, with 70% upper-middle-income countries, 26% LMIC and none from low-income countries (2020: 389). Forty-five of the articles used quantitative methods, 17 used qualitative methods and eight were mixed methods. I undertook a search for the terms 'religion', 'religious', 'faith' and 'worship' in each of the 70 articles, which revealed that out of the 45 quantitative studies only one mentioned any of these terms, when referring to instructions to interviewees about how to think about their neighbourhood – including religious institutions (Chor et al. 2016: 3); out of the 17 qualitative studies, only two mentioned one or more of these terms (Kolopaking et al. 2011; Maxfield et al. 2016), and out of the seven mixed methods studies none mentioned any of these terms. None mentioned PWs and the specific role that they play in the food environment.

Kolopaking et al. (2011) focus on maternal self-efficacy in the home food environment among low-income mothers of nutritionally at-risk children in an urban area of Jakarta, Indonesia. Out of a total number of 19 participants, 17 were Muslim and two were Christian. One of the questions they were asked was, 'How do you think your culture/religious belief influence your attitude toward food and eating?' (2011: 183). Kolopaking et al. report that the women 'believed that they should trust in God's will…Some of the mothers fasted regularly on Mondays and Thursdays, which is part of an Islamic religious ritual to improve mental strength. They thanked God for what they received in their lives' (2011: 185). The authors specifically note that more research on the 'religious approach' to food is needed. Maxfield et al. (2016) focus on globalisation and food prestige among Indian adolescents and note how 'Food habits reproduce class distinctions' as well as reinforcing 'membership across ethnic, religious, gendered, and social categories' (2016: 342). However, while much scholarship on food in India has 'tied food's status-connoting properties to its role as a transducer of pollution in the caste system' (2016: 345), they note that wealthy urbanites 'are often far more interested in knowing what is 'cool' to eat than in traditional socio-moral or religious proscriptions about spiritual pollution… Even traditional Hindu religious prohibitions against meat consumption blur as one moves up or down the socioeconomic ladder' (2016: 345).

While there is a paucity of research on this topic and none that focusses on PWs, faith-based and secular practitioners are beginning to collaborate in this area, particularly since the inception of the Sustainable Development Goals (SDGs) in 2015, where SDG 2 is to achieve zero hunger by 2030.

### 10.3.1 Case Study 2: The World Food Programme – Inter-Religious Engagement for Zero Hunger

The WFP – 'the world's largest humanitarian agency'[2] – was established in 1961 and is the food assistance wing of the United Nations (est. 1945). Today, four core humanitarian principles of humanity, impartiality, neutrality and operational independence guide the work of the UN, including the WFP.[3] The UN as well as secular

---

[2] https://www.wfp.org/history.

[3] https://time.com/wp-content/uploads/2015/02/oom-humanitarianprinciples_eng_june12.pdf.

development and humanitarian NGOs have been cautious about engaging with faith actors, for fear of compromising these principles, to the extent that this has resulted in what many see as a disproportionate response to concerns over proselytisation (Tomalin 2013). This has led to the exclusion of religious leaders and faith-based organisations from many aspects of humanitarianism and development at the global level, when these actors are important providers of aid, education and health at the national and local level. Over the past decade or so, this bias has started to recede, not least because the rise of Islamist terrorist organisations has reinforced the idea that understanding religion is important for foreign policy. Today, the voices of religious leaders are increasingly sought by the UN and other agencies, and faith-based organisations compete for donor funding, as long as they keep their faith in the background. However, many continue to be suspicious of the motives of religious organisations involved in humanitarian and development work. In 2017, David Beasley, a governor of South Carolina between 1995 and 1999, became the new Executive Director of the WFP. In an article entitled 'The UN World Food Program Boss, Mixing Work With Religion?', he is criticised for not keeping his personal religious beliefs separate from his work (Leimbach 2018). People who were interviewed for the article say that 'it really does make people uneasy', that 'Religious parochialism could interfere with the UN's primary mission of providing food aid' and 'It's completely inappropriate… Doing so flies in the face of UN norms' (Leimbach 2018).

Such concerns notwithstanding, the WFP increasingly partners with faith actors and in 2016 made a pledge to 'seek enhanced partnership with religious actors' at an event addressed by Pope Francis (WFP 2016a: 1). On 12–13 June 2016, to launch this initiative, religious scholars and leaders were invited to a meeting in Rome 'to discuss how best to join forces to achieve Zero Hunger by 2030 – as stipulated in the Sustainable Development Goals (SDGs)' (WFP 2016a: 1). In preparation for the meeting, 24 religious leaders were invited to share their 'faith statements' beforehand. As the then Executive Director of the WFP Ertharin Cousin wrote in the preface to the faith statements booklet,

> Eliminating hunger…. requires fully harnessing strategic partnerships, including with religious communities, faith-inspired organisations, governments, international organisations, and other stakeholders… The moral imperative of feeding the hungry and caring for the poor lie at the heart of the world's major religions… Religious leaders and communities offer enormous potential to galvanize global political will, catalyse local action and achieve lasting change in the lives of vulnerable people
>
> *WFA (2016b)*

Most of the faith statements came from religious leaders who were senior figures in faith-based organisations and networks to tackle hunger and related humanitarian issues. Organisations included Religions for Peace, World Council of Churches, Fahmina Institute, Indonesia, and the International Network of Engaged Buddhists. There were ten Christian individuals/organisations, three Muslim, two each were Hindu, Buddhist, Japanese religions and interfaith, one each were Sikh, Baha'i and Jewish, and one was the Alliance to End Hunger formed by Lutheran NGO, Bread for the World, 'as a platform for both secular and faith organisations to join together in the fight against hunger.'[4] A few things are worth noting that raise questions about how representative and impactful such global events can be. First, out of the 24, only four were women and nine were from LMICs – Sengal, Ghana, Indonesia, India (x2), Thailand, Sri Lanka, Kenya and Venezuela. Second, the predominance of Christian organisations in the faith-based development/humanitarian space is well known, reflecting the colonial history of Christianity. Third, as is common with other UN events, this one involved high-level religious leaders who were already well known at the international level. For such initiatives to move beyond symbolic gestures, it is necessary that efforts are made to localise them, alongside better understanding how local religious dynamics shape food choice and access, as well as how faith resources, including PWs, can be leveraged towards zero hunger.

## 10.4 CONCLUSIONS

This chapter has demonstrated that PWs form part of the social environment that shapes people's access to and food choice, as well as playing a role as food environments themselves, where they provide food aid for those in need. While the core business of PWs comprises religious activities for their membership or congregation, they also reach out to those beyond their immediate communities, providing services and support that have important implications for people's health and well-being. In both HICs and LMICs the existing impact of PWs in this regard, as well as potential for the future, has not yet become the focus of a robust research agenda, despite evidence that national and global public health bodies are beginning to take the role of religion and faith actors more seriously. In both HICs and LMICs, PWs can play a role in reducing inequalities and diet and health. In LMICs, it is important that moves by global food and health bodies to partner with religious leaders and faith-based organisations also pay attention to the role of local faith communities and their places of worship in food aid and dietary health.

## REFERENCES

Boltri JM, Davis-Smith YM, Seale JP, Shellenberger S, Okosun IS, Cornelius ME. (2008) Diabetes prevention in a faith-based setting: results of translational research. *J Public Health Manag Pract* 14: 29–32.

Buta B, Brewer L, Hamlin DL, Palmer MW, Bowie J, Gielen A. (2011) An innovative faith-based healthy eating program: from class assignment to real-world application of PRECEDE/PROCEED. *Health Promot Pract* 12(6): 867–875.

Chor D, Cardoso LO, Nobre AA, Griep RH, Fonseca MDM, Giatti L, Bensenor I, Molina MDB, Aquino EML, Diez-Roux A, et al. (2016) Association between perceived neighbourhood characteristics, physical activity and diet quality: results of the Brazilian Longitudinal Study of Adult Health (ELSA-Brasil). *BMC Public Health* 16: 751.

City of Bradford Metropolitan District Council (2012). 2011 census release 2.1: key statistics for local authorities bradford district. https://ubd.bradford.gov.uk/media/1275/2011-census-second-release-11-december-summary-note.pdf.

---

[4] https://alliancetoendhunger.org/about-us/who-we-are/.

Cloke P, May J, Williams A. (2017). The geographies of food banks in the meantime. *Prog Hum Geogr* 41(6): 703–726.

Corcoran N, Bone A, Everett C. (2013). Using settings. In: Corcoran, N. (Ed.) *Communicating Health: Strategies for Health Promotion.* Sage: London, pp. 112–113.

Department of Health (2001) *National Service Framework for Diabetes.* Department of Health: London.

Dooris M. (2005) Healthy settings: challenges to generating evidence of effectiveness. *Health Promot Int* 21(1): 55–65.

Ghouri N. (2005) Health fair in a mosque: putting policy into practice. *Public Health* 119: 197–201.

Gunderson G, Cochrane J. (2012) *Religion and the Health of the Public: Shifting the Paradigm.* Palgrave Macmillan: Basingstoke.

Joint Public Issues Team (2014) Faith in Foodbanks: resources for churches. A resource from the Baptist Union of Great Britain, the Methodist Church, the United Reformed Church and Church Action on Poverty. http://www.jointpublicissues.org.uk/wp-content/uploads/Faith-in-Foodbanks-Report.pdf.

Kolopaking R, Bardosono S, Fahmida U. (2011) Maternal self-efficacy in the home food environment: a qualitative study among low-income mothers of nutritionally at-risk children in an urban area of Jakarta, Indonesia. *J Nutr Educ Behav* 43(3): 180–188.

Kraft K. (2015) Faith and impartiality in humanitarian response: lessons from Lebanese evangelical churches providing food aid. *Int Rev Red Cross* 97(897–898): 395–421.

Leimbach, D. (2018) The UN world food program boss, mixing work with religion? January 31, 2018, *PassBlue.* https://www.passblue.com/2018/01/31/the-un-world-food-program-boss-mixing-work-with-religion/.

Maxfield A, Patil S, Cunningham SA. (2016) Globalization and food prestige among Indian adolescents. *Ecol Food Nutr* 55(4): 341–364.

Maynard M, Baker G, Rawlins E, Anderson A, Harding S. (2009) Developing obesity prevention interventions among minority ethnic children in schools and places of 80 worship: The DEAL (DiEt and Active Living) study. *BMC Public Health* 9(1): 480.

Maynard, M, Baker, G, Harding, S. (2017) Exploring childhood obesity prevention among diverse ethnic groups in schools and places of worship: recruitment, acceptability and feasibility of data collection and intervention components. *Preventive Medicine Reports*, 6: 130–136.

Newlin K, Dyess S, Allard E, Chase S, Melkus G. (2012) A methodological review of faith-based health promotion literature: advancing the science to expand delivery of diabetes education to Black Americans. *J Relig Health* 51(4): 1075–1097.

NHS (2012) National Child Measurement Programme: England, 2011/12 school year. The Health and Social Care Information Centre. https://digital.nhs.uk/data-and-information/publications/statistical/national-child-measurement-programme/2011-12-school-year.

Nooney J, Woodrum E. (2002) Religious coping and church-based social support as predictors of mental health outcomes: testing a conceptual model. *J Sci Study Religion* 41(2): 359–368.

November L. (2014) The impact of faith-based organisations on public health and social capital. Faith Action. https://www.faithaction.net/wp-content/uploads/2014/09/FaithAction-Public-Health-Report.pdf.

Power M, Small N, Doherty B, Stewart-Knox B, Pickett KE. (2017) "Bringing heaven down to earth": the purpose and place of religion in UK food aid. *Soc Enterp J* 13(3): 251–267.

Rao N, Eastwood S, Jain A, Shah M, Leurent B, Harvey D, Robertson L, Walters K, Persaud J, Mikhailidis D, Nair D. (2012). Cardiovascular risk assessment of South Asians in a religious setting: a feasibility study. *Int J Clin Pract* 66(3): 262–269.

Salonen AS. (2016) Food for the soul or the soul for food: users' perspectives on religiously affiliated food charity in a Finnish city. University of Helsinki, Helsinki. https://helda.helsinki.fi/handle/10138/166534.

Singh J. (2015) From the temple to the street: how Sikh kitchens are becoming the new food banks. The Conversation. https://theconversation.com/from-the-temple-to-the-street-how-sikh-kitchens-are-becoming-the-new-food-banks-44611.

Tomalin, E, Russell, A, Sadgrove, J. (2015) Places of Worship as Settings for Black and Minority Public Health in Leeds. Leeds City Council: England.

Tomalin, E, Sadgrove, J, Summers, R. (2019) Health, faith and therapeutic landscapes: Places of worship as Black, Asian and Minority Ethnic (BAME) public health settings in the United Kingdom, *Social Science & Medicine,* 230: 57–65. doi:10.1016/j.socscimed.2019.03.006.

Tomalin E, Starkey C. (2017). Buddhist buildings in England: the construction of underrepresented faith heritages in a multicultural and post-Christian setting. *Int J Herit Stud* 23(2): 156–172.

Tomalin E. (2013) *Religions and Development.* Routledge: London and New York.

Turner V. (1969). *The Ritual Process: Structure and Anti-Structure.* Cornell University Press: Ithaca New York.

Turner CA, Walls H, Herforth A, Drewnowskie A, Coates J, Kalamatianou S, Kadiyala S. (2018) Concepts and critical perspectives for food environment research: a global framework with implications for action in low- and middle-income countries. *Global Food Sec* 18: 93–101.

Turner C, Kalamatianou S, Drewnowski A, Kulkarni B, Kinra S, and Suneetha Kadiyala Food (2020) Environment research in low- and middle-income countries: a systematic scoping review. *Adv Nutr* 11(2): 387–397.

WFP (2016a) Inter-religious engagement for zero hunger summary report from events at the World Food Programme, 12–13 June 2016. https://www.partner-religion-development.org/fileadmin/Dateien/Resources/Knowledge_Center/2016_WFP_Summary_Report_Inter-religious_engagement_for_Zero_Hunger_12-13_June_2016.pdf.

WFP (2016b) Voices of faith: statements from religious leaders and actors Inter-religious engagement for Zero Hunger 13 June 2016 at WFP HQ, Rome. https://www.bread.org/sites/default/files/religious_leaders_final_enlow.pdf.

WHO (1986) The Ottawa Charter for Health Promotion. https://www.who.int/healthpromotion/conferences/previous/ottawa/en/.

# 11 Food Insecurity, Poverty and the Very Low-Income Food Environment

*Madeleine S. Power*
University of York

*Suzy L. Liddell*
The Trussell Trust

*Mariko Koide*
United Nations officer, United Nations Relief and Works Agency for Palestine Refugees in the Near East

**CONTENTS**



## 11.1 INTRODUCTION

The very low-income food environment, whether in the UK or globally, can be defined as a context in which individuals and households experience 'food insecurity'. According to the Food and Agriculture Organisation (FAO) of the United Nations, 'a person is food insecure when they lack regular access to enough safe and nutritious food for normal growth and development and an active healthy life' (FAO, 2020). The

DOI: 10.1201/9781003043720-11

FAO measures food insecurity using the Food Insecurity Experience Scale (FIES), according to which an individual can be categorised as severely food insecure, moderately food insecure or experiencing mild food insecurity/food security; and monitors hunger or 'undernourishment' using the Prevalence of Undernourishment indicator. In 2020, nearly 690 million people were estimated to be undernourished globally, or 8.9% of the world population – up by 10 million people in 1 year and by nearly 60 million since 2014; a marked reversal of the decades-long decline in hunger in the world, as measured using the prevalence of undernourishment. The number of people affected by severe food insecurity shows a similar upwards trend since 2014. In 2019, close to 750 million were exposed to severe levels of food insecurity (FAO et al., 2020). According to the FAO, the reasons for the observed increase in food insecurity and undernourishment globally since 2014 are multiple. Whilst much of the recent increase in food insecurity can be attributed to the greater number of conflicts, often exacerbated by climate-related shocks; even in some peaceful settings, food security has deteriorated as a result of economic slowdowns threatening access to food for the poorest households (FAO et al., 2020).

Today, food insecurity is prevalent in both the Global South and the Global North. There is clear evidence that food insecurity has increased across Europe since the 2007–2008 global financial crisis, with the sharpest rise in countries with more liberalised economies and higher economic inequality, such as the UK (Davis and Geiger, 2017). According to the Family Resource Survey (2019–2020), 8% of UK households are food insecure, with low household food security (4%) or very low household food security (4%) (Department for Work and Pensions, 2021). A large body of research documents that the primary cause of food insecurity is low income and poverty; however, poverty is not necessarily synonymous with food insecurity: in the United States, a high proportion of households reporting food security are poor, and a portion of households with incomes above the poverty line are food insecure (Gundersen et al., 2011). The work of Gundersen et al. (2011) and Wight et al. (2014) suggests that the relationship between poverty and food insecurity may in fact be dependent upon the measure of income used. For example, the analyses by Wight et al. (2014) indicate that a more inclusive measure of income and resources (a supplemental poverty measure) reveals a stronger association between poverty and food insecurity than the US official poverty measure. In the UK, there are currently estimated to be 14 million people living in poverty, including 8 million working-age adults, 4 million children and 2 million pensioners (JRF, 2020).

Consistent with international evidence (Knowles et al., 2016), households with young children in the UK are at greater risk of food insecurity than the general population (FAO et al., 2017). Food insecurity has considerable health and developmental implications for children, including lower vegetable intake and higher added sugar intake (Eicher-Miller and Zhao, 2018), and poorer academic performance (Jyoti et al., 2005). The impacts of food insecurity on health, well-being and diet among adults are manifold and severe. Food insecurity is a cause and consequence of poor mental and physical health (Power et al., 2017b; Power et al., 2018b) and associated with overweight, obesity (Adams et al., 2003) and diet quality: research among UK women finds that food insecure mothers were more likely to be overweight and had dietary intakes of poorer quality, with fewer vegetables and higher consumption of sugar-sweetened drinks (Yang et al., 2018). In line with evidence of a strong relationship between food insecurity and poor health, international literature finds that household food insecurity can place a significant additional burden on health care services (Tarasuk et al., 2018) and UK research suggests that the use of food banks is particularly prevalent among individuals who report mental health problems (MacLeod et al., 2019).

COVID-19 has precipitated a significant and sustained increase in household food insecurity since March 2020 (Loopstra, 2020), which is projected to continue (OBR, 2020). In July 2020, roughly 16% of adults – equivalent to 7.8 million people – reduced meal sizes or skipped meals due to insufficient income for food; this figure, which remained stable between April and July 2020, is roughly double the rate of food insecurity before COVID-19 (Food Standards Agency, 2021). Community-based and charitable food aid has been essential in responding to rapid rises in food insecurity since March 2020 (IFAN, 2021); however, the sustainability of this support and its effectiveness in addressing food insecurity among varied groups has been questioned (Power et al., 2020). It is unclear whether food aid, largely reliant on donations, will be able to continue to respond to likely increases in food insecurity amidst the continued social and economic fallout of COVID-19.

## 11.2 UK RESPONSE TO FOOD INSECURITY

In the UK, food insecurity has become a third sector priority only in the past decade, reflecting the relative 'newness' of food insecurity as distinct from poverty in the British context. The apparent increase in food insecurity, particularly since 2010, has been accompanied by a rapid growth in community-based and charitable responses to hunger and destitution (Lambie-Mumford, 2017). Many of these responses are in the form of food banks which in the UK are defined as 'agencies that enact the transfer of grocery-type foods free of charge to individuals in need' (Loopstra and Tarasuk, 2015). Food banks are largely run as independent charities, set up to meet local needs for emergency food, and some form part of a national food bank network. The two main food bank membership networks in the UK are the Trussell Trust (TT) and the Independent Food Aid Network (IFAN). Food banks usually provide a parcel of 3 days' worth of dry food to be consumed at home. All food banks in the TT network and over 60% of independent food banks require a person to have a professional referral in order to access emergency food (Loopstra et al., 2019).

Evidence suggests that growth in the use of food banks since 2010 is closely related to austerity policies. In the UK, cuts to working-age social security from 2010 (Lambie-Mumford and Green, 2017) have led to excessive waiting times for benefits, delays in receiving payments, increased debt and loan repayments, and benefit sanctions, which have rendered many people destitute. The roll-out of a new benefits system known as Universal Credit has been especially detrimental to household food insecurity in the UK, precipitating sudden and severe financial losses for many families (Reeves and Loopstra, 2021). Such cuts to the welfare state have occurred against a backdrop of wider insecurity and inequality: of rising living costs; of low paid and insecure work and of stagnating wages in the middle of the income range, accompanied by rising incomes at the top (Bourquin et al., 2019).

Approximately 95% of people referred to a food bank in the TT network are classed as destitute (Bramley et al., 2021), making these the most vulnerable people in society and the most at risk of experiencing food insecurity. The demography of food bank use in the UK is similar to the demography of food insecurity; financial difficulties, such as redundancies, loss of working hours and in-work poverty, as well as long-term health conditions and welfare reforms are implicated in food bank use (MacLeod et al., 2019). However, it is increasingly well established that food bank use is a poor proxy for food insecurity (Pybus et al., 2020).

## 11.3 FOOD AID IN THE UK

The IFAN estimates that in addition to more than 2,400 UK food banks, there are over 3,000 independent food aid providers distributing meals and other forms of food aid (IFAN, 2021). These include soup kitchens, Pay-As-You-Feel cafes, community kitchens, community supermarkets and community gardens. Whilst the majority of this food aid provision is run by charities, projects can vary considerably in their activities and size, in their funding, staffing and commercial arrangements and in their aims (Lambie-Mumford et al., 2014). For instance, community supermarkets may provide low-cost food which can be chosen by customers, whilst community cafes may offer universal, open-access provision – thereby avoiding the stigma associated with means-tested support – and encourage sociability between service users through communal meals.

There are over 1,000 independent food banks in the UK (IFAN, 2021). These organisations operate according to both third-party referral systems and self-referral, and tend to be more flexible than food banks in the TT network in the quantity and type of food distributed: 45% of independent food banks distribute food parcels with more than 3 days' worth of food per person, with an additional 10% not restricting food parcel content (Loopstra et al., 2019). Although food banks generally provide food for the short term, typically for 3 days, some households may rely on them for more regular contributions (Garratt, 2017), heightening the importance of the quality of the food within the food bank parcel. Garratt (2017) found that over half of households visiting West Cheshire food bank between 2013 and 2015 received only one food parcel, and these households accounted for one quarter of food parcels distributed over this period. A further quarter of food parcels were received by 7% of households who received six or more food parcels in a year, suggesting that in some food banks, the distribution of total food parcels may be concentrated among a small number of households which receive emergency food on multiple occasions.

The most high-profile provider of food aid in the UK, the TT network of food banks, has grown rapidly from 12 a year between 2003 and 2008 to roughly 400 food banks operating out of 1,200 food bank centres today. The following section presents a detailed overview of the TT, outlining the characteristics of those using its services, the nutritional content of its food banks parcels, and its work to end the need for food banks in the UK.

### 11.3.1 The Trussell Trust Charity

The TT supports 56% of all registered food banks across the UK (IFAN, 2021), which equates to over 426 food banks operating out of over 1,200 food bank centres (Trussell-Trust, 2020); the charity has been giving out emergency food since 1997, when they set up Salisbury food bank to help local people in the community who were hungry (Trussell-Trust, 2021). Food banks in the TT network predominantly operate according to a referral system in which an individual in need of food is referred by a third-party agent (doctor, social worker, health visitor or an organisation such as Citizens Advice) to the food bank. The food banks are often run by local volunteers who weigh, sort and distribute the emergency food, as well as process referral voucher data and signpost people to local support services.

Since 2017, the number of new food banks joining the TT network has stabilised (Loopstra and Lalor, 2017), but the number of food parcels distributed continues to rise. The increase in the number of emergency food parcels given out by TT over the past decade has risen from 61 k in 2010/2011 to 1.6 m in 2018/2019 (Sosenko et al., 2019). The latest statistics for 2020/2021 show that TT has given out 2.5 m food parcels, a 33% increase on the previous year (Trussell-Trust, 2021). In 5 years from 2016 to 2021, food bank use in the TT network increased by 128%. In April of the 2020 COVID-19 pandemic, TT saw an 89% increase in the number of food parcels given out compared to the same period in 2019, with a 107% increase in food parcels going to children and a 52% increase in people needing a food bank for the very first time (Trussell-Trust, 2020).

Data collected from TT referral vouchers indicate that the most frequent reasons for a person being referred to a food bank are due to issues associated with the benefit system, such as delays or reductions to payments, along with experiencing ill health, a difficult life situation and a lack of formal support (Trussell-Trust, 2021). The average number of times a person visits a food bank in the TT network is estimated to be twice a year (Trussell-Trust, 2021) – with evidence showing that 370,000 UK households were supported by food banks in the TT network, including 840,000 unique individuals, with 520,000 adults and 320,000 children (Bramley et al., 2021).

Certain groups of individuals and types of households are more likely to use food banks. According to the TT State of Hunger report (Bramley et al., 2021), disability has a high association with food bank referrals, with 62% of working-age people referred to a food bank in 2020 classed as disabled. Mental health is also a significant risk factor for needing to use a food bank, with 72% of all households referred reporting poor mental health. Demographically, the people most likely to need to use a food bank are aged between 25 and 54 years (84%), particularly those aged 35–44 (35%), with low use among people aged 65 and over (4%). People living in either socially rented or privately rented accommodation (74%) are more likely to need to use a food bank than homeowners (3%) whilst 20% are homeless. Single adults living alone (42%) and single parents (18%) with the majority of whom are female (84%) are also widely overrepresented.

TT data taken during the coronavirus pandemic showed 71% of people referred to food banks in the TT network identified as White British, and 9% identifying as Black or Black British, triple the UK population rate (Trussell-Trust, 2020). However, there is some evidence to suggest that ethnicity minority groups are generally under-represented in UK food aid (Power et al., 2017a). Whilst it remains uncertain whether this is attributable to the potentially exclusionary practices of food aid organisations or to approaches among ethnic minority communities towards food charity, emerging evidence suggests that some ethnic minorities may avoid food aid out of shame, embarrassment and cultural preferences to manage food insecurity within the community (Power et al., 2018a).

### 11.3.2 The Food and Nutritional Content of Food Parcels in the UK

A typical emergency food parcel distributed by a food bank in the TT network is composed of ambient, canned and packaged foods designed to last a person for 3 days. Food is donated by the public, which means food items and stock levels can see regular variance and inconsistency. Food parcels have undergone a nutritional analysis review finding the sugar content of the parcels exceeding government recommendations resulting in a recommendation for raw sugar to be removed from the list of items that compose a parcel (Hughes and Prayogo, 2018). As a consequence of this review, many food banks provide sugar as a non-standard, 'help yourself' option, should the food bank receive donations of this item. This provides the element of choice, which is often something removed from people who are unable to afford to buy food. Food banks try to provide choice of the food items they have available to them as much as possible and will ask a person about their choices and preferences of flavours from all items on the packing list (Trussell-Trust, 2018b). Food banks will also ask about access to cooking facilities, and if they are able to, will provide items such as a tin opener or heat flask for soup. The items that make up a standard TT food parcel are shown in Figure 11.1.

**Food Allocation Form: One Person**

| Volunteer: | Voucher No: | Date: |
|---|---|---|
| | | |

| Item | Allocation | Amount given |
|---|---|---|
| Cereal | 1 small | |
| Soup (can/packet) | 2 standard | |
| Beans/spaghetti in sauce | 2 small | |
| Tomatoes/pasta sauce | 2 small | |
| Vegetables | 2 small | |
| Meat | 2 small | |
| Or Vegetarian | 2 small | |
| Fish | 1 small | |
| Fruit | 2 small | |
| Rice pudding/custard | 1 standard | |
| Biscuits | 1 small packet | |
| Pasta/rice/noodles | 500g | |
| Tea or coffee | 40 bags/small jar | |
| Long-life juice | 1 litre | |
| Milk UHT | 1 litre | |

**Extra items when available**

| | | |
|---|---|---|
| Sauces | 1 packet | |
| Chocolate | 1 small bar | |
| | | |
| | | |

| | |
|---|---|
| **Client signature to confirm food received:** | |

**Additional requests:**

| | COMMENTS |
|---|---|
| Cooking facilities? | |
| Vegetarian? | |
| Any other dietary requirements? | |
| Children's ages? | |

| ITEM | | REQUIRED | ISSUED |
|---|---|---|---|
| Cat/Dog? | Size? | | |
| Washing Powder? | | | |
| Washing up liquid? | | | |
| Toilet rolls? | | | |
| Toiletries | Soap or Shower gel? | | |
| | Deodorant? | | |
| | Toothpaste? | | |
| | Toothbrush? | | |
| | Shampoo? | | |
| | Feminine hygiene? | | |
| | Shaving foam? | | |
| | Razors? | | |

**FIGURE 11.1** The food allocation list for one person, listing key food items making up a food parcel plus extra items and additional considerations. (Reprinted with permission from The Trussell Trust, https://www.trusselltrust.org/2018/06/08/whats-trussell-trust-foodbank-parcel/.)

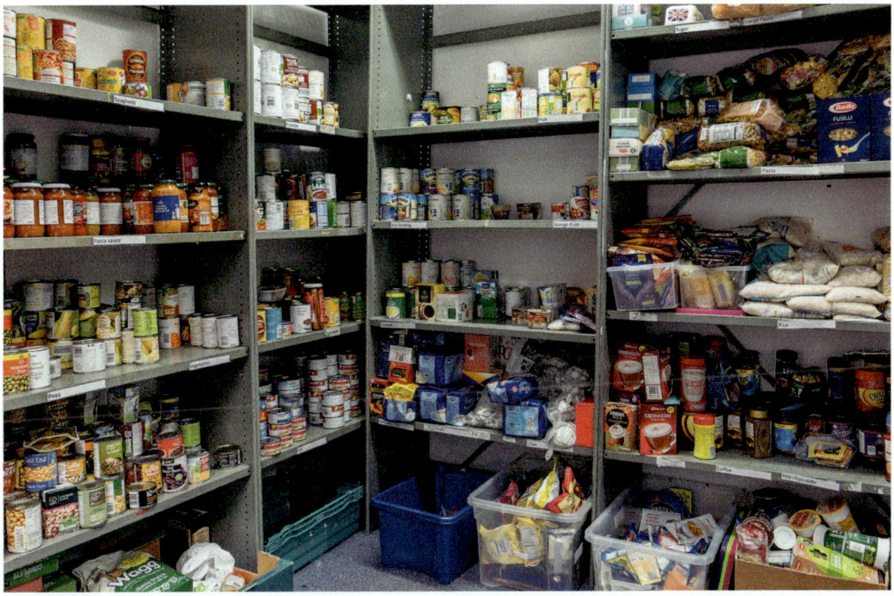


**FIGURE 11.2** Foodbank supplies in a foodbank in the UK. (Reprinted with permission from Shutterstock, available from https://www.shutterstock.com/image-photo/rotherham-england-uk-february-14-2019-1342132301.)

In addition to a standard food parcel, many food banks will also offer fresh foods, such as fruits, vegetables, eggs and bread (see Figure 11.2). However, this is dependent on whether a food bank is able to provide these foods safely and is often limited to food banks with adequate facilities, refrigeration and the resources to manage a fresh food scheme (Trussell-Trust, 2018b) as well as what food is donated (see Figure 11.3).

The estimated average cost of a food bank food parcel is £17.66 (Furey and Caraher, 2018), equating to £44.1 m of publicly donated food being distributed in 1 year based on latest TT food parcel figures. In addition, a 2017 study by The TT and IFAN found that TT and independent food bank volunteers contribute more than 4 million hours of unpaid work each year to help feed their local communities. This equates to over £30.8 m worth of hours spent to help tackle UK hunger (Trussell-Trust, 2017). These combined contributions demonstrate the huge costs that food banks and the general public are working to alleviate. However, it also highlights the instability of relying on donated time and food; with the increase in food bank use rising year after year, it is clear that the food bank model is increasingly unsustainable.

### 11.3.3 Charitable Initiatives to Reduce Food Bank Use and Food Insecurity

Both The TT and IFAN believe that food banks and food aid should not be needed in the UK and that everyone should be able to afford their own food.

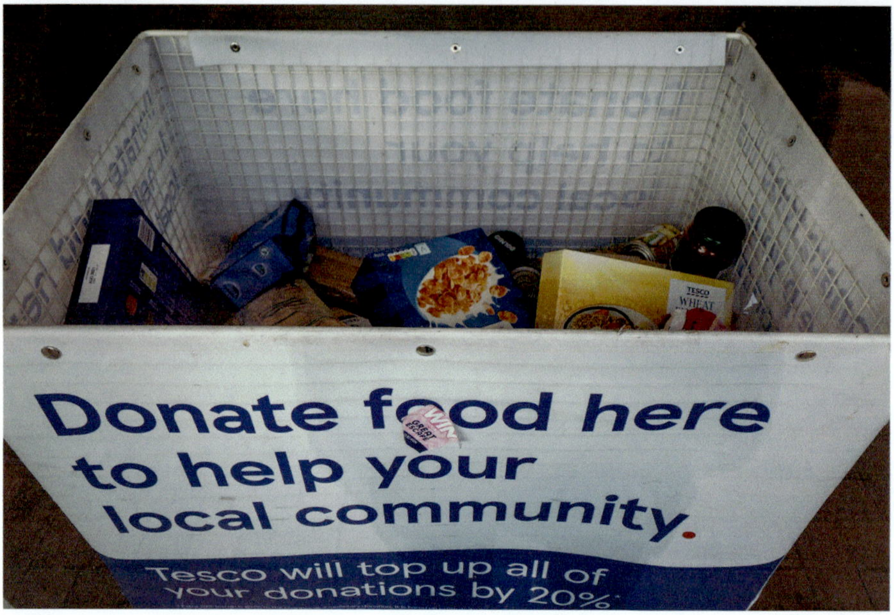
Donate food here
to help your
local community.
Tesco will top up all of
your donations by 20%
WIN
GREAT
ESCAPE
TESCO
WHEAT

**FIGURE 11.3** Donation box in a supermarket in the UK. (Reprinted with permission from Shutterstock available from https://www.shutterstock.com/image-photo/london-uk-1216-container-tesco-supermarket-1876971844.)

The TT vision is for a UK without the need for food banks, with their strategic approach to achieving this centred around campaigning for local and national policy change to eradicate destitution. Initiatives include the development of a national helpline with Citizens Advice to provide instant advice to those facing crisis and help maximise people's income and give instant food bank referrals, and the provision of financial grants for food banks to help them fund services that tackle the root causes of poverty in their community (Trussell-Trust, 2020). The strategy also acknowledges the need for public support and looks to increase their collaboration with people who have lived experience of poverty, harness celebrity, corporate, media and individual support to increase the awareness of the situations people face and reduce the stigma associated with food bank use and destitution. The provision of food is not a strategic priority, instead financial and local support, service provision and a protective welfare system are thought to be key to ensuring individuals are lifted from destitution and do not require emergency food aid.

## 11.4 GLOBAL RESPONSE TO FOOD INSECURITY

Food insecurity has been a key priority among the international humanitarian community since the 1970s, underpinned by the Universal Declaration on the Eradication of Hunger and Malnutrition, endorsed by the General Assembly resolution of the UN in 1974 (UN, 1974). It declared that "Every man, woman and child has the inalienable right to be free from hunger and malnutrition in order to develop fully and maintain

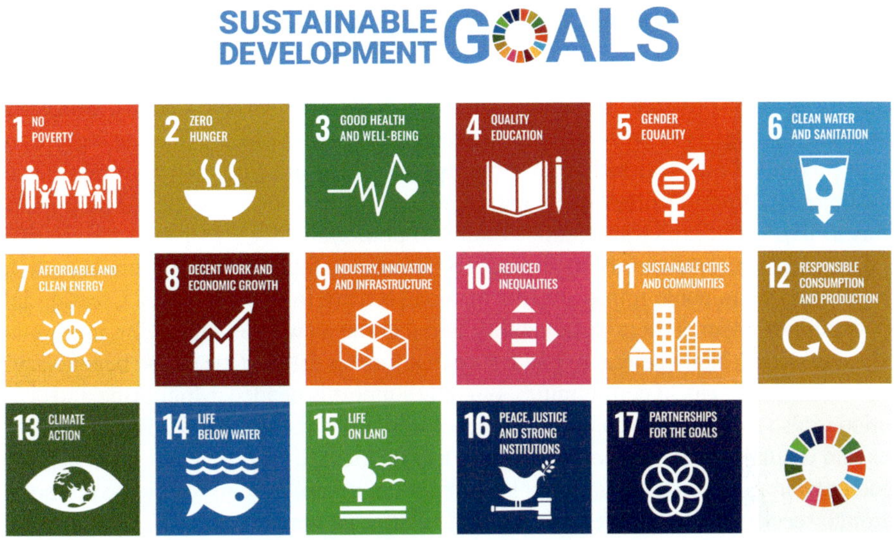
SUSTAINABLE DEVELOPMENT GOALS
1 NO POVERTY
2 ZERO HUNGER
3 GOOD HEALTH AND WELL-BEING
4 QUALITY EDUCATION
5 GENDER EQUALITY
6 CLEAN WATER AND SANITATION
7 AFFORDABLE AND CLEAN ENERGY
8 DECENT WORK AND ECONOMIC GROWTH
9 INDUSTRY, INNOVATION AND INFRASTRUCTURE
10 REDUCED INEQUALITIES
11 SUSTAINABLE CITIES AND COMMUNITIES
12 RESPONSIBLE CONSUMPTION AND PRODUCTION
13 CLIMATE ACTION
14 LIFE BELOW WATER
15 LIFE ON LAND
16 PEACE, JUSTICE AND STRONG INSTITUTIONS
17 PARTNERSHIPS FOR THE GOALS

**FIGURE 11.4** The United Nations Sustainable Development Goals, 2018. (Reprinted from the United Nations according to the guidelines, https://www.un.org/sustainabledevelopment/wp-content/uploads/2019/01/SDG_Guidelines_AUG_2019_Final.pdf. Available from https://sdgs.un.org/goals.)

their physical and mental faculties (UN, 1974)". In 2015, all the UN Member States adopted the 17 Sustainable Development Goals (SDGs) and made commitments to tackle these by 2030 as shown in Figure 11.4. However, the fact remains that an estimated 750 million people globally are faced with severe levels of food insecurity, leading to the high prevalence of malnutrition (FAO, 2020).

Refugees are among the most vulnerable populations to food insecurity whilst basic rights such as access to shelter, clean water and education are hindered. In 2019, 25.9 million people were recorded as refugees, defined as people who are forced to flee their homes, often due to war or famine, and cross a border (UNHCR, 2019).

Food insecurity increases the risk of malnutrition. Malnutrition attributed to inadequate food intakes leaves people more susceptible to preventable diseases, adding to financial burdens on the family and pushing them into a negative cycle of poverty. Moreover, women and children are more often vulnerable to food insecurity; and lack of appropriate nutritional intakes among pregnant and lactating mothers has a huge impact on child-birth outcomes and child development. Continuous support is needed to refugee populations in order to assure their human rights are met, including access to sufficient amounts of nutritious food, in order to improve nutritional status. Responses to food insecurity in the Global South have, in recent years, transitioned from provision of traditional food baskets to financial assistance with food, including food vouchers and cash distribution. This section provides information on issues faced by refugee populations and specifically focuses on Palestinian refugees based in Gaza.

## 11.5 FOOD INSECURITY IN REFUGEE SETTINGS

Food security in refugee settings is related to multiple issues, and therefore, food security is only possible if realised through multi-sectoral approaches. Since the number of refugees is steadily increasing and the situations are increasingly even more prolonged and entrenched, it remains critical for international communities to continuously support vulnerable populations including refugees to enable all populations to live with dignity and realise their full potential.

Long-term economic stability in refugee settings is a foundation to ensure household income and sustainable improvements in food security in the long term. Creating job opportunities ensures their sustainability and income as well as improving nutritional values to meals. Nonetheless, to make sure that food assistance meets the beneficiary's needs and benefits local communities, ongoing support is needed. Monitoring and evaluation is also important to enable all stakeholders to understand the needs of communities and ensure implementation is effective and efficient. In addition to food or cash for food provision, fortification and supplementation of micronutrients should be promoted through services such as maternal and child health cares in the cases where micronutrient deficiencies are public health concerns. This is particularly true for especially vulnerable groups such as pregnant mothers, adolescents and children under 5 years of age.

### 11.5.1 Gaza: A Case Study

Among the large number of food insecure populations, the Palestinian population has faced a high level of food insecurity in the occupied Palestinian territory. In 2018, it is reported that approximately one third of the Palestinian population, 1.6 million people, are affected by food insecurity according to the national estimate, whilst half of the population are registered as refugees (PCBS, 2018b). Food insecurity is more prevalent in the Gaza strip, where 68.5% of household experience food insecurity (PCBS, 2018b).

Food insecure households among Palestine refugees in Gaza receive food baskets including some basic food items provided by international agencies. Daily meals usually consist of cereals and tubers (rice, bread, potatoes, and other grains), oil and sugar in food insecure households (PCBS, 2012). Breakfast typically contains bread and plant-based protein foods (see Figure 11.5). These food items are included in food baskets and thus more likely to be consumed on a daily basis. Food insecure households consume meat and eggs, dairy products, vegetables and fruits less frequently compared to food secure households (PCBS, 2012). This can be explained by the fact that these are not always included in food baskets or limited in its quantity. The quantity and quality of food baskets follows the criteria such as nutritional values, and local food habits, as well as taking into consideration availability and logistics. Food basket providers have strived to improve the quality of food baskets by adding more nutritious foods such as lentils, chickpeas and canned sardines for good sources of proteins to replace energy needed due to reduced amounts of sugar (UNRWA, 2017). Food fortification is also ensured for items such as wheat flour.

These strategies are expected to improve nutritional values of food commodity and are very critical, given that both under and over-nutrition are prevailing in Gaza.

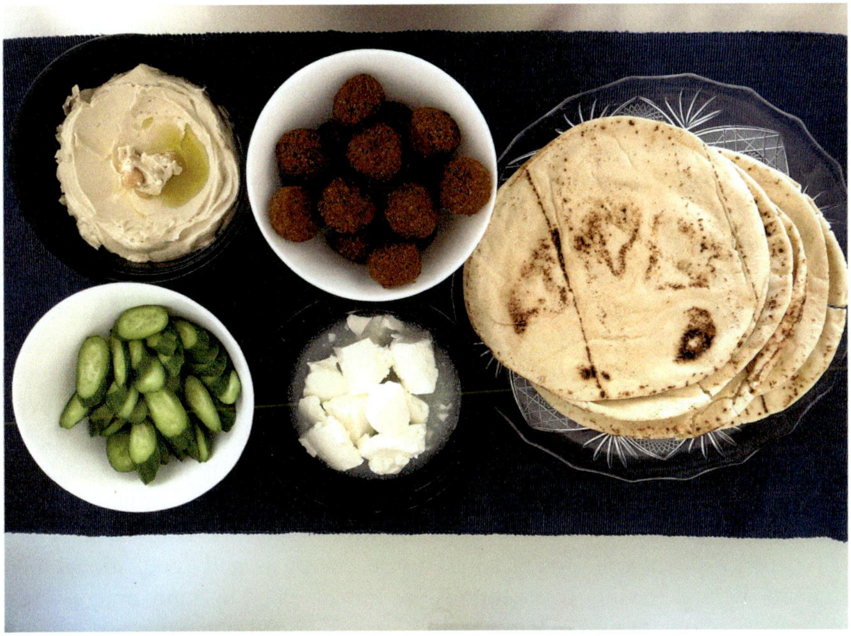

**FIGURE 11.5** A traditional breakfast in Gaza.

In 2019, it is reported that anaemia prevalence was 35.6% among pregnant women, 45.7% among lactating mothers and 54.7% among children under 3 years of the age in the refugee population in Gaza (UNRWA, 2019). At the same time, non-communicable diseases, namely type 2 diabetes and hypertension, are steadily increasing among refugees, especially those over 40 years old. Besides, more than 50% of those with diabetes or/and hypertension had risk factors including obesity, physical inactivity and raised cholesterol level.

A lack of a healthy diet can exacerbate poor health among refugees. Households report purchasing cheaper and lower quality types of food, skipping meals and/or reducing the quantity of meals to cope with food insecurity (PCBS, 2018b). There is no stable access to electricity, which makes fresh food deteriorate quickly. People need to visit a market regularly and purchase canned or processed food that does not need cooking. This is considered as a coping strategy to save energy whilst living in poverty. Despite 69% of households reporting that they received at least one type of assistance from any source including relatives and international organisations, it was still necessary to instigate strategies to cope with food insecurity and to make ends meet.

### 11.5.2 Successes and Challenges in Gaza and Other Contexts

Provision of food baskets remains crucial to ensuring basic energy intake for refugee households. Over the years, however, food aid has shifted globally from the traditional food basket to food assistance with "cash" in different forms, ranging from food vouchers to cash distribution and electronic funds. These strategies aim to empower beneficiaries with more flexibility to meet their needs. For example, food vouchers can be redeemed at contracted local retail shops where beneficiaries can purchase what they need. This is also beneficial to local communities, boosting the local economy and proving to be efficient and effective as an intervention (WFP, 2019). This shift in approach enables organisations to not only tackle food insecurity as emergency interventions but also tailor beneficiary's needs from a long-term perspective. Nevertheless, fragile economies and volatile food prices in local markets necessitate caution in transitioning from the traditional form of food baskets to other modalities.

Social and health equity is also an important factor for food security. In Gaza, female-headed households were predominantly unemployed and reported as one of the most vulnerable groups (PCBS, 2012). This group is thus targeted for timely assistance which has had the impact of lifting food security level of this vulnerable group close to other types of households (PCBS, 2012). More intensive assistance such as providing animals or poultry together with training is also provided, which aims to provide skills to ensure food and create income, helping reduce food insecurity in the medium term.

The school feeding programme is another key intervention aiming to improve the diet quality of children and adolescents. Providing nutritious foods such as biscuits fortified with vitamins and minerals boosts energy as well as nutritional intakes of students. School feeding interventions are implemented in many emergency and stable settings globally and report not only health-related outcomes but a range of impacts such as improved enrolments and attendances (WFP, 2019). Evaluation shows that the WFP school feeding programme significantly reduced school drop out by 3.5% and increased school attendance by 5% on average in 2019, which is also critical to prevent child labour and early marriage.

Nevertheless, despite much effort and funding invested in improving food security in refugee communities, there is still a large gap between need and assistance. This holds true in Gaza, where, even after receiving assistance, some households still face poverty and food insecurity (PCBS, 2018a). Some vulnerable groups may be excluded from assistance, falling further into food insecurity. Secondly, other factors are worsening the nutritional status of many vulnerable people such as limited access to clean water and health care, which undermine health status. Moreover, larger households face more food insecurity. In Gaza, large households are more likely to fall into poverty and spend less money on food per capita (PCBS, 2018a). Employment directly impacts on food security whilst status of labour such as regular or irregular employees is a significant factor.

In summary, the issues in refugee settings are immensely complex where poverty, population/household size and economic stability among many other factors need to be considered. More importantly, food assistance predominantly relies on international funds, affecting the availability of food assistance and leaving refugees susceptible to food insecurity.

## 11.6 CONCLUSION

Food insecurity has increased sharply in the UK since the 2007–2008 financial crisis and in the Global South since 2014, reversing a downwards trend in global hunger throughout the latter half of the 20th century. Non-governmental food systems may address immediate symptoms of food insecurity – hunger – through the direct provision of food and, in the Global South, cash grants. Household food insecurity is, nevertheless, ultimately dependent on economic stability, including adequate incomes from employment and social security systems. In the absence of adequate employment and social security to guarantee food security, it is important to ensure that food assistance meets the needs of beneficiaries and reduces rather than exacerbates health inequalities.

## REFERENCES

Adams, E. J., Grummer-Strawn, L. & Chavez, G. 2003. Food insecurity is associated with increased risk of obesity in California women. *The Journal of Nutrition,* 133, 1070–1074.

Bourquin, P., Cribb, J., Waters, T. & Xu, X. 2019. Living standards, poverty and inequality in the UK: 2019. London: Institute for Fiscal Studies.

Bramley, G., Treanor, M., Sosenko, F., Littlewood, M. 2021 State of hunger: Building the evidence on poverty, destitution and food insecurity in the UK. Trussell Trust.

Davis, O. & Geiger, B. B. 2017. Did Food Insecurity rise across Europe after the 2008 Crisis? An analysis across welfare regimes. *Social Policy and Society,* 16, 343–360.

Department for Work and Pensions. 2021. Family Resources Survey: financial year 2019 to 2020, U. Government, Editor.

Eicher-Miller, H. A. & Zhao, Y. 2018. Evidence for the age-specific relationship of food insecurity and key dietary outcomes among US children and adolescents. *Nutrition Research Reviews,* 31, 98–113.

FAO. 2020. Hunger and food insecurity [Online]. Food and Agriculture Organisation of the United States Available: http://www.fao.org/hunger/en/ [Accessed 7 January 2021].

FAO, IFAD, UNICEF, WFP & WHO 2017. The State of Food Insecurity and Nutrition in the World 2017. Building resilience for peace and food security. Rome: FAO.

FAO, IFAD, UNICEF, WFP & WHO 2020. The State of Food Security and Nutrition in the World 2020. Transforming food systems for affordable healthy diets. Rome: FAO.

Food Standards Agency 2021. The COVID-19 consumer research (https://www.food.gov.uk/research/research-projects/the-covid-19-consumer-research).

Furey, S. & Caraher, M. 2018. The differential cost of an emergency food parcel and a consensually acceptable basket of healthy food. *4th World Congress on Health Economics, Health Policy and Health care Management*, Zurich, Switzerland: Ulster University.

Garratt, E. 2017. Please sir, I want some more: an exploration of repeat foodbank use. *BMC Public Health,* 17, 828.

Gundersen, C., Kreider, B. & Pepper, J. 2011. The economics of food insecurity in the United States. *Applied Economic Perspectives and Policy,* 33, 281–303.

Hughes, D. & Prayogo, E. 2018. A nutritional analysis of the Trussell Trust emergency food parcel. Trussell Trust. https://www.trusselltrust.org/wp-content/uploads/sites/2/2018/06/Food_Parcel_Report_April_2018.pdf

IFAN. 2021. Mapping the UK's independent food banks [Online]. Independent Food Aid Network. Available: https://www.foodaidnetwork.org.uk/independent-food-banks-map [Accessed 6 July 2021].

JRF 2020. UK poverty 2019/2020. York: Joseph Rowntree Foundation.

Jyoti, D. F., Frongillo, E. A. & Jones, S. J. 2005. Food insecurity affects school children's academic performance, weight gain, and social skills. *The Journal of Nutrition,* 135, 2831–2839.

Knowles, M., Rabinowich, J., Ettinger De Cuba, S., Cutts, D. B. & Chilton, M. 2016. "Do you wanna breathe or eat?" Parent perspectives on child health consequences of food insecurity, trade-offs, and toxic stress. *Maternal and Child Health Journal,* 20, 25–32.

Lambie-Mumford, H. 2017. *Hungry Britain: The Rise of Food Charity.* Bristol: Bristol Policy Press.

Lambie-Mumford, H. & Green, M. A. 2017. Austerity, welfare reform and the rising use of food banks by children in England and Wales. *Area,* 49, 273–279.

Lambie-Mumford, H., Crossley, D., Jensen, E., Verbeke, M. & Dowler, E. 2014. Household food security in the UK: A review of food aid. Department for Environment, Food & Rural Affairs.

Loopstra, R. & Lalor, D. 2017. Financial insecurity, food insecurity, and disability: The profile of people receiving emergency food assistance from the Trussell Trust Foodbank Network in Britain. Trussell-Trust.

Loopstra, R. & Tarasuk, V. 2015. Food bank usage is a poor indicator of food insecurity: Insights from Canada. *Social Policy and Society,* 14, 443–455.

Loopstra, R. 2020. Vulnerability to food insecurity since the COVID-19 lockdown preliminary report. London.

Loopstra, R., Goodwin, S., Goldberg, B., Lambie-Mumford, H., May, J. & Williams, A. 2019. A survey of food banks operating independently of The Trussell Trust food bank network. London: Independent Food Aid Network.

Macleod, M. A., Curl, A. & Kearns, A. 2019. Understanding the prevalence and drivers of food bank use: Evidence from deprived communities in Glasgow. *Social Policy and Society,* 18, 67–86.

OBR. 2020. Coronavirus analysis [Online]. London: Office for Budget Responsibility. Available: https://obr.uk/coronavirus-analysis/ [Accessed 7 January 2021].

PCBS. 2012. Socio: Economic and food security survey. Ramallah – Palestine: Palestinian Central Bureau of Statistics. https://documents.wfp.org/stellent/groups/public/documents/ena/wfp259657.pdf

PCBS 2018a. Living standards in the Palestinian territory. Expenditure, consumption, poverty, 2017. Ramallah – Palestine: Palestinian Central Bureau of Statistics. https://www.pcbs.gov.ps/post.aspx?lang=en&ItemID=3115

PCBS 2018b. Socio-economic food security survey 2018 preliminary results. Ramallah – Palestine: Palestinian Central Bureau of Statistics. https://fscluster.org/sites/default/files/documents/sefsec_2018_-_food_security_analysis_preliminary_results.pdf

Power, M., Doherty, B. O. B., Small, N., Teasdale, S. & Pickett, K. E. 2017a. All in it together? Community food aid in a multi-ethnic context. *Journal of Social Policy,* 46, 447–471.

Power, M., Uphoff, E., Kelly, B. & Pickett, K. E. 2017b. Food insecurity and mental health: an analysis of routine primary care data of pregnant women in the Born in Bradford cohort. *Journal of Epidemiology and Community Health,* 71, 324–328.

Power, M., Small, N., Doherty, B. & Pickett Kate, E. 2018a. Hidden hunger? Experiences of food insecurity amongst Pakistani and white British women. *British Food Journal,* 120, 2716–2732.

Power, M. S., Small, N., Doherty, B., Stewart-Knox, B. & Pickett, K. E. 2018b. Is food insecurity associated with maternal health among UK ethnic groups? An exploration of women in the BiB cohort. *European Journal of Public Health,* 28, 661–663.

Power, M., Doherty, B., Pybus, K. & Pickett, K. 2020. How COVID-19 has exposed inequalities in the UK food system: The case of UK food and poverty [version 2; peer review: 5 approved]. *Emerald Open Research,* 2, 11.

Pybus, K., Power, M. & Pickett, K. E. 2020. We are constantly overdrawn, despite not spending money on anything other than bills and food': a mixed-methods, participatory study of food and food insecurity in the context of income inequality. *Journal of Poverty and Social Justice*, 29, 21–45.

Reeves, A. & Loopstra, R. 2021. The continuing effects of welfare reform on food bank use in the UK: The roll-out of universal credit. *Journal of Social Policy*, 50, 788–808.

Sosenko, F., Littlewood, M., Bramley, G., Fitzpatrick, S., Blenkinsopp, J. & Wood, J. 2019. State of hunger: A study of poverty and food insecurity in the UK. Trussell Trust.

Tarasuk, V., Cheng, J., Gundersen, C., De Oliveira, C. & Kurdyak, P. 2018. The relation between food insecurity and mental health care service utilization in Ontario. *Canadian Journal of Psychiatry,* 63, 557–569.

Trussell-Trust. 2017. Volunteers across the UK giving 'at least £30 million' a year in unpaid work to support foodbanks [Online]. Trussell Trust. Available: https://www.trusselltrust.org/2017/10/17/foodbank-volunteers-30-million-unpaid-work/ [Accessed 25.01 2021].

Trussell-Trust. 2018a. Food allocation form [Online]. Trussell Trust. Available: https://www.trusselltrust.org/wp-content/uploads/sites/2/2018/06/singlepersonpackinglist.png [Accessed 25.01.2021].

Trussell-Trust. 2018b. What's in a Trussell Trust foodbank parcel and why? [Online]. Trussell Trust. Available: https://www.trusselltrust.org/2018/06/08/whats-trussell-trust-food-bank-parcel/ [Accessed 25.01.2021].

Trussell-Trust 2020. Annual report and accounts. Trussell Trust. https://www.trusselltrust.org/annual-reports/

Trussell-Trust. 2021. End of year stats [Online]. Trussell Trust. Available: https://www.trusselltrust.org/news-and-blog/latest-stats/end-year-stats/ [Accessed 7 July 2021].

UN 1974. Resolution 3348 (Xxix): Universal declaration on the eradication of hunger and malnutrition. 28th: 1973–1974 ed.: United Nations.

UNHCR 2019. Figures at a Glance. Geneva: United Nations High Commissioner for Refugees.

UNRWA 2017. Annual operational report 2017. Amman: United Nations Relief and Works Agency for Palestine Refugees in the Near East.

UNRWA 2019. Annual report health department 2019. Amman: United Nations Relief and Works Agency for Palestine Refugees in the Near East.

WFP 2019. 2019 annual performance report for 2019. Rome: United Nations World Food Programme (WFP).

Wight, V., Kaushal, N., Waldfogel, J. & Garfinkel, I. 2014. Understanding the link between poverty and food insecurity among children: Does the definition of poverty matter? *Journal of Children & Poverty,* 20, 1–20.

Yang, T. C., Sahota, P., Pickett, K. E. & Bryant, M. 2018. Association of food security status with overweight and dietary intake: exploration of White British and Pakistani-origin families in the Born in Bradford cohort. *Nutrition Journal,* 17, 48.

# 12 Nutrition Communication in Public Health and the Media

*Cassandra H. Ellis*
Nutrition Society

*Charlotte E.L. Evans*
University of Leeds

**CONTENTS**



## 12.1 INTRODUCTION

The wider food environment does not just include the food available in different physical spaces but also includes nutrition information which could originate from a number of different sources. Nutrition information plays a role in guiding people to make food choices but perhaps is often given less emphasis compared to food marketing by food companies. This chapter provides a discussion of the quality and impact of nutritional information in the public domain including information from public health bodies in newspapers and social media.

DOI: 10.1201/9781003043720-12

In the UK, the majority of people obtain nutritional information from the media which includes printed newspapers, television, online news and, in the last decade, social media. A 2017 report from a UK supermarket found that almost a quarter of young people refer to social media for dietary advice, and based on this advice, 50% think that cutting out a food group (e.g. gluten or dairy) can create a healthy lifestyle. As these are key sources of information, the quality of all nutrition-related reporting plays a fundamental role in population health. However, research highlights poor-quality reporting, and in the case of social media, it is largely unregulated. Misinformation and disinformation, or what is more colloquially termed 'fake news', also challenges adherence to nutrition guidelines as it creates erroneous beliefs and polarises opinion. It also erodes the public's trust in science and creates a perception that nutrition scientists 'cannot make up their minds'. Social media campaigns such as Change4Life in the UK reach a large number of people and are also discussed.

## 12.2 HEALTH AND NUTRITION COMMUNICATION

Public health messaging plays an important role in behaviour change in many countries around the globe including the UK. The application of evidence into practice and influencing public health policy through public health messaging is a key aspect of Public Health England (2018), including through the social media campaign, Change4Life.

### 12.2.1 History of Health and Nutrition Communication in the UK

Health communication has been integral in the UK for over a century, starting with communication framed around the importance of personal hygiene and moderate eating and drinking to support the war effort (Figure 12.1).

Advertising agencies were used to create campaigns with engaging slogans and images; examples of which can be found at the Imperial War Museum (https://www.iwm.org.uk/learning/resources/second-world-war-posters). Early campaigns focused on consuming less wheat and meat, reducing food waste and consuming less alcohol, although the latter had less to do with health risk or war-time rationing, and was instead used as propaganda to encourage workplace productivity. The Second World War saw nutrition campaigns focus on nutrients with potatoes promoted for energy, carrots for vision (vitamin A) and leafy vegetables as nutrient powerhouses in order to feed the nation and support the war effort. By the 1960s, there was a marked shift towards the challenges of affluence, and health communication began to consider obesity for the first time in 1975. However, the emphasis was on physical appearance, with the relationship between weight gain and disease risk being a secondary message. More recently, public health campaigns in the UK have focused on reducing the risk of non-communicable diseases.

### 12.2.2 Social Marketing Campaigns

Different types of public health communication exist which can be broadly categorised as informed decision-making interventions (such as food labelling

| Year | Health Communication |
|---|---|
| 1914 | First World War begins |
| 1917 | Department for Information established. *Focused on reductions of food and alcohol, and improved sexual health and personal hygiene to aid the war effort.* |
| 1918 | Food rationing *(sugar, meat, flour, butter, margarine and milk).* |
| 1918 | First World War ends |
| 1939 | Second World War begins |
| 1940 | Ministry of Food established to provide a nutritionally adequate diet to war time Britain. *Promotion through leaflets and radio announcements, they educated the public on reducing food waste, encouraged healthy eating and growing own food.* |
| 1942 | Rationing reinstated to most foods, except fruit and vegetables. |
| 1945 | Second World War ends |
| 1948 | UK National Health Service established. |
| 1954 | Food rationing ends |
| 1960 | Communications focus on vaccinations against communicable diseases. |
| 1964 | Cohen Report published *recommending that public health communications use advertising and journalistic methods* |
| 1965 | Advertising smoking on television announced illegal. |
| 1968 | Health Education Council established. |
| 1970 | Anti-smoking campaigns now linked with disease risk and celebrities used to for health communication |
| 1975 | 'Is your body coming between you and the opposite sex?' *Obesity messaging focused towards weight and physical appearance, disease risk was secondary.* |
| 1990 | HIV and Aids promotion coupled with promotion of safer sexual practices. |
| 1992 | Raising awareness of sugars intake and oral health. |
| 1994 | 'Balance of Good Health', UK dietary guidelines (early Eatwell Guide). |
| 2003 | '5 a day' message introduced *in response to WHO recommendations that 400g of fruit and vegetables per day has a protective effect.* |
| 2007 | Smoking in public places banned. |
| 2009 | Change4Life launched - *a UK social marketing plan to address obesity.* |
| 2013 | Public Health England (PHE) established. |
| 2012 | Start4Life launched *in acknowledgment of the lifespan approach.* |
| 2016 | UK Eatwell Guide - *update to the 2007 Eatwell Plate to include making sustainable choices for planetary health.* |
| 2016 | 'One You' *launched by PHE to target middle age and older adults.* |

**FIGURE 12.1** Timeline of health communication in the UK.

covered in Chapter 13), persuasion-oriented interventions and advocacy interventions. Persuasion-oriented interventions are used to encourage a specific behaviour such as encouraging the wearing of helmets for cycling or improving dietary behaviour. Advocacy encompasses larger and more comprehensive social marketing campaigns such as reducing smoking. Andreas in the 1990s defined social marketing campaigns as the "application of commercial marketing technologies to the analysis, planning, execution and evaluation of programs designed to influence the voluntary behaviour of target audiences in order to improve their personal welfare" (Piggin and Lee, 2011). There are benefits in using this approach as complex messages can be conveyed and behaviour change techniques applied to large populations whilst also adapting the materials for different groups of consumers (Piggin and Lee, 2011). Communication concerned primarily with providing clear messages around managing risk, and crisis management is also an important tool in public health, which we have experienced first-hand during the COVID-19 epidemic, leading to dramatic changes in our behaviour such as social distancing and wearing masks. This type of communication also includes food poisoning outbreaks.

A review of health communication commissioned by the European Centre for Disease prevention and control (ECDC) (https://www.ecdc.europa.eu/en/health-communication) highlighted the need for good quality research into health communication and evaluation in order to assist in the development and evaluation of effective campaigns (Piggin and Lee, 2011). The necessary steps in designing and assessing a campaign include identifying specific target audiences and their needs; evaluating the message; pilot testing the messages; guiding message development; identifying appropriate communication channels that are more likely to reach and influence the target audience; monitoring progress of the campaign and evaluating the effectiveness of the campaign on target audiences and public health.

In 2017, the World Health Organization (WHO) published the Strategic Communications Framework for effective communications (World Health Organization (WHO), 2017). The WHO principles for effective communications are based on a framework consisting of six principles: accessible, actionable, credible and trusted, relevant, timely and understandable.

### 12.2.3 Case Study: UK Change4Life Social Marketing Campaign

The Change4life campaign in the UK was implemented in 2009 and informed by a published document Healthy Weight, Healthy Lives: a cross government strategy for England published by the Department of Health (DoH) in 2008 as well as a consumer insight report (Department of Health, 2008). The aim of the campaign is to "drive, coax, encourage and support people... [to] eat well, move more and live longer". One of the central goals of the campaign is to reduce childhood obesity. Between 2009 and 2011, £75 million of funding was provided by DoH (Piggin and Lee, 2011) and £14m per year between 2011 and 2014 (Department of Health (DoH), 2011). The design of the Change4Life campaign was guided by the theoretical framework developed by WHO, UNICEF and FAO, the Communication for Behavioural Impact (COMBI) framework (World Health Organization (WHO), 2012). The six main steps involve defining the behaviour objectives, market analysis, refining objectives, preparing plans and budget and monitoring and evaluation. Although this framework was originally produced to be used for communication during outbreaks of communicable diseases, it is suitable for a wide range of public health communications including reducing risks of non-communicable diseases such as obesity. Guidelines for the Change4Life campaign include the use of simple messaging, branding with identifiable colours and fonts and an accessible and fun tone. Controversially, the decision was made early on that the word obesity would not appear in any of the Change4Life campaign's marketing materials as it is a sensitive issue for parents; this is discussed by Piggin and Lee (2011).

Evaluating social marketing campaigns is a challenge and evaluation of Change4Life has mostly focused on awareness of the campaign and perceived behaviour change rather than actual behaviour change and short-term outcomes rather than long term. Nevertheless, improvements in children's snacks in terms of fats and sugars due to the Change4life campaign have been reported (Wrieden and Levy, 2016).

## 12.3 NUTRITION IN THE MEDIA

In the 21st century, there is a plethora of nutrition information available to consumers from sources other than public health communications. Through print media, television, internet and social media, consumers are continually exposed to nutritional information. Some of the information disseminated through these media channels has come from scientific studies that have been published in reputable scientific journals and reported by journalists, but much of the information available has no scientific basis, or the science has been misinterpreted by journalists, or in the case of social media, misinterpreted by the public.

### 12.3.1 Newspapers

Printed newspapers have been a key source of information in the UK since the 17th century when the printing press was invented making it easier and cheaper to print material in large quantities for distribution. Originally printed to share news, an increase in education and literacy led to new publications being created in the early 20th century which shared more popular stories such as sports and features. The increase in publications has led to more feature-style content which tends to focus on issues of human interest, lifestyle, health (including nutrition) and personal improvement which typically have an entertaining storytelling narrative rather than a scientific basis. Where nutrition is covered as news, journalists often tend to be concerned with what is novel, what affects the public and public health challenges and there is an over-emphasis on pieces of information that contradict a large amount of existing evidence and provide a sensational headline (Goldacre, 2008). This drive for a sensational story to entertain readers could be why research has found that nutrition reporting in print news is not always evidence based, is poor quality, biased and does not always reflect current nutritional guidelines (Kininmonth et al., 2017). However, a survey of readers reported that the general public want to be provided with good quality news once there is consensus among nutrition professionals (Goldberg and Hellwig, 1997).

A small number of studies have reported on the quality of newspaper articles related to health in general or nutrition specifically. A study of 141 nutrition-related articles in five popular UK print newspapers over a period of 6 weeks which used a validated quality assessment tool (Robinson et al., 2013) found that the news articles were typically satisfactory quality (Kininmonth et al., 2017). The mean quality score varied by newspaper; however, these differences could be explained by different factors related to newspaper articles. Articles that were larger in size and were written by a named journalist, often a health correspondent, tended to be better quality, while articles about obesity tended to be lower in quality (compared with articles on cardiovascular disease, type 2 diabetes or cancers). Common reasons for poor-quality articles were a lack of information on study design, statistics and/or limitations and little background or context provided. Fewer but higher-quality articles in the news may be preferable to larger numbers of poor quality articles.

As internet penetration has increased, consumers have switched to digital content. Consequently, print newspaper circulation has declined over the last decade, with a reported 53% decrease in circulation since 2012 (OFCOM, 2019). This has resulted in more people reading nutrition articles on online newspaper websites which can be shared although this generally happens less often than on other social media sites.

### 12.3.2 Blogs

In addition to news media, there has been a proliferation of professional bloggers over the last two decades, many of whom have thousands of followers, but no formal nutritional science training. It is reported that blogs do not encourage healthy diets and only 6% of American food bloggers have nutrition degrees, despite offering nutrition advice (Garza et al., 2019). A recent study found that blogs shared through the microblogging platform Twitter were of poorer quality, were less likely to cite journals and authors and were less likely to include references compared to online news reports and press releases. Conversely, blogs were more likely to be shared and to inspire comment compared to other articles analysed (Ellis et al., 2020). However, there is little research available in this area related to nutrition.

### 12.3.3 Online Social Media

Social media presents opportunities and challenges for sharing news, information and opinion. The development of a range of social media platforms including Facebook, Twitter and Instagram has changed the way millions of individuals interact with information, making the internet more interactive and creating a shift from the user being a passive consumer, to the user being an active participant (Obar, 2015). This creates a virtual space that supports information sharing which research suggests can also influence health behaviours (Grilli et al., 2002).

Facebook remains the most popular social network (Figure 12.2) and usage of social media continues to grow globally with 4.4 billion people with one or more social media accounts in 2019 (DataReportal, 2019). Weibo and We Chat are the most popular channels in the People's Republic of China as there are restrictions on using Facebook and Twitter. All the social media channels share similar characteristics allowing users to share text, pictures, images and videos with their networks, and to tag other users and create conversations.

Whilst social media can potentially reduce knowledge translation gaps and create communities of best practice, it is unclear whether this is applicable to nutrition information. There is evidence to suggest social media can empower people to

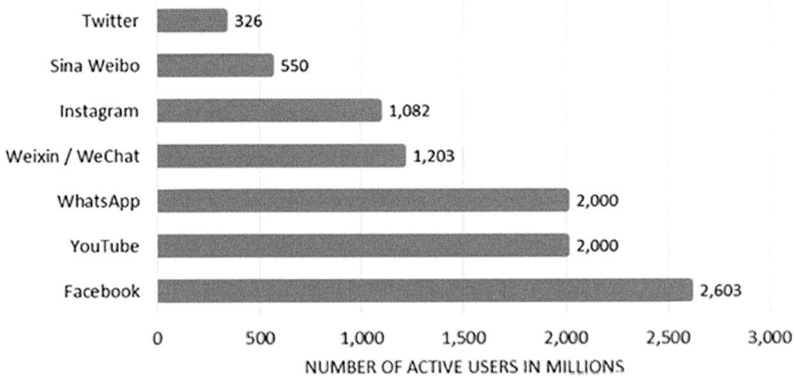


**FIGURE 12.2** Most popular social networks worldwide as of July 2020, ranked by number of active users (in millions) using data from Data Reportal. (Available from https://datareportal.com.)

develop healthier lifestyles; however, other studies have found that it is not viewed as a useful source of health information within some groups (Khobzi et al., 2019). It is likely that the source of health information is important as this affects how users evaluate the information and how likely they are to propagate the information through their own networks (DeAndrea and Vendemia, 2016). However, it is often difficult to know whether the source has reported the science correctly or whether the information shared is evidence based. Likes and shares could be seen as affirmation through reinforcement increasing the perception that it is evidence based. This information can be in contrast to public health messages and dietary guidelines further supporting the perception of confused messaging from scientists. This is particularly prevalent in the current era of 'fake news'.

## 12.4 FALSE INFORMATION AND 'FAKE NEWS'

A lack of trust in the information provided by scientists and medical experts can lead to the sharing of false information. In nutritional science, the erosion of trust is most evident when new, unexpected results undermine previously understood links between food and/or nutrients and disease risk. Reporting new evidence in the media (remembering that journalist are looking for novel information) may appear to suggest that a given nutrient is harmful one moment, then healthy, then harmful again (Mozaffarian and Forouhi, 2018). This has been seen recently as evidence has changed in relation to dietary cholesterol found in eggs and can erode the public's confidence in nutritional science and dietary guidelines.

Worryingly, a 2017 survey by the Academy of Medical Sciences (AMS) reported that only 37% of the public trust the evidence from medical research. Question marks over funding, conflict of interest and author accountability can damage the public's trust in science and lead the public to believe that conclusions in science are ever-changing. In addition, the time period between the scientific development and policy changes can create the appearance of controversy which is exacerbated by media reporting creating public confusion (Garza et al., 2019). This may have an impact on the effectiveness of health communication across all media but particularly in social media.

Misinformation, disinformation or 'fake news', whilst not exclusive to nutritional science, poses a threat to the public understanding of nutritional information and adherence to dietary guidelines. Interest in misinformation by far predates the digital age and can be traced back to research into how and why rumours spread published in 1947 (Allport and Postman, 1947). In today's connected world, information is consumed at a rate previously unknown; however, this information is not always true. Both truths and untruths can be shared through social media networks with minimum quality control. The colloquial term for untruths is 'fake news', but the definition is broader than this with research identifying three distinct categories of information behaviour: information, disinformation and misinformation (Fallis, 2015). These are looked at in turn.

### 12.4.1 Misinformation

An early definition of misinformation was information that might not be true but remains informative (Fox, 1983). Later, different types of misinformation were defined, including concealment, ambivalence, distortion and falsification, although this did not differentiate between misinformation and disinformation (Zhou and Zhang, 2007). Karlova and Lee added to the debate saying misinformation may also be inaccurate, uncertain, vague or ambiguous, suggesting that information which is incomplete may also be a form of deception, which would instead qualify as disinformation (Karlova and Lee, 2011). Misinformation tends to be 'accidental', but the informativeness of it may depend on the relationship between the speaker and the receiver, for example, if the receiver knows the information is incorrect (Karlova and Fisher, 2013).

The recent SARS-CoV-2 pandemic provides a very real example of scientific misinformation that led to the WHO expressing their concerns. From injecting disinfectant to drinking cow urine, the public were exposed to a wide range of false and potentially harmful information to 'cure' COVID-19 symptoms. One study investigating COVID-19 rumours reported 82% of claims were false and estimated that 800 people died and a further 5,876 were hospitalised as a result of drinking highly concentrated alcohol after believing rumours on social media that it would kill the virus (Islam et al., 2020).

### 12.4.2 Disinformation

Disinformation is 'deliberately false information' and does not necessarily need to be inaccurate, but it must be misleading and deliberately deceptive. The intentions behind creating and sharing such information are difficult to define; however, cited reasons include social motivation, benevolent reasons or personally motivated, antagonistic reasons (Karlova and Fisher, 2013).

Fallis (2015) identifies three important identifiers of disinformation: it is information, it is misleading and it is intentionally misleading. Instances of disinformation include deceptive advertising, government propaganda, falsified photographs, internet frauds and fake websites and blogs. It has been argued that disinformation could be more informative than misinformation because the implication is deliberate; however, if people believe disinformation, it can do significant harm, threatening information integrity.

### 12.4.3 Fake News

Fake news is a colloquial term and is often used interchangeably with misinformation and disinformation making comparisons across research challenging. Fake news sits within the larger context of misinformation and disinformation; and researchers have defined it as a form of falsehood intended to primarily deceive people by mimicking the look and feel of real news. Informativeness depends on the situation as different situations instil different meanings, and these meanings are interpreted depending on the knowledge of the receiver (Buckland, 1991). This could underpin why fake news is challenging to define and identify.

### 12.4.4 Sharing False Information

Karlova and Fisher's 2013 model (Figure 12.3) shows how misinformation and disinformation can evolve through social networks and diffusion. Through personal

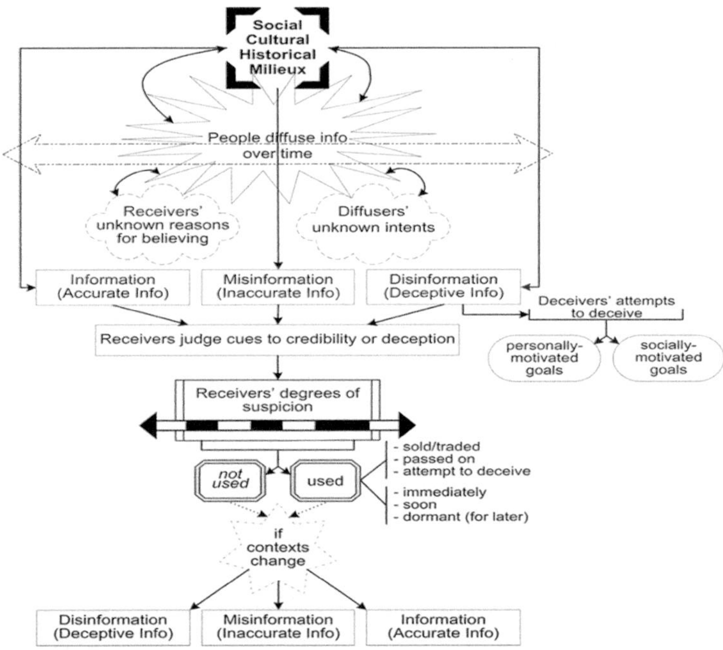


**FIGURE 12.3** Social diffusion model of information, misinformation and disinformation. Reproduced under licence CC BY-NC-ND 3.0 (Karlova and Fisher, 2013).

experience and context, receivers make judgements about the truth of the information and make a decision on the information and whether to propagate. Considering the motivations for sharing misinformation, Karlova and Fisher state that many individuals may enjoy sharing information and news, even though they may not believe such information themselves as they take pleasure in disseminating it through their social networks. In this way, misinformation and disinformation diffuse across social groups. Social media supports making dissemination easier, wider and faster.

Other explanations suggest confirmation bias, whereby individuals find information which supports their beliefs to be more persuasive. Algorithms and personalised browsing support this theory as users are more likely to be exposed to content which aligns with pre-existing attitudes and browsing behaviours. Individuals may also share news because they do not recognise it is false as they fail to think analytically about the information they are reading.

Alternatively, false news articles could be shared because they tend to be more novel and therefore spread faster than real news (Vosoughi et al., 2018). Sentiment analysis suggests that false news articles inspire fear, disgust and surprise which could make individuals more likely to share (Vosoughi et al., 2018). Some of these motivations are supported by earlier findings by Chen et al. who investigated the top reasons that students share misinformation (Table 12.1). Personality research suggests that extroverts are more likely to knowingly share misinformation as a way of socialising and seeking opinions which is independent of gender.

Information literacy, the ability to identify, locate, evaluate and effectively use information have been cited as key to identifying misinformation and disinformation (Karlova and Fisher, 2013). Knowledge of the source of information provides context and can inform the interpretation and validity judgements. Types of source information include who the author is, when the document was published, and the quality controls in place. This information can be used to evaluate the quality of the information, its trustworthiness and its interpretation. Intervention studies have found that knowledge on the dangers of sharing misinformation can reduce the number of likes and shares; however, other studies have reported that it does not deter participants

**TABLE 12.1**
**Top Five Reasons for Sharing Misinformation on Social Media by Gender**

| Rank | Men | Women |
|---|---|---|
| 1 | The information can be a good topic for conversation | The information can be a good topic for conversation |
| 2 | The information is interesting | The information is interesting |
| 3 | Sharing helps me get other people's opinions regarding the information/event | The information is new and eye-catching |
| 4 | The information is new and eye-catching | Sharing helps me interact with other people |
| 5 | The information is current | I can express my opinion by sharing that information |

*Source*: Reprinted with permission from Elsevier (Chen et al., 2015).

from sharing, suggesting that knowledge does not necessarily translate to behaviour and that stronger interventions are needed.

### 12.4.5 Media as a Propagandist

Industries as well as public health policy makers are involved in communicating messages which can be picked up by the media. The food industry has been accused of using similar tactics to the tobacco industry to influence policy through heavy promotion and public relations investment, and by distorting the science (see Chapter 7). The objective of the tobacco strategy was to fund new research to refute the detrimental effects of tobacco on health focusing on other carcinogens, such as asbestos causing controversy and scientific uncertainty. In having access to the science and in reporting the controversy to the public, the media play a key role as a propagandist altering public belief and impacting policy makers (Weatherall et al., 2018). By emphasising the importance of individuals making healthy choices rather than industries' role in creating unhealthy environments, the responsibility shifts to the consumer. This strategy can also be mapped to nutrition communication on social media (which in turn means the public), as the propagandist, with influence over the public and policy makers (Frederick et al., 2016). The media can shape public opinion through media framing, which exerts pressures on policy makers mobilising policy change (Roland 2018).

In the case of nutrition, the media may selectively share a biased sample of the evidence with the public and policy makers, dividing opinion from scientific consensus. Sensational headlines and novel or contradictory evidence capitalise on scientific uncertainty and do not favour scientific clarity. Missing details such as references, quotes from the author, the strength of the evidence and its application to humans are often omitted further reducing clarity. Evidence of media framing to affect policy was seen in the USA in response to banning sugar-sweetened beverage (SSB) cup sizes over 16 oz, with suggestions that the news media delayed policy development and implementation (Donaldson et al., 2015).

## 12.5 CONCLUSIONS AND RECOMMENDATIONS

In order to improve the quality of available nutritional information, high-quality social marketing campaigns are needed based on established theoretical frameworks as well as robust standards for reporting nutritional studies in the news media, whether in print or online. In a bid to improve science reporting within Science, Technology, Engineering and Mathematics (STEM) in the UK, the Science Media Centre, on behalf of the Academy of Medical Sciences, has created a labelling system to be used by press officers and journalists to assess how robust a study is and its application to the population (Science Media Centre, 2018). Learned societies such as The UK Nutrition Society (www.nutritionsociety.org) have a role in publishing and disseminating high-quality nutritional science and in working closely with organisations like the Science Media Centre to ensure that experts are contacted for media quotes and advice. In addition, more research is needed on the quality of information shared on social media and the steps that need to be taken to ensure that it is easy to determine the source and quality of online nutritional information.

## REFERENCES

Allport, G. W., & Postman, L. 1947. *The Psychology of Rumor,* New York: Holt, Rnehart & Winston.

Buckland, M. 1991. Information as thing. *Journal of the American Society for Information Science,* 42, 351.

Chen, X., Sin, S.-C. J., Theng, Y.-L. & Lee, C. S. 2015. Why students share misinformation on social media: motivation, gender, and study-level differences. *The Journal of Academic Librarianship,* 41, 583–592.

Datareportal. 2019. Global digital overview [Online]. Available: https://datareportal.com/reports/digital-2019-global-digital-overview [Accessed January 2020].

Deandrea, D. C. & Vendemia, M. A. 2016. How affiliation disclosure and control over user-generated comments affects consumer health knowledge and behavior: A randomized controlled experiment of pharmaceutical direct-to-consumer advertising on social media. *Journal Medical Internet Research,* 18, e189.

Department of Health (DoH). 2011. Change4Life: Three year social marketing strategy.

Department of Health (DoH). 2008. Healthy weight, healthy lives: A cross government strategy for England [Online]. Available: http://www.dh.gov.uk/en/Publicationsandstatistics/Publications/PublicationsPolicyAndGuidance/DH_082378 [Accessed 2008/07/17].

Donaldson, E. A., Cohen, J. E., Truant, P. L., Rutkow, L., Kanarek, N. F. & Barry, C. L. 2015. News media framing of New York City's sugar-sweetened beverage portion-size cap. *American Journal Public Health,* 105, 2202–2209.

Ellis, C., Evans, C. & Moore, J. 2020. Systematic assessment of obesity information on the microblogging platform Twitter. *Proceedings of the Nutrition Society*, 79(OCE3), E791.

Fallis, D. 2015. What is disinformation? *Library Trends,* 63, 401–426.

Fox, C. J. 1983. *Information and Misinformation: An Investigation of the Notions of Information, Misinformation, Informing, and Misinforming.* Westport, CT: Greenwood.

Frederick, D. A., Saguy, A. C., Sandhu, G. & Mann, T. 2016. Effects of competing news media frames of weight on antifat stigma, beliefs about weight and support for obesity-related public policies. *International Journal of Obesity (London),* 40, 543–549.

Garza, C., Stover, P. J., Ohlhorst, S. D., Field, M. S., Steinbrook, R., Rowe, S., Woteki, C. & Campbell, E. 2019. Best practices in nutrition science to earn and keep the public's trust. *The American Journal of Clinical Nutrition,* 109, 225–243.

Goldacre, B. M. 2008. *Bad Science*. New York: Harper Collins.

Goldberg, J. P. & Hellwig, J. P. 1997. Nutrition research in the media: the challenge facing scientists. *Journal of the American College of Nutrition,* 16, 544–550.

Grilli, R., Ramsay, C. & Minozzi, S. 2002. Mass media interventions: effects on health services utilisation. *Cochrane Database of Systematic Reviews*, 2002(1), CD000389.

Islam, M. S., Sarkar, T., Khan, S. H., Mostofa Kamal, A.-H., Hasan, S. M. M., Kabir, A., Yeasmin, D., Islam, M. A., Amin Chowdhury, K. I., Anwar, K. S., Chughtai, A. A. & Seale, H. 2020. COVID-19: Related infodemic and its impact on public health: A global social media analysis. *The American Journal of Tropical Medicine and Hygiene*, 103(4), 1621–1629.

Karlova, N. A. & Lee, J. H. 2011. Notes from the underground city of disinformation: A conceptual investigation. *Proceedings of the American Society for Information Science and Technology,* 48, 1–9.

Karlova, N. A. & Fisher, K. 2013. A social diffusion model of misinformation and disinformation for understanding human information behaviour. *Information Research,* 18(1), paper 573.

Khobzi, H., Lau, R. Y. K. and Cheung, T. C. H. 2019. The outcome of online social interactions on Facebook pages: A study of user engagement behavior. *Internet Research,* 29, 2–23.

Kininmonth, A., Jamil, N., Almatrouk, N. & Evans, C. 2017. Quality assessment of nutrition coverage in the media: A 6-week survey of five popular UK newspapers. *BMJ Open,* 7(12): e014633.

Mozaffarian, D. & Forouhi, N. G. 2018. Dietary guidelines and health: Is nutrition science up to the task? *BMJ,* 360, k822.

Obar, J. A. 2015. Social media definition and the governance challenge: An introduction to the special issue. *Telecommunications Policy,* 39, 745–750.

OFCOM. 2019. News consumption in the UK: 2019 [Online]. Available: https://www.ofcom.org.uk/__data/assets/pdf_file/0027/157914/uk-news-consumption-2019-report.pdf [Accessed].

Piggin, J. & Lee, J. 2011. 'Don't mention obesity': Contradictions and tensions in the UK Change4Life health promotion campaign. *Journal of Health Psychology,* 16, 1151–1164.

Public Health England. 2018. A century of public health marketing [Online]. Available: https://publichealthengland.exposure.co/100-years-of-public-health-marketing[AccessedApril 2019 2019].

Robinson, A., Coutinho, A., Bryden, A. & Mckee, M. 2013. Analysis of health stories in daily newspapers in the UK. *Public Health,* 127, 39–45.

Roland, D. 2018. Social media, health policy, and knowledge translation. *Journal of the American College of Radiology,* 15, 149–152.

Science Media Centre. 2018. A new labelling system for medical research press releases [Online]. Available: https://www.sciencemediacentre.org/a-new-labelling-system-for-medical-research-press-releases/ [Accessed July 2020].

Vosoughi, S., Roy, D. & Aral, S. 2018. The spread of true and false news online. *Science* 359, 1146.

Weatherall, J. O., O'connor, C. & Bruner, J. P. 2018. How to beat science and influence people: Policymakers and propaganda in epistemic networks. *The British Journal for the Philosophy of Science*, 71(4), 1157–1186.

World Health Organization (WHO) 2012. Communication for behavioural impact (COMBI). https://apps.who.int/iris/handle/10665/75170

World Health Organization (WHO) 2017. WHO strategic communications framework for effective communications. https://www.who.int/mediacentre/communication-framework.pdf

Wrieden, W. L. & Levy, L. B. 2016. 'Change4Life smart swaps': Quasi-experimental evaluation of a natural experiment. *Public Health Nutrition,* 19, 2388–2392.

Zhou, L. & Zhang, D. 2007. An ontology-supported misinformation model: Toward a digital misinformation library. *IEEE Transactions on Systems, Man, and Cybernetics - Part A: Systems and Humans,* 37, 804–813.

# 13 Nutrition Labelling on Food Products and Menus

*Sally G. Moore*
University of Leeds

*Yael Benn*
Manchester Metropolitan University

**CONTENTS**



## 13.1 INTRODUCTION

Nutrition label information on food products is needed by consumers to help them navigate the rapidly changing provision of food products with our current food environments, including processed foods, ready-to-eat products and menu items offered in out-of-home settings (i.e. cafés and restaurants). Nutrition label information is considered a tool for consumers to use to promote healthier eating and "wise" food choices, amidst the increasing global prevalence of obesity (CAC, 2011). Using nutrition labels to choose products lower in fat, saturates, sugar and salt is now a public health recommendation within UK food-based dietary guidance (PHE, 2016).

## 13.2 LEGISLATION, POLICY AND PREVALENCE

Legislation mandating that products declare nutrition information within Nutrition Facts Panels has been in place in the US since the implementation of their Nutrition Labelling and Education Act (FDA, 1995). More recently, European legislation mandated that nutrition information appears on pre-packaged products sold in EU countries, including the UK, although such information has been displayed

DOI: 10.1201/9781003043720-13

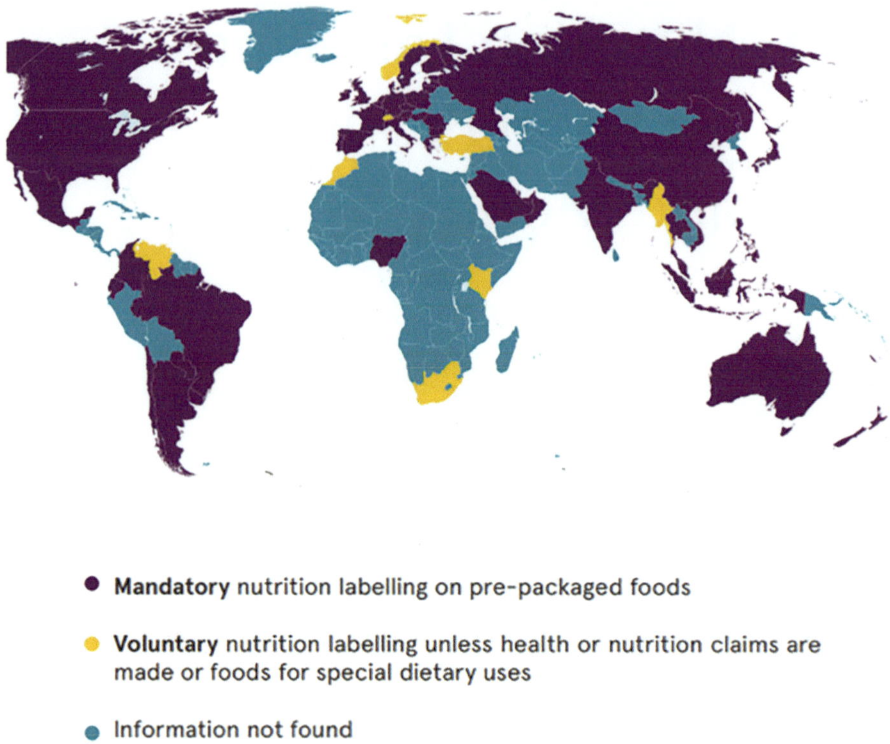


**FIGURE 13.1** Global overview of mandatory and voluntary nutrition labelling available free to use from the European Food Information Council (EUFIC), 2018 at www.eufic.org.

voluntarily for many years and was required if the product made any claims (EC, 2011). An audit of food products conducted in European countries prior to 2010 showed an average of 85% of products declared back-of-pack nutrition labelling (Bonsmann et al., 2010). The availability of nutrition label information on products can therefore be considered widespread across much of global marketplaces (EUFIC, 2018) (Figure 13.1).

In order to provide nutrition label information, manufacturers are expected to analyse their product's nutritional composition before declaring this data in the format required by food labelling legislation. Mandatory nutrition declarations will appear alongside other "food label" information (e.g. ingredients, cooking instructions), and are usually tabulated on the back (or side) of pre-packed products. Nutrition information elements that are required to be declared include energy (i.e. kcals/kJ) as well as the content of specific nutrients: the types and format of which differ according to the relevant legislation (see Figure 13.2). Declared amounts of fat, saturated fat, carbohydrates, sugars, protein and salt appears "per 100g" and/or "per serving" of the product. Nutrition labels may also include information on the contributions of a serving of the product to recommended daily amounts of energy or nutrients, usually called "Daily Values" (DV) in the US, or "Reference Intakes" (RI) in the EU/UK (formerly Guideline Daily Amounts, GDAs) (DoH, 2016).

(a)

**Nutrition**

| Typical values | 100g contains | Each slice (typically 44g) contains | % RI* | RI* for an average adult |
|---|---|---|---|---|
| Energy | 985kJ<br>235kcal | 435kJ<br>105kcal | 5% | 8400kJ<br>2000kcal |
| Fat | 1.5g | 0.7g | 1% | 70g |
| of which saturates | 0.3g | 0.1g | 1% | 20g |
| Carbohydrate | 45.5g | 20.0g | | |
| of which sugars | 3.8g | 1.7g | 2% | 90g |
| Fibre | 2.8g | 1.2g | | |
| Protein | 7.7g | 3.4g | | |
| Salt | 1.0g | 0.4g | 7% | 6g |

This pack contains 16 servings

*Reference intake of an average adult (8400kJ / 2000kcal)

(b)

**Nutrition Facts**

8 servings per container

**Serving size 2/3 cup (55g)**

**Amount per serving**

**Calories 230**

| | % Daily Value* |
|---|---|
| **Total Fat** 8g | **10%** |
| Saturated Fat 1g | **5%** |
| *Trans* Fat 0g | |
| **Cholesterol** 0mg | **0%** |
| **Sodium** 160mg | **7%** |
| **Total Carbohydrate** 37g | **13%** |
| Dietary Fiber 4g | **14%** |
| Total Sugars 12g | |
| Includes 10g Added Sugars | **20%** |
| **Protein** 3g | |
| Vitamin D 2mcg | 10% |
| Calcium 260mg | 20% |
| Iron 8mg | 45% |
| Potassium 235mg | 6% |

* The % Daily Value (DV) tells you how much a nutrient in a serving of food contributes to a daily diet. 2,000 calories a day is used for general nutrition advice.

(c)

NUTRITION INFORMATION

Servings per package: 3.00

Serving size: 25.00 g

| | Average Quantity per Serving | Average Quantity per 100 g |
|---|---|---|
| Energy | 496 kJ | 1980 kJ |
| Protein | 0.8 g | 3.3 g |
| Fat, total | 9.3 g | 37.0 g |
| - saturated | 1.9 g | 7.7 g |
| Carbohydrate | 7.6 g | 30.5 g |
| - sugars | 0.0 g | 0.1 g |
| Sodium | 10 mg | 41 mg |

**FIGURE 13.2** Examples of back-of-pack nutrition label formats, which include mandatory elements, commonly used in the UK (a), US (b) and Australia (c).

Additionally, alternative versions of nutrition information may also be (mostly voluntarily) provided on food labels, in line with those forms of expression allowed under the country's food labelling legislation (EUFIC, 2018). Nutrition signposting schemes, as these label versions have become known, include information panels or logos positioned on the "front-of-pack" which often provide a visual interpretation of the amounts of specific nutrients and/or energy provided per serving or other quantity of the product (Figure 13.3). Examples of "nutrient-level" front-of-pack schemes include the EU Reference Intakes or the UK Multiple Traffic Lights, both of which show (numerical or colour-coded) interpretations of the content of nutrients of public health concern (i.e. energy, fat, saturated fat, sugars and salt) (DoH, 2016). Other "summary indicator" front-of-pack nutrition label schemes tend to provide an overall

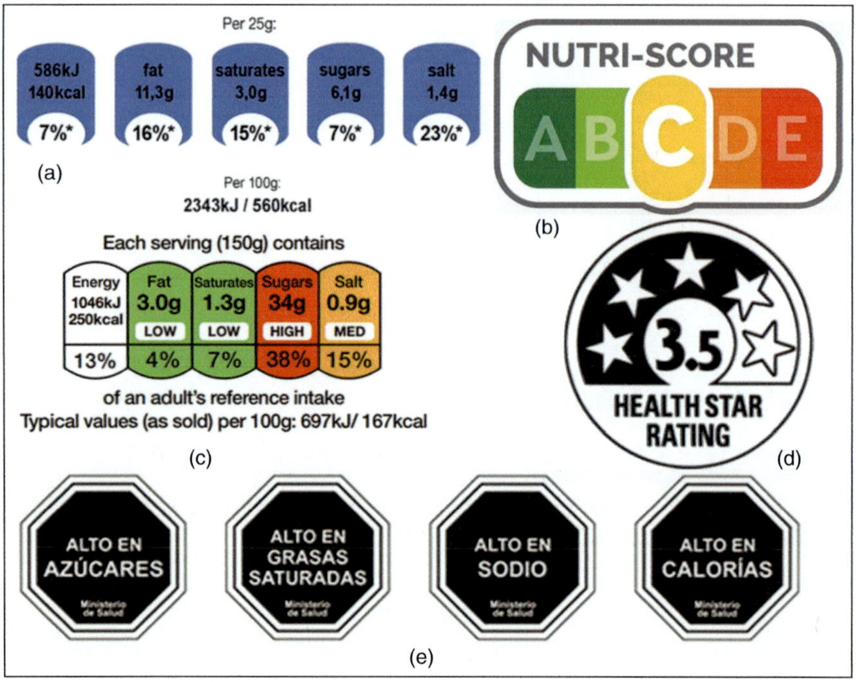


**FIGURE 13.3** Examples of current front-of-pack nutrition label signposting schemes from around the world. (a) EU Reference Intakes, (b) Nutri-Score, (c) Current UK Multiple Traffic Lights, (d) Australian Health Star Rating, (e) Chilean Warning Symbols.

assessment of the product's nutritional quality or healthfulness. Such schemes include the French Nutri-Score, the Australian Health Star Rating and the Scandinavian Keyhole or Choices logos (Bonsmann et al., 2020). Another front-of-pack scheme known as "warning symbols", is currently mandatory in Chile and indicates the presence of "high" levels of calories, saturated fat, sugar or sodium. Most front-of-pack schemes are underpinned by a criterion which determines the levels of nutrients which are considered "high" etc. or provides an overall product "score" or "rating". This may be a nutrient profile model or algorithm used to compute the product's overall nutritional quality or healthfulness classification (Bonsmann et al., 2020).

Front-of-pack labels vary in their provision across products and countries. Within Europe, the UK was previously found to have the highest prevalence of (several different formats of) front-of-pack labels (82% of audited products) (Bonsmann et al., 2010). In 2018, up to 20% of French products displayed Nutri-Score, and uptake of the Health Star Rating label is now growing in Australia (Jones et al., 2018). Although not as prevalent on products as back-of-pack nutrition labels, voluntary adoption of front-of-pack labelling is increasing (Bonsmann et al., 2020).

Also increasing is the provision of energy or "calorie" labelling on restaurant menus and within out-of-home food settings (i.e. cafés, counter sales, take-away outlets) (EUFIC, 2018). Several countries now have policies on menu labelling in restaurants or other food outlets (Rincón-Gallardo Patiño et al., 2020). In New York

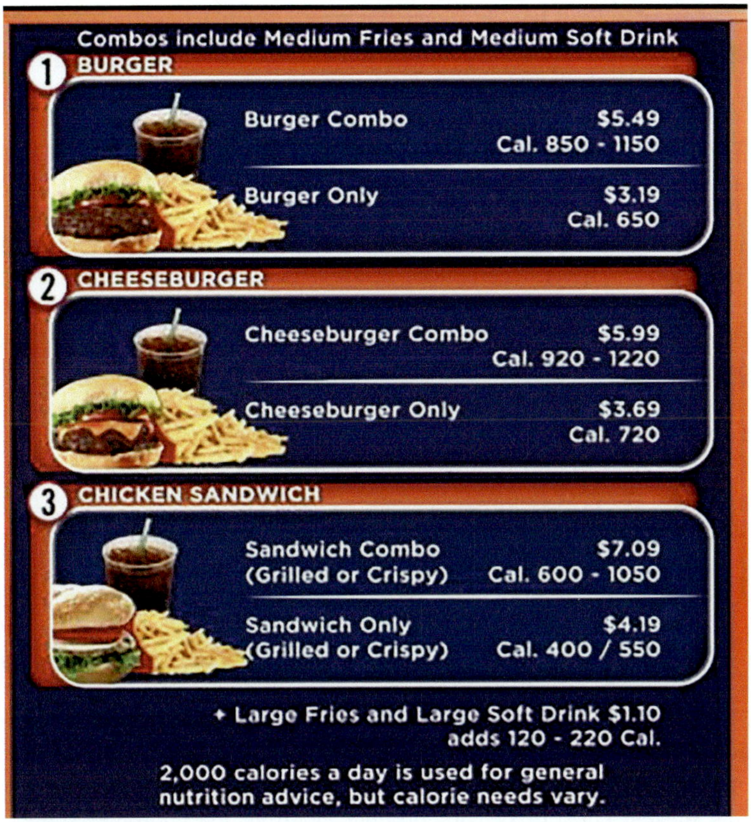
Combos include Medium Fries and Medium Soft Drink
1 BURGER
Burger Combo $5.49
Cal. 850 - 1150
Burger Only $3.19
Cal. 650
2 CHEESEBURGER
Cheeseburger Combo $5.99
Cal. 920 - 1220
Cheeseburger Only $3.69
Cal. 720
3 CHICKEN SANDWICH
Sandwich Combo (Grilled or Crispy) $7.09
Cal. 600 - 1050
Sandwich Only (Grilled or Crispy) $4.19
Cal. 400 / 550
+ Large Fries and Large Soft Drink $1.10
adds 120 - 220 Cal.
2,000 calories a day is used for general nutrition advice, but calorie needs vary.

**FIGURE 13.4** Illustration of restaurant calorie menu labelling. Source: US Food and Drug Administration.

and other US states, mandatory calorie labelling has been required in multi-outlet restaurant chains since 2010 (see Figure 13.4). In Taiwan, fast food restaurants and other outlets have been required to display energy content as well as information for caffeine and sugar since 2015 (Rincón-Gallardo Patiño et al., 2020). The presentation of menu labelling information currently provided in the UK is to become mandatory and comprises of energy content (i.e. kcal/kJ) accompanied by information on Reference Intakes (RI) (DHSC, 2018).

## 13.3 IMPACT OF NUTRITION LABEL INFORMATION ON CONSUMERS' DIETS

The impact of nutrition labels on consumers' food choices depends on consumers using them appropriately to inform their food selection and purchase decisions. Practically, there are several ways in which consumers may use the provided nutrition label information to choose products and eat a healthier diet. These include using the "per 100g" or "per serving" information elements to evaluate a product's nutrient content levels and overall healthfulness (i.e. using "high"/"low" nutrient thresholds) or to compare two products. Consumers may also use the provided "per serving" nutrient values to track their own intakes of energy or nutrients in line with recommended daily intakes (i.e. DV/RI values) (Cowburn and Stockley, 2005).

Review evidence suggests that reading nutrition labels is associated with healthier diets, as measured by food frequency questionnaires and 24-hour recalls (Anastasiou et al., 2019). A meta-analysis of studies conducted in various countries since 1990 found that food labelling decreased consumer's intakes of energy and total fat, as well as unhealthy options (Shangguan et al., 2018). However, review evidence of consumer's purchase choices is less convincing in terms of the impact of back-of-pack and other forms of nutrition information. An examination the effects of US mandatory labelling legislation since the early 1990s suggests this information has only modestly influenced consumers' purchase behaviours (Patterson et al., 2017).

More promising evidence on the impact of nutrition labelling reflects the evolution of (front-of-pack) nutrition labelling formats, their increasing availability on products and the growing research concerning such newer label types. A meta-analysis of studies encompassing various labelling formats and front-of-pack schemes suggested that nutrition labels could be expected to increase the number of people selecting a healthier food product by about 18% and decrease calorie choice/intakes by 3.5% (Cecchini and Warin, 2015). Further review evidence focussed specifically on front-of-pack labels now suggests these significantly reduce purchased content of sugar and sodium (Croker et al., 2020).

A variety of approaches have been used to evaluate the impact of nutrition labels on consumer food choices, including experimental and real-world research. There are acknowledged limitations with the ecological validity of experimental studies that simply present consumers with product labelling via computer screens (Vyth et al., 2012). However, studies conducted in the real world need to overcome other limitations, including product-level differences across in-store label display and the tendency for consumers to over-report their use of labelling (Grunert et al., 2010). New and novel research methods have been employed to quantify label viewing/use in real-world settings, including with smart phone label-viewing apps and wearable cameras.

Observations of consumers' actual label use behaviours favour front over back-of-pack nutrition labelling. For example, in a study of UK consumers, 66% of supermarket label readers were found to have looked at front-of-pack information, whereas only 11.6% looked "elsewhere" on the pack (Grunert et al., 2010). Furthermore, consumers who frequently used (Health Star Rating or Traffic Light) front-of-pack labels via a smartphone app were more likely to have significantly healthier food purchases, compared with nutrition information panel users (Ni Mhurchu et al., 2017). A recent Danish longitudinal study of households' "home-scan" purchasing data has found that consumers' use of the front-of-pack (i.e. the Keyhole and wholegrain logos) but not back-of-pack nutrition labels resulted in small improvements in diet quality (Rønnow, 2020).

Similar to on-pack nutrition labels, evaluations of the effects of menu calorie labelling on consumer purchases have also produced mixed findings. A recent meta-analysis of the effects of various menu labelling formats has found that this information significantly reduced calories "purchased" by –47 calories (Crockett et al., 2018).

Similarly, a study evaluating (voluntary) calorie labelling within several UK workplace canteens showed a significant reduction (6.6%) in calories purchased by staff on the day after implementation (Vasiljevic et al., 2018). However, this effect was only found within one of the six included canteens and appeared to diminish over time. There may be limitations to the impact of menu labelling, but it is promising that the number of consumers who report seeing and using calorie labels on menus has increased in line with the growing availability of this information between 2007 and 2014 (Feng and Fox, 2018).

It is likely that consumers' use of menu labelling will depend on the setting, eating occasion and type of information provided. In terms of setting, evidence suggests that providing menu information results in a greater effect on the healthiness of foods purchased in cafeterias, compared to restaurants (Fernandes et al., 2016). In relation to eating occasion, calorie menu labelling together with contextual information on daily intakes was found to result in study participants consuming around 250 fewer calories across dinner and subsequent eating occasions, compared to groups provided with no information or calorie information alone (Roberto et al., 2010).

An alternative pathway for nutrition labels to impact on consumers' nutritional intakes is via product reformulation. Declaration of nutrition information on products by manufacturers is now thought to influence whether and how (pre-packed and menu) products are reformulated (Rincón-Gallardo Patiño et al., 2020; Shangguan et al., 2018). Reformulation of recipes can improve these products' nutritional composition by, for example, reducing levels of energy or specific nutrients of public health concern (e.g. sugars, salt, saturated fat). Motivations for product reformulation initiatives include the desire to avoid declaring "red" traffic lights on products' front-of-pack nutrition labels. Evidence from New Zealand suggests that the reformulation of products to lower their energy and sodium content was greater for products with (compared to those without) the Health Star Rating front-of-pack nutrition labels during a 2-year (2014–2016) time frame (Mhurchu et al., 2017). In restaurants, menu labelling is associated with decreases in the calorie content of menu options and an increase in "healthier" options (Saelens et al., 2012).

## 13.4 VARIATIONS IN CONSUMER UNDERSTANDING AND USE OF NUTRITION LABEL INFORMATION

Global evidence suggests that around 50% of consumers report using nutrition labels, with frequent label users likely to be female and those who possess higher levels of education and income (Campos et al., 2011). Use of nutrition labels has been outlined as a process comprising of several internal and external influences which result in an individual consumer evaluating a product and making a food choice or purchase decision (Figure 13.5) (Grunert et al., 2010). First, consumers must be "exposed" to nutrition label information, including via the (mandatory) display of these labels. In addition, a key influence on the attention consumers pay to this information appears to be the location and format of nutrition labels on product packaging (Bialkova and van Trijp, 2010). Consumers' personal motivations including their desire to attain nutrition goals or adhere to dietary restrictions are key to them viewing and utilising

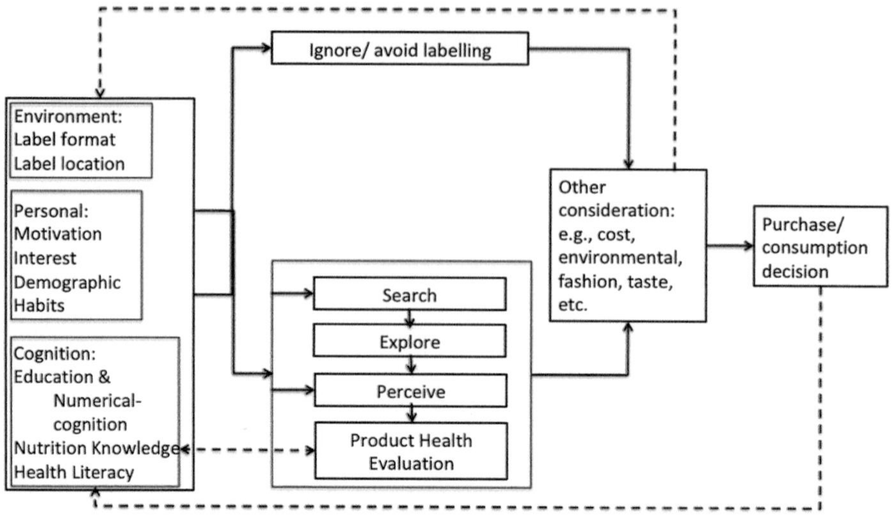


**FIGURE 13.5** A conceptual framework of consumer use of nutrition labels, including influences. (Extended from Grunert et al. (2010) and Nabec (2017).)

this information. A general lack of motivation to engage with labels (or lack of interest in healthy eating) is currently considered a major "bottle neck" to consumers' use of this information (Grunert et al., 2010).

After perceiving the provided nutrition label information, consumers then need to read, locate and understand the elements presented on it. Consumers tend to look for (locate) nutritional elements they wish to avoid such as fat, calories, sugars or salt content, and may be more inclined to view information positioned towards the top of the label rather than the bottom (Graham et al., 2012). Understanding the intended meaning of the information, which includes accurately locating and interpreting specific elements of label data, is important since these tasks will form the basis of consumers' product evaluations (Grunert et al., 2010). Most consumers appear to be able to locate specific information (i.e. per 100 g), but research has revealed a general lack of understanding of specific elements of nutrition information including "serving size" and label terminology reflecting recommended daily amounts such as "percent daily values (DV)", "Reference Intakes" (RI) or "Guideline Daily Amounts" (Cowburn and Stockley, 2005). This is of potential importance since the display and use of the "per 100 g" or "Guideline Daily Amounts" label elements are thought to influence consumers' evaluation of a product's healthfulness (Raats et al., 2015). In addition, it is possible that poor levels of understanding of labelled serving size information may partly explain why there is a lack of evidence regarding this label element's impact on consumers' dietary intakes (Anastasiou et al., 2019).

Although tempting, it should not be assumed that consumers who claim to frequently use nutrition labels, or who are highly personally motivated to do so, are those who fully understand and properly interpret the information provided. Nutrition information may not be fully understood, even among frequent label users (Sharif et al., 2014). Furthermore, consumers themselves may not realise that they lack proper understanding of nutrition label information. As highlighted by a large European Study, 77% of consumers claimed to understand the term "Guideline Daily Amounts" although only 33% were able to give the correct meaning (Gregori et al., 2014).

In general, those least likely to properly understand nutrition label information include older adults, as well as consumers with lower incomes or educational attainment (Campos et al., 2011). Besides numeracy, levels of health literacy (defined as an individual's "...ability to identify, interpret and use information related to health") is now also a clear determinant of nutrition label use and understanding (Persoskie, 2017). In addition, the possession of basic nutrition knowledge (i.e. of the concepts and processes related to nutrition and health) is also thought to support the correct understanding and interpretation of nutrition label information (Grunert et al., 2010). Overall, there is clearly a requirement for consumers to possess specific skill and knowledge attributes in order to properly understand nutrition labels, and therefore for this information to be effective at informing food choices.

To help reduce the potential for inequalities in the use and understanding of nutrition label information and increase the effect of labelling on consumers' food choices, there exists a role for educating consumers about "how to use" nutrition labels. Such education is required by labelling legislation, including the US 1990 Nutrition Labelling and Education Act (FDA, 1995). Nutrition label education, including web-based "training" or sessions delivered by dietitians, is likely to improve consumer understanding and intended use of this information (Moore et al., 2018). However, there is presently a need to identify the types of population education and awareness initiatives that are most effective at encouraging consumer use and understanding of nutrition labelling (EUFIC, 2018).

Improving consumers' use and understanding of nutrition labels is an often-cited rationale for proposals to implement or mandate specific front-of-pack label formats (Bonsmann et al., 2020). To this end, which front-of-pack label formats should be displayed on food products is the subject of much cross-sector discussion, as reflected by the recent UK Government consultation on nutrition labelling following exit from the EU (Brexit) (DHSC, 2020). The public health policy preference is for a consistent single front-of-pack scheme, including at EU level, since the existence of multiple different versions of front-of-pack labels in the marketplace is thought to create consumer confusion (Bonsmann et al., 2020). As such, much research has been performed with consumers to determine the most "effective" front-of-pack nutrition label in terms of understanding and using this information to accurately identify the "healthier" product choice, including with consumers considered "nutritionally at risk" and who possess little pre-existing nutrition knowledge (Ducrot et al., 2015).

In terms of menu labelling, differences also exist between consumer groups in their understanding and use of this information. High-frequency users of menu labelling include those from sociodemographic groups who are likely to possess low health literacy and educational attainment levels (Feng and Fox, 2018). In addition, the impact of menu labelling (i.e. decreases in calories purchased) has been found to be greater in higher socioeconomic groups (Sarink et al., 2016). Socioeconomic characteristics of consumers who use labels frequently are important to consider, since these may influence the ability to understand and "act" on menu labels. For example, label uses may not fully understand or be unable to "act" on the recommendations of the label information, particularly if this involves paying higher prices for healthier items (Green et al., 2015). Accompanying contextual information on calorie recommendations may also be required for labelling to impact food choices given that a third of surveyed UK consumers did not know their recommended calorie intakes (NatCen, 2017).

In real life, nutrition labels are not the only influence on consumers' product evaluations and purchase choices. This information will, at best, be integrated with other influences that occur both on pack and within the retail environment, including price, brand, marketing messages and other claims (Nabec, 2017). Hence, in order to navigate the variety and complexity of the provided product information, consumers need to prioritise the types of information (e.g., organic vs sugar content) they use. Overall, for the provided nutrition information to impact on health and promote healthy eating, consumers need to possess high levels of knowledge, understanding and individual agency (use of personal resources) (Adams et al., 2016).

## 13.5 ONLINE PRODUCT NUTRITION INFORMATION

In the UK and other EU countries, it is mandatory to provide product nutrition information for food products sold online (i.e. distance selling) (EC, 2011). Many retailers now declare this information at point-of-purchase within product information webpages, usually as tables providing back-of-pack nutrition label information and using images of front-of-pack labels (for an example, see Figure 13.6). Evidence is emerging on how the provided information is used by consumers and can influence food choices (Jilcott Pitts et al., 2018).

Evidence from studies undertaken with consumers within "mock" online supermarkets suggest that providing this information could help consumers to choose healthier products (Jilcott Pitts et al., 2018). In contrast, research within a real-life online supermarket has shown that implementation of traffic light front-of-pack nutrition labels on various products had no impact on sales of healthier foods (Sacks et al., 2011). Furthermore, online product nutrition information was found to be poorly attended to in a study examining shoppers' actual viewing (measured using eye-tracking) of product webpages, as displayed within a UK retailer's website (Benn et al., 2015). In this study, both quantitative and qualitative data collected from participants revealed that shopping (online or offline) requires high cognitive load (e.g. sticking to a budget, remembering who in the household eats what) and involves decisions that are beyond the food itself but extend to the consumer's other, wider values (e.g., environmental).

Two aspects of the presentation of online "virtual" nutrition information that could potentially influence its use by consumers include its location and presentation format. Both aspects are known to influence consumer attention to on-pack labels yet have been shown to vary considerably across and within major UK supermarket websites (Stones, 2016). In these environments, some mandatory (back-of-pack) nutrition label information also appears to be located "below the fold" of the product webpage, requiring consumers to scroll down in order to view this information (Stones, 2016) or to click on the item and go to another page (Benn et al., 2015). It is possible that online shoppers could purchase a product without viewing nutrition

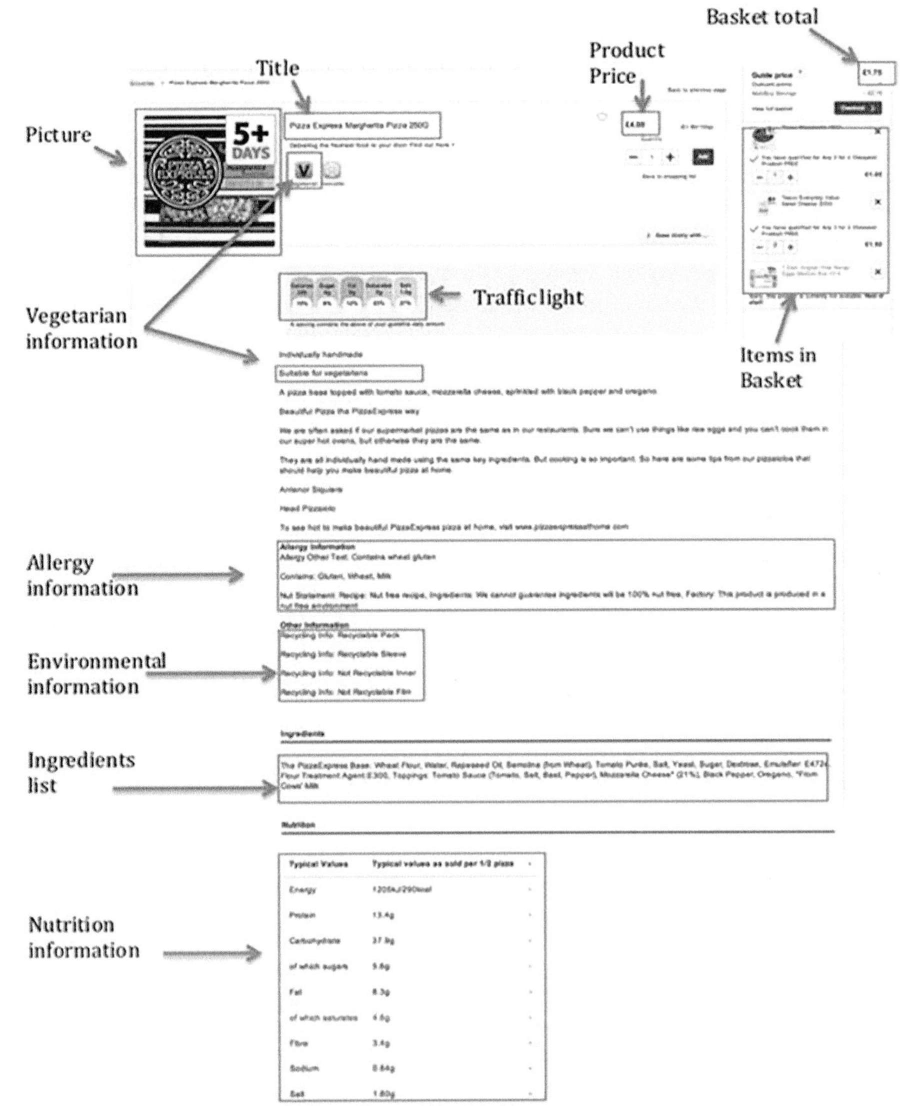


**FIGURE 13.6** A UK retailer's online supermarket product information webpage, with annotations of specific information elements. (From Benn et al. (2015).)

label information. Overall, it is understandable that product nutrition information is overlooked by online food consumers who instead appear to use product images and categories claims (organic, fresh), or their familiarity with existing product attributes, to inform their choices (Benn et al., 2015).

Advances in technology can help reduce the requirement for consumers to consult product nutrition information. Websites and apps can now present consumers with a (filtered) list of products according to their personalised preferences. For example, products may be ordered by nutritional values or listed by attribute (e.g. low saturated fat, high fibre). Online supermarket websites can also suggest specific "tailored" food swaps to shoppers, including products lower in saturated fat (Jilcott Pitts et al., 2018). With these technologies, product nutrition label information is being utilised within "behind-the-scenes" algorithms to provide consumers with interpretive, realistic product listings which they can control. The application of product nutrition information in these ways may therefore encourage consumers' (indirect) use of labels, according to their personal motivations and circumstances. Whether the presentation of nutrition information in these virtual formats, combined with consumers' use of these technologies, can impact on real-world purchase choices remains to be fully evaluated.

## 13.6 CONCLUSIONS

Although the provision of nutrition and menu labelling has increased, there is a need to improve the efficacy of this information on consumers' food choices and purchases, including when shopping online. To improve population-level health via nutrition labelling, policy makers must appreciate the specific nature and effects of both mandatory and voluntary nutrition labelling in individual countries. Improving the design format of front-of-pack nutrition information and adopting menu labels, whilst making the provision of both mandatory, could help reduce the disparities in consumers' understanding and use of this information. To increase the impact of nutrition labelling on consumers' diets, corresponding initiatives are needed such as consumer-targeted nutrition label education and industrial product reformulation to improve declared values. Furthermore, developing personalised technologies could reduce the need for shoppers to actively consult online (or on-pack) nutrition labels whilst still enabling their use of this information. Evidence on the effects of such online tools, including product listings, is now required.

## REFERENCES

Adams, J., Mytton, O., White, M., Monsivais, P., 2016. Why are some population interventions for diet and obesity more equitable and effective than others? The role of individual agency. *PLoS Med.* 13, e1001990. doi: 10.1371/journal.pmed.1001990.

Anastasiou, K., Miller, M., Dickinson, K., 2019. The relationship between food label use and dietary intake in adults: A systematic review. *Appetite* 139, 280–291. doi: 10.1016/j.appet.2019.03.025.

Benn, Y., Webb, T.L., Chang, B.P.I., Reidy, J., 2015. What information do consumers consider, and how do they look for it, when shopping for groceries online? *Appetite* 89, 265–273. doi: 10.1016/j.appet.2015.01.025.

Bialkova, S., van Trijp, H., 2010. What determines consumer attention to nutrition labels? *Food Qual. Prefer.*, Eighth Pangborn Sensory Science Symposium, 21, 1042–1051. doi: 10.1016/j.foodqual.2010.07.001.

Bonsmann, S., Genannt, S., Celemín, L.F., Larrañaga, A., Egger, S., Wills, J.M., Hodgkins, C., Raats, M.M., 2010. Penetration of nutrition information on food labels across the EU-27 plus Turkey. *Eur. J. Clin. Nutr.* 64, 1379–1385. doi: 10.1038/ejcn.2010.179.

Bonsmann, S.G., Marandola, G., Ciriolo, E., van Bavel, R., Wollgast, J., 2020. JRC science for policy report. Front-of-pack nutrition labelling schemes: a comprehensive review. European Commission (Text). European Commission.

CAC, 2011. Codex Alimentarius Commission. Guidelines on Nutrition Labelling, CAC/GL 2-1985. Revisions 1993 and 2011. Amendment 2003, 2006, 2009, 2010 and 2012. Annex adopted 2011. Food and Agriculture Organization of the United Nations/World Health Organization, Rome.

Campos, S., Doxey, J., Hammond, D., 2011. Nutrition labels on pre-packaged foods: a systematic review. *Public Health Nutr.* 14, 1496–1506. doi: 10.1017/S1368980010003290.

Cecchini, M., Warin, L., 2015. Impact of food labelling systems on food choices and eating behaviours: a systematic review and meta-analysis of randomized studies. *Obes. Rev.* 17, 201–210. doi: 10.1111/obr.12364.

Cowburn, G., Stockley, L., 2005. Consumer understanding and use of nutrition labelling: a systematic review. *Public Health Nutr.* 8, 21–28. doi: 10.1079/PHN2004666.

Crockett, R.A., King, S.E., Marteau, T.M., Prevost, A.T., Bignardi, G., Roberts, N.W., Stubbs, B., Hollands, G.J., Jebb, S.A., 2018. Nutritional labelling for healthier food or non-alcoholic drink purchasing and consumption. *Cochrane Database Syst. Rev.* doi: 10.1002/14651858.CD009315.pub2.

Croker, H., Packer, J., Russell, S.J., Stansfield, C., Viner, R.M., 2020. Front of pack nutritional labelling schemes: a systematic review and meta-analysis of recent evidence relating to objectively measured consumption and purchasing. *J. Hum. Nutr. Diet. Off. J. Br. Diet. Assoc.* doi: 10.1111/jhn.12758.

DHSC, 2018. Department of Health and Social Care. Consultation on mandating calorie labelling in the out-of-home sector.

DHSC, 2020. Department of Health and Social Care. Building on the success of front-of-pack nutrition labelling in the UK: a public consultation. UK Government and Food Standards Agencies.

DoH, 2016. Department of Health. Guide to creating a front of pack (FoP) nutrition label for pre-packed products sold through retail outlets.

Ducrot, P., Méjean, C., Julia, C., Kesse-Guyot, E., Touvier, M., Fezeu, L.K., Hercberg, S., Péneau, S., 2015. Objective understanding of front-of-package nutrition labels among nutritionally at-risk individuals. *Nutrients* 7, 7106–7125. doi: 10.3390/nu7085325.

EC (European Commission) 2011. Regulation (EU) No 1169/2011 of the European Parliament and of the Council of 25 October 2011 on the provision of food information to consumers. Official Journal of the European Union L304/18, OJ L.

EUFIC, 2018. Global update on nutrition labelling from the European Food Information Council.

FDA, 1995. US Food and Drug Administration. Guide to nutrition labeling and education act requirements FDA August 1994 [WWW Document]. *Nutr. Labeling Educ. Act NLEA Requir.* 894–295. https://www.fda.gov/iceci/inspections/inspectionguides/ucm074948.htm (accessed 8.29.2018).

Feng, W., Fox, A., 2018. Menu labels, for better, and worse? Exploring socio-economic and race-ethnic differences in menu label use in a national sample. *Appetite* 128, 223–232. doi: 10.1016/j.appet.2018.06.015.

Fernandes, A.C., Oliveira, R.C., Proença, R.P.C., Curioni, C.C., Rodrigues, V.M., Fiates, G.M.R., 2016. Influence of menu labeling on food choices in real-life settings: a systematic review. *Nutr. Rev.* 74, 534–548. doi: 10.1093/nutrit/nuw013.

Graham, D.J., Orquin, J.L., Visschers, V.H.M., 2012. Eye tracking and nutrition label use: A review of the literature and recommendations for label enhancement. *Food Policy* 37, 378–382. doi: 10.1016/j.foodpol.2012.03.004.

Green, J.E., Brown, A.G., Ohri-Vachaspati, P., 2015. Sociodemographic disparities among fast-food restaurant customers who notice and use calorie menu labels. *J. Acad. Nutr. Diet.* 115, 1093–1101. doi: 10.1016/j.jand.2014.12.004.

Gregori, D., Ballali, S., Vögele, C., Gafare, C.E., Stefanini, G., Widhalm, K., 2014. Evaluating food front-of-pack labelling: a pan-European survey on consumers' attitudes toward food labelling. *Int. J. Food Sci. Nutr.* 65, 177–186. doi: 10.3109/09637486.2013.854743.

Grunert, K.G., Wills, J.M., Fernández-Celemín, L., 2010. Nutrition knowledge, and use and understanding of nutrition information on food labels among consumers in the UK. *Appetite* 55, 177–189. doi: 10.1016/j.appet.2010.05.045.

Jilcott Pitts, S.B., Ng, S.W., Blitstein, J.L., Gustafson, A., Niculescu, M., 2018. Online grocery shopping: promise and pitfalls for healthier food and beverage purchases. *Public Health Nutr.* 21, 3360–3376. doi: 10.1017/S1368980018002409.

Jones, A., Shahid, M., Neal, B., 2018. Uptake of Australia's health star rating system. *Nutrients* 10. doi: 10.3390/nu10080997.

Mhurchu, C.N., Eyles, H., Choi, Y.-H. 2017. Effects of a voluntary front-of-pack nutrition labelling system on packaged food reformulation: The health star rating system in New Zealand. *Nutrients* 9. doi: 10.3390/nu9080918.

Moore, S.G., Donnelly, J.K., Jones, S., Cade, J.E. 2018. Effect of Educational Interventions on Understanding and Use of Nutrition Labels: A Systematic Review. Nutrients 10(10), 1432. doi: 10.3390/nu10101432.

Nabec, L., 2017. Improving dietary behaviour with nutrition labelling: Towards a research agenda that serves consumer well-being. *Rech. Appl. En Mark. Engl. Ed.* 32, 71–97. doi: 10.1177/2051570716685522.

NatCen, 2017. Engagement with labelling: informing the Calorie Wise scheme prepared for: Food Standards Agency. Food and You Waves 1–4 Briefing paper 3.

Ni Mhurchu, C., Volkova, E., Jiang, Y., Eyles, H., Michie, J., Neal, B., Blakely, T., Swinburn, B., Rayner, M., 2017. Effects of interpretive nutrition labels on consumer food purchases: the Starlight randomized controlled trial. *Am. J. Clin. Nutr.* 105, 695–704. doi: 10.3945/ajcn.116.144956.

Patterson, M., Bhargava, S., Loewenstein, G., 2017. An unhealthy attitude? New insight into the modest effects of the NLEA. *J. Behav. Econ. Policy* 1, 15–26.

Persoskie, A., 2017. US consumers' understanding of nutrition labels in 2013: The importance of health literacy. *Prev. Chronic. Dis.* 14. doi: 10.5888/pcd14.170066.

PHE, 2016. Public Health England. From Plate to Guide: What, why and how for the eatwell model.

Raats, M.M., Hieke, S., Jola, C., Hodgkins, C., Kennedy, J., Wills, J., 2015. Reference amounts utilised in front of package nutrition labelling; impact on product healthfulness evaluations. *Eur. J. Clin. Nutr.* 69, 619–625. doi: 10.1038/ejcn.2014.190.

Rincón-Gallardo Patiño, S., Zhou, M., Da Silva Gomes, F., Lemaire, R., Hedrick, V., Serrano, E., Kraak, V.I., 2020. Effects of menu labeling policies on transnational restaurant chains to promote a healthy diet: A scoping review to inform policy and research. *Nutrients* 12, 1544. doi: 10.3390/nu12061544.

Roberto, C.A., Larsen, P.D., Agnew, H., Baik, J., Brownell, K.D., 2010. Evaluating the impact of menu labeling on food choices and intake. *Am. J. Public Health* 100, 312–318. doi: 10.2105/AJPH.2009.160226.

Rønnow, H.N., 2020. The effect of front-of-pack nutritional labels and back-of-pack tables on dietary quality. *Nutrients* 12, 1704. doi: 10.3390/nu12061704.

Sacks, G., Tikellis, K., Millar, L., Swinburn, B., 2011. Impact of "traffic-light" nutrition information on online food purchases in Australia. *Aust. N. Z. J. Public Health* 35, 122–126. doi: 10.1111/j.1753-6405.2011.00684.x.

Saelens, B.E., Chan, N.L., Krieger, J., Nelson, Y., Boles, M., Colburn, T.A., Glanz, K., Ta, M.L., Bruemmer, B., 2012. Nutrition-labeling regulation impacts on restaurant environments. *Am. J. Prev. Med.* 43, 505–511. doi: 10.1016/j.amepre.2012.07.025.

Sarink, D., Peeters, A., Freak-Poli, R., Beauchamp, A., Woods, J., Ball, K., Backholer, K., 2016. The impact of menu energy labelling across socioeconomic groups: a systematic review. *Appetite* 99, 59–75. doi: 10.1016/j.appet.2015.12.022.

Shangguan, S., Afshin, A., Shulkin, M., Ma, W., Marsden, D., Smith, J., Saheb-Kashaf, M., Shi, P., Micha, R., Imamura, F., Mozaffarian, D., 2018. A meta-analysis of food labeling effects on consumer diet behaviors and industry practices. *Am. J. Prev. Med.* doi: 10.1016/j.amepre.2018.09.024.

Sharif, M.Z., Rizzo, S., Prelip, M.L., Glik, D.C., Belin, T.R., Langellier, B.A., Kuo, A.A., Garza, J.R., Ortega, A.N., 2014. The association between nutrition facts label utilization and comprehension among latinos in Two East Los Angeles Neighborhoods. *J. Acad. Nutr. Diet.* 114, 1915–1922. doi: 10.1016/j.jand.2014.05.004.

Stones, C., 2016. Online food nutrition labelling in the UK: how consistent are supermarkets in their presentation of nutrition labels online? *Public Health Nutr.* 19, 2175–2184. doi: 10.1017/S1368980015003110.

Vasiljevic, M., Cartwright, E., Pilling, M., Lee, M.-M., Bignardi, G., Pechey, R., Hollands, G.J., Jebb, S.A., Marteau, T.M., 2018. Impact of calorie labelling in worksite cafeterias: a stepped wedge randomised controlled pilot trial. *Int. J. Behav. Nutr. Phys. Act.* 15, 41. doi: 10.1186/s12966-018-0671-7.

Vyth, E.L., Steenhuis, I.H.M., Brandt, H.E., Roodenburg, A.J.C., Brug, J., Seidell, J.C., 2012. Methodological quality of front-of-pack labeling studies: a review plus identification of research challenges. *Nutr. Rev.* 70, 709–720. doi: 10.1111/j.1753-4887.2012.00535.x.

# 14 Commercial Marketing Food Environment for Young People

*Vivica I. Kraak*
Virginia Polytechnic Institute and State University

*Emma Boyland*
University of Liverpool

**CONTENTS**



## 14.1 INTRODUCTION

Over the past two decades, a robust body of evidence has accrued to link an array of advertising and marketing practices used by transnational food, beverage, chain restaurant, entertainment and digital technology firms to create food environments that have influenced the attitudes, preferences, choices and eating behaviours of children, adolescents and their adult parents (Boyland et al. 2016). The evidence has primarily focused on the micro-level impacts of unhealthy food marketing on young people's cognitive and dietary outcomes and trends in marketing practices rather than the macro-level impacts that have shaped social and cultural norms for

DOI: 10.1201/9781003043720-14

entire populations (Cairns, 2019). Despite compelling evidence that comprehensive government statutory restrictions and stronger voluntary industry commitments may improve marketing practices, progress has been limited in many countries in terms of substantially changing, regulating or banning advertising and marketing practices. These include practices that use emotional appeals to target parents of infants and toddlers to market specialized formulas and products (Harris & Pomeranz, 2020); and children and adolescents, aged 2 up to age 18 years (World Cancer Research Fund International, 2020).

Food environments have evolved to exploit the biological, psychological, social and economic vulnerabilities of children and their parents to reinforce preferences and demand for unhealthy food and beverage products (Roberto et al., 2015). Unhealthy high in fat, sugar and salt/sodium (HFSS) food and beverage products are tasty, convenient, accessible and affordable, oftentimes more so than minimally processed foods such as fruits and vegetables, whole grains and plant-based proteins that are recommended by governments to support healthy eating patterns. The consequences for young people have fostered poor diet quality by encouraging a higher risk of overeating, obesity and diet-related chronic non-communicable diseases at an early age (Lobstein et al., 2015). The World Obesity Federation (2019) estimated that 254 million children between the ages of 5 and 19 years in 191 countries will have obesity by 2030 and children who are obese at ages 6–7 years show cardiometabolic risks as early as 11–12 years, which justifies urgent actions to address these risks in young children (Lycett et al., 2020).

The commercial marketing foodscape that has evolved in many countries has enabled a permissive public policy environment for private-sector actors to use integrated marketing communications (IMC) strategies and techniques to socially normalize and create demand for unhealthy HFSS food and beverage products purchased and consumed by young people and their families. The effects of food and beverage marketing on children's dietary patterns and health are described here. Secondly, a conceptual framework is used to discuss how IMC strategies and techniques are systematically applied by private-sector actors, often in partnership with non-profit organizations across diverse settings and media platforms to systematically shape the cognitive, behavioural and health outcomes of children and adolescents.

Thirdly, best-practice recommendations are discussed that have been issued by United Nations (UN) organizations and other authoritative bodies for the industry to restrict the marketing of unhealthy HFSS products to children and adolescents from birth up to age 18 years. This chapter discusses private-sector actors and sectors (i.e., food and beverage manufacturers, chain restaurants, retailers, entertainment and digital technology firms) that engage in transnational advertising and marketing of food and beverage brands and products to young people. Thereafter, it summarizes evidence of the limitations of industry actors' voluntary commitments and self-regulatory programmes to market healthy food and beverage products to children. It concludes with recommendations for diverse actors to use marketing to create healthy food environments for young people globally that align with the targets set by the World Health Organization (WHO) and UN system to ensure healthy lives for all by 2030.

## 14.2 EVIDENCE FOR FOOD AND BEVERAGE MARKETING EFFECTS ON YOUNG PEOPLE'S DIET AND HEALTH

Infants and young children have a biological preference for HFSS products (Mennella, 2014). Children's frequent, repeated and long-term exposure to advertising and marketing messages that encourage the consumption of highly processed or "ultra-processed," energy-dense and nutrient-poor food and beverage may trigger environmental cues that reward, stimulate or reinforce addictive-like eating behaviours that result in overeating and excessive energy intake, especially by children and adolescents who have less inhibitory control and dietary constraint (Gearhardt et al., 2020).

Children recognize food brand logos more often as they get older, and their knowledge of fast food and sugary beverage brands is linked to a higher body mass index (Cornwell et al., 2014). Adolescents and teenagers are targeted by food and beverage firms that have not committed to comprehensive responsible marketing pledges that protect adolescents aged 13–18 years from the aggressive marketing of unhealthy HFSS food and beverage products between 2006 and 2020 (Kraak et al., 2019; Kraak et al., 2020). Many transnational firms work with other industry actors (i.e., advertising, marketing and public relations firms, and industry trade associations) at national and global levels as well as non-profit organizations to systematically apply IMC strategies and techniques to promote primarily HFSS food and beverage products. Examples are discussed in the next section. One of the reasons that adolescents and young adults are cognitively vulnerable to advertising and marketing messages is because the human brain does not fully develop until 25 years (Crone et al., 2008). Furthermore, they have greater discretionary income spent on food and beverage brands and products, and their peer groups are a strong influence on their dietary preferences and choices (Truman and Elliott, 2019).

## 14.3 EVIDENCE FOR SYSTEMATIC IMC PRACTICES TARGETED TO YOUNG PEOPLE

The globalization of the food supply and expansion of transnational food and beverage industry actors has affected most high-, middle- and low-income countries worldwide (Shekar and Popkin, 2019). IMC strategies are used by commercial businesses in the marketplace to reach customers to build brand awareness, brand loyalty and brand equity (Kraak et al. 2019). Figure 14.1 shows a conceptual framework that outlines IMC strategies (i.e., advertising, direct marketing, public relations and sales promotion) used to reach target audiences based on their age, gender, ethnicity, race, culture or other characteristics (Kraak et al., 2019).

A brand is a proprietary visual, emotional and cultural image associated with a company, corporation or product (American Marketing Association, 2020). Branding is the name or symbol that legally identifies a company, organization or product for consumers to differentiate it in the marketplace (American Marketing Association, 2020). Co-branding is a marketing relationship or partnership between two or more companies, and/or a company, non-profit organizations, or government agency to associate one or more brands with products or services to build brand loyalty among

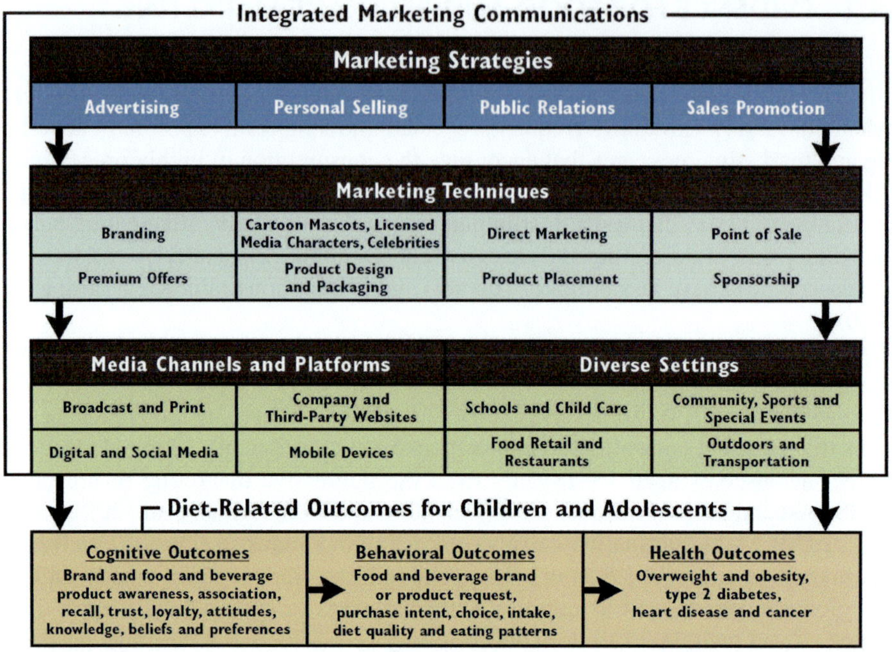


**FIGURE 14.1** Conceptual model of integrated marketing communication strategies targeted to children and adolescents to promote HFSS food and beverage products linked to obesity and diet-related non-communicable diseases. (Available from Kraak et al. (2019) under licence CC BY 4.0, https://creativecommons.org/licenses/by/4.0/.)

customers to maximize revenues and profits (Kraak et al., 2019). Figure 14.1 categorizes various IMC techniques (i.e., branding, cartoon media characters, mascots, celebrities and influencers, packaging, product placement, premiums, sponsorship and child-targeted emotional appeals) through diverse media channels and platforms (i.e., print, television broadcast, digital, mobile devices and social media applications) and through diverse settings (i.e., schools, sporting events, food retail and restaurants, transportation and billboards) used by industry actors to create consistent and compelling messages to influence the diet-related cognitive, behavioural and health outcomes of children and adolescents (Kraak et al., 2019).

Co-branding has been used extensively to promote unhealthy HFSS food and beverage products to young people through sports sponsorship (Dixon et al., 2019); mascots and licensed characters (Kraak & Story, 2015); movie characters and toys (Dixon et al., 2017); celebrities and influencers (De Veirman et al., 2019; Zhou et al., 2019) and product packaging (Elliott and Truman, 2020; Smith et al., 2019).

Digital marketing has emerged recently as an important IMC technique to reach young people by promoting brands and products through digital platforms, mobile apps and electronic devices connected to the Internet (Kraak et al., 2020). The WHO (2016) defines digital marketing as "a promotional activity, delivered through a digital medium, that seeks to maximize impact through creative and/or analytic methods to build engagement and facilitate emotional persuasion (i.e., e-word of-mouth, influencers, online games and virtual environments); or analyze emotions, responses, preferences, behaviours and location to target vulnerable groups or individuals." Comprehensive reviews of digital marketing trends and techniques to influence the brand choices and HFSS product consumption of young people are beyond the scope of this chapter but available (De Veirman et al., 2019).

## 14.4 BEST-PRACTICE RECOMMENDATIONS TO REDUCE YOUNG PEOPLE'S EXPOSURE TO FOOD MARKETING

In May 2010, in World Health Assembly, Resolution WHA63.14 was endorsed by 193 member states of the UN that provided 12 recommendations for governments to restrict the marketing of unhealthy food and non-alcoholic beverage products to children (WHO, 2010). In 2012, WHO published a monitoring and evaluation framework for members to implement Resolution WHA63.14, and encouraged governments and civil society organizations to monitor all advertising and marketing practices targeted to children (WHO, 2012). Other goals and targets have been provided by subsequent UN and WHO documents and agreements from 2015 to 2020, including the WHO's Global Action Plan for Prevention and Control of Non-Communicable Diseases, 2013–2020; the UN Decade of Action on Nutrition, 2016–2025; and the UN Sustainable Development Goals 2030 Agenda. These documents have emphasized the importance of national governments fulfilling their international agreements and obligations by using a human rights framework to develop and implement comprehensive guidelines that will protect children and adolescents, birth up to age 18 years, and foster healthy food environments (Kraak et al., 2019; Kraak et al. 2020).

Nutrient profiling is a useful approach for policymakers to identify products that should be restricted in advertising and marketing to children. Table 14.1 describes the nutrient-profiling models released by the six WHO Regional Offices worldwide between 2015 and 2019 to guide member states in the development, implementation, and monitoring and evaluation of comprehensive policies to restrict the marketing of unhealthy HFSS food and beverage products to children and adolescents (Kraak et al., 2019).

These models include the WHO Regional Office for Europe (2015) formerly based in Copenhagen, Denmark, that has moved to Moscow, Russia, to provide technical assistance to 53 countries; Pan American Health Organization, WHO (2016) based in Washington, DC, United States that provides technical assistance to 35 countries; WHO Regional Office for the Western Pacific (2016) based in Manila, Philippines, that provides technical assistance to 37 countries; WHO Regional Office for South-East Asia (2016) headquartered in New Delhi, India, that provides technical assistance to 11 countries; WHO Regional Office for the Eastern Mediterranean (2017) based in Cairo, Egypt, that provides technical assistance to 22 countries and territories and the WHO Regional Office for Africa (2019) based in Brazzaville, Congo, that provides technical assistance to 46 countries.

Evaluations have compared these WHO nutrient-profiling guidelines (i.e., WHO Europe versus PAHO/WHO's NOVA classification guidelines for processed and ultra-process foods); compared them to government-recommended guidelines (i.e., Australia's Health-Star Rating versus PAHO's NOVA classification) and industry

**TABLE 14.1**
**Nutrient Profiling Models of Six World Health Organization (WHO) Regional Offices to Guide States to Restrict Unhealthy Food and Beverage Marketing to Children, 2015–2019**

| | WHO African Region (2019) *Brazzaville, Congo* | WHO Eastern Mediterranean Region (2017) *Cairo, Egypt* | WHO Regional Office for Europe (2015) *Copenhagen, Denmark* | PAHO/WHO Region of Americas (2016) *Washington, DC* | WHO Regional Office South-East Asia (2017) *New Delhi, India* | WHO Regional Office Western Pacific (2016) *Manila, Philippines* |
|---|---|---|---|---|---|---|
| Member states | 46 countries | 22 countries | 53 countries | 35 countries | 11 countries | 27 countries |
| Permitted food and beverage categories | Fresh and frozen vegetables and animal products | Fresh and frozen fruit, vegetables and legumes | Fresh and frozen meat, poultry, fish and similar; Fresh and frozen fruit, vegetables and legumes | Unprocessed or minimally processed foods | Fresh and frozen fruit, vegetables and legumes | Fresh and frozen fruit, vegetables and legumes |
| Food and beverage categories | 18[a] | 18 | 17 | 3[b] | 18[a] | 18[c] |
| Nutrients of concern ($n = 8$) | | | | | | |
| Total fat | | | | | | |
| Total sugars | | | | | | |
| Added sugars or free sugars | | | | | | |
| Non-sugar sweeteners or other non-nutritive sweeteners | n/a | | | | n/a | |

(*Continued*)

**TABLE 14.1 (*Continued*)**

**Nutrient Profiling Models of Six World Health Organization (WHO) Regional Offices to Guide States to Restrict Unhealthy Food and Beverage Marketing to Children, 2015–2019**

| | WHO African Region (2019) *Brazzaville, Congo* | WHO Eastern Mediterranean Region (2017) *Cairo, Egypt* | WHO Regional Office for Europe (2015) *Copenhagen, Denmark* | PAHO/WHO Region of Americas (2016) *Washington, DC* | WHO Regional Office South-East Asia (2017) *New Delhi, India* | WHO Regional Office Western Pacific (2016) *Manila, Philippines* |
|---|---|---|---|---|---|---|
| Energy | | | | | | |
| Saturated fat | | | | | | |
| Sodium or salt | | | | | | |
| Trans-fats | n/a | n/a | n/a | | | n/a |
| Prohibited food and beverage categories | Products that do not comply with the nutrient criteria including food products that contain >1% of total energy in the form of industrially produced trans-fatty acid (1% of energy = 20 kcal = 2.2 g trans-fat) | Products that do not comply with the nutrient criteria including chocolate and sugar confectionery, energy bars, and sweet toppings and deserts; fruit juices, energy drinks; edible ices; cakes, sweet biscuits and pastries; other sweet baked goods and dried mixes for making such goods | Products that do not comply with the nutrient criteria including chocolate, sugar confectionery, energy bars and sweet toppings and desserts; pastries; croissants; cookies/biscuits; sponge cakes; wafers; fruit pies; sweet buns; chocolate-covered biscuits; cake mixes and batters; juices, energy drinks and edible ices | Products that do not comply with the NOVA classification criteria including those classified as processed or ultra-processed | Products that do not comply with the nutrient criteria | Products that do not comply with the nutrient criteria including chocolate and sugar confectionery, energy bars and sweet toppings and desserts; cakes, sweet biscuits and pastries, and other sweet bakery products and dry mixes for making such; energy drinks, tea and coffee |

*Source:* Adapted from Kraak et al. (2019) and the WHO Regional Office reports (2015–2019).

*n/a:* not available.

[a] Based on the WHO's and FAO's CODEX Alimentarius categories.

[b] PAHO's NOVA classification categories: (i) minimally processed foods (unprocessed foods); (ii) culinary ingredients; (iii) processed foods (products manufactured by industry with two or three ingredients); and (iv) ultra-processed foods (industrial formulations manufactured with several taste and flavour-enhancing ingredients).

[c] Seventeen categories included in the European nutrient-profiling model, with criteria added for products made from soybeans.

guidelines (i.e., WHO Europe and the Children's Food & Beverage Advertising Initiative) (Labonté et al. 2017). The results suggest wide variation across the WHO, government and industry nutrient-profiling models. For example, Wootan et al. (2019) compared the WHO Europe guidelines with the CFBAI industry targets in 2015 and found that nearly half (49%) of the products allowed under the industry's guidelines exceeded level for sweeteners, a quarter (25%) exceeded the sodium levels and 6% exceeded calories. Moreover, only two out of 34 multi-component children's meals met the WHO Europe targets that would be allowed to be marketed under the industry's more permissive guidelines (Wootan et al., 2019). Nutrient profiling systems have limitations as some may provide a health halo for ultra-processed food products compared to more holistic ways of classifying foods that align with healthy eating patterns. These results raise important considerations for policymakers who must select a suitable nutrient-profiling model that is not too strict or ambiguous, but realistic for industry actors to reformulate or develop new and healthy products meeting recommended nutrient targets.

Adhering to the strict PAHO/WHO NOVA classification would require major restructuring of food systems and marketing practices to ensure full compliance. However, there is growing evidence that the consumption of highly processed or ultra-processed foods and beverages (i.e., chocolate, ice cream, cake, cookies (biscuits), sweets, sugary beverages, salty snacks, fries or chips and pizza) in various settings may trigger environmental cues that promote addictive eating behaviours in certain vulnerable individuals, including children and adolescents, which are reinforced through advertising and other IMC strategies shown in Figure 14.1 (Gearhardt et al., 2020).

By 2020, less than a third (31%) or 60 of 194 countries had reported implementing a national policy to restrict the marketing of unhealthy foods and beverages to children, of which half of the countries were located in the European region, and a majority of voluntary industry self-regulatory policies were in high-income countries (WHO, 2020). Only three of six WHO regional offices have conducted evaluations of corporate food and beverage marketing trends targeting young people in their regions, and most countries had adopted voluntary or selected statutory restrictions (WHO, 2020). Box 1 describes a case study for the UK government that implemented a national policy to restrict the marketing of unhealthy food and beverage products to children through media. Table 14.2 provides a timeline of UK food and beverage marketing regulatory policies, 2003–2020. The final section describes actions that diverse institutional actors can take to develop, implement, monitor and evaluate policies to protect and promote healthy dietary choices and healthy food environments for children and adolescents in countries and worldwide.

## 14.5 CASE STUDY: UK NATIONAL POLICIES TO RESTRICT THE MARKETING OF UNHEALTHY FOOD AND NON-ALCOHOLIC BEVERAGE PRODUCTS TO CHILDREN

The UK is one of the few countries in the world to restrict unhealthy food and non-alcoholic beverage advertising to children both on television and online using government-led and industry self-regulation approaches and to evaluate the

**TABLE 14.2**
**Timeline of UK Food and Beverage Marketing Regulatory Policies, 2003–2020**

| Year | Key Actions |
|---|---|
| 2003 | The Food Standards Agency commissioned report concludes that food advertising has both brand- and category-level effects on consumption in children (Hastings et al., 2003). |
| | Secretary of State for Culture, Media and Sport asks Ofcom, the UK communications regulator, to consider the need for proposals to strengthen the rules on television food advertising aimed at children. |
| 2004 | UK Health Department published the White Paper "Making Healthy Choices Easier" (2004) and warns of legislation if the food industry did not act to improve "the balance of food and drink advertising and promotion to children". |
| 2006 | Ofcom concluded that advertising has a "modest, direct effect on children's food choices and a larger but unquantifiable indirect effect on children's food preferences, consumption and behaviour" (Livingstone, 2006). |
| | UK Government mandates Ofcom to act through legislation to protect children's diet and health. |
| 2007 | Ofcom announced new scheduling restrictions and content rules to be introduced in a phased approach between 2007 and 2009 (Ofcom, 2007) |
| 2008 | Ofcom published first, interim, evaluation of TV advertising regulation effectiveness (Ofcom, 2008) |
| 2010 | Ofcom published second and final evaluation of TV advertising regulation effectiveness (Ofcom, 2010) |
| 2015 | House of Commons Health Committee (2015) undertook an inquiry into childhood obesity that resulted in the report titled, "Brave and Bold Action" that recommended tougher controls on marketing and advertising of unhealthy food and drink |
| 2016 | UK Government published a childhood obesity plan that does not feature food marketing controls. The UK's Committee of Advertising Practice introduced new rules restricting digital advertising of HFSS foods and non-alcoholic beverages in children's media and where children make up more than 25% of the audience to commence in 2017 (CAP, 2016). |
| 2018 | Following a further Health and Social Care Committee inquiry into childhood obesity, the UK Government published an updated childhood obesity plan (Chapter 2) that committed to conducting a consultation to introduce a 9:00 pm watershed for advertising of HFSS products on television and online |
| 2019 | UK Government launched a consultation on the introduction of further HFSS advertising restrictions on television and online and published a green paper titled, "Advancing our health: prevention in the 2020s," which contained a third childhood obesity plan that committed to following up on the advertising consultation |
| 2020 | UK Government announced a new obesity strategy that included a ban on television and online advertising for food high in fat, sugar and salt before 9:00 pm to be implemented by the end of 2022 |

impact of these policies. Table 14.2 provides a timeline of UK food and beverage marketing regulatory policies from 2003 through 2020. The UK government has committed to further strengthen the regulations that were updated in 2021 (UK Government, 2021) to implement effective policies to restrict online and digital marketing of unhealthy food and beverage products to children to protect their diet and health.

### 14.5.1 Television Food Advertising Regulation

In 2003, the UK Food Standards Agency commissioned a report that concluded food advertising produced both brand- and category-level effects on children's dietary choices and intake (Hastings et al., 2003). Based on a comprehensive commissioned review (Livingstone, 2006), the UK Ofcom concluded that advertising had a large but unquantifiable indirect effect on children's food preferences, consumption and behaviours (Ofcom, 2008), which justified the UK government to take regulatory actions to protect children's health.

In 2007, the UK became the first country in the European region to introduce legally binding regulations specifically targeting the television advertising of foods and non-alcoholic beverages HFSS to children. The principal aim of these restrictions was to "reduce the exposure of children to HFSS advertising, as a means of reducing opportunities to persuade children to demand and consume HFSS products" (Ofcom, 2008: p. 1). The regulations preceded the WHO 2010 recommendations by 3 years and were pioneering due to the comprehensive nature of the restrictions and the substantial step-change from previous controls, self-regulatory codes from the Broadcasting Committee of Advertising Practice, which had largely focused on preventing misleading advertising.

The UK regulations included scheduling restrictions that banned HFSS food and beverage advertising (determined by a nutrient profile model that allocated scores to products) on dedicated children's television channels and in and around any programming "of particular appeal" to children under 16 years, where the proportion of children in the viewing audience is at least 20% higher than in the general population. Content rules also prohibited the use of particular marketing strategies for HFSS food and beverage product advertisements targeted directly at pre-school or primary school children, such as the use of promotional characters (licensed only as brand-equity characters or brand mascots were exempt) and premium offers such as free toys, celebrity endorsers and nutritional or health claims, and stated that advertisements must not encourage excessive consumption of any food or drink product or appeal to emotions such as fear or self-confidence so as to "reduce children's emotional engagement with unhealthy advertisements" (Ofcom, 2008; p. 8).

The official evaluation of the effectiveness of the restrictions concluded that in 2009, compared with 2005 before the regulations came into force, children in the UK saw ~37% less HFSS advertising or 4.4 billion fewer impacts with ten impacts being equivalent to ten people viewing a single advertisement, or one person seeing the advertisement ten times (Ofcom, 2010). This was reportedly driven by the virtual elimination of HFSS advertising spots from children's airtime. However, this review determined that HFSS advertising around programming in adult airtime, such as soap operas and entertainment shows that were not directed at but often watched by children in large numbers, had substantially increased.

### 14.5.2 Digital Food Advertising Regulations

In 2017, the UK's Committee of Advertising Practice (CAP) introduced new rules for digital advertising of HFSS foods and non-alcoholic beverages. The updated codes, administered by an industry self-regulatory body called the Advertising Standards

Authority, banned advertising for HFSS products in "children's media" online (e.g. a website aimed at children) or other content for which children under 16 years make up more than 25% of the audience (e.g., a YouTube influencer video with general appeal but also a substantial child audience) (ASA, 2019).

The onus was placed on marketers to demonstrate that these audience thresholds were not breached. The definition of HFSS food and beverage products was based on using the same nutrient profile model for television, and these rules were seen to harmonize non-broadcast regulation with broadcast that was a step towards media neutrality. The ASA conducted two evaluations of online self-regulation effectiveness in 2019, which identified 947 breaches in a 2-week period on YouTube channels targeted to children (ASA, 2019); and 2020 that further identified breaches over a 3-month period, including 78 different HFSS advertisements from 29 advertisers appearing within child-focused content (e.g., 24 websites and 5 YouTube channels) (ASA, 2020).

It is important to note that these evaluations only examined websites that attracted "disproportionately high" child audiences and were not a comprehensive assessment of the full range of online content children that engage in such as social media and signed-in environments. Several complaints have been raised by non-governmental advocacy organizations, including the Children's Food Campaign (Sustain) and the Obesity Health Alliance, about perceived non-compliance with the online rules, with some complaints ultimately being upheld by the ASA. For example, where materials were found to be HFSS and directed at children or dismissed, where influencer content was deemed to not focus on themes of "particular appeal" to under 16s, and where <25% of followers worldwide were registered as under 18 years, despite the influencers in question having been nominated for, and winning, a number of major children and teen media awards (WHO Europe, 2016).

### 14.5.3 What Next for UK Food Marketing Regulatory Policy?

In July 2020, the UK Department of Health and Social Care published a policy paper that stated the intention to "ban HFSS products being shown on TV and online before 9:00 pm… and introduce a total HFSS advertising restriction online. It is our intention to implement both TV and online measures at the same time" and new restrictions for online marketing were released in 2021 (UK Government, 2021). Health impact modelling suggests that a 9 pm television watershed would reduce the number of children (5–17 years) with obesity by 4.6%, and children with overweight and obesity by 3.6%, resulting in a health-related net monetary benefit of £7.4 billion to society (Mytton et al. 2020). However, a government-commissioned evaluation of the potential impact of a 9 pm watershed online found an underestimation of the scale of children's exposure to marketing on digital devices at least tenfold or more (Tatlow-Golden and Parker, 2020).

## 14.6 PRIVATE-SECTOR ACTORS INVOLVED IN FOOD AND BEVERAGE MARKETING TO YOUNG PEOPLE

A myriad of private-sector actors, business sectors and actor networks are engaged in marketing activities to promote food and beverage brands and products to young people. Table 14.3 describes major transnational industry actors involved in food and

**TABLE 14.3**
**Examples of Major Transnational Industry Actors Involved in Food and Beverage Marketing to Children and Adolescents Using Data from Kraak et al. (2019) and Kraak et al. (2020)**

| Industry Trade Associations and Alliances | Food and Beverage Manufacturers | Chain Restaurants | Retailer Firms | Entertainment Firms | Digital Technology Firms |
|---|---|---|---|---|---|
| International Food & Beverage Alliance (IFBA) (*12 members*) | Coca-Cola Company | McDonald's Corporation | Walmart | DreamWorks Animation | Alphabet Inc. (Android Enterprise, Google and YouTube and YouTube Kids) |
| European Union (EU) Platform for Action on Diet, Physical Activity and Health (*22 members in 27 countries*) | Danone | Starbucks | Costco | Sesame Workshop | Amazon Global, Inc. (Twitch Prime) |
| International Chamber of Commerce (ICC) | Ferrero | Subway | 7-Eleven Holdings | Viacom (*Nickelodeon*) | Facebook, Inc. (Facebook, Instagram, Messenger, Oculus and WhatsApp) |
| World Federation of Advertisers (WFA) & Consumers Goods Forum (CGF) | General Mills, Inc. | Yum! Brands, Inc. (*KFC, Pizza Hut* and *Taco Bell*) | Lidl Kaufland | Walt Disney Company | Microsoft Corporation (LinkedIn and Skype) |
| | Grupo Bimbo | Domino's Pizza | Aldi | Warner Brothers Entertainment, Inc. | Reddit (Reddit) |
| | Kellogg Company | Burger King (*Hungry Jacks*) | Carrefour | | Snap, Inc. (Snapchat) Twitter (Twitter) |
| | Mars Incorporated | | Aeon | | |
| | Mondelez International | | Tesco | | |
| | Nestle S.A. | | Target | | |
| | PepsiCo, Inc. | | | | |
| | Unilever | | | | |

beverage marketing to children and adolescents through voluntary commitments, codes of conduct and self-regulatory programmes in countries and regions worldwide (Kraak et al., 2019; Kraak et al., 2020). An in-depth analysis of their networks and interactions is needed to inform future accountability actions. Evaluations have examined the effectiveness of self-regulatory programmes and policies developed by food and beverage manufacturers, chain restaurants, entertainment firms, digital technology firms and sectors or trade associations through alliances and networks at national, regional and global levels (Kraak et al., 2019; Kraak et al., 2020).

An accountability evaluation of the IFBA's Global Marketing Communications Policy (2009–2019) showed several weaknesses to adequately protecting children from the aggressive marketing of unhealthy HFSS food and beverage products (Kraak et al., 2019). Before August 2021, the IFBA policy failed to use a children's rights-based approach, as recommended by the United Nations (Garde et al., 2018) and did not cover the wide range of digital marketing and media in voluntary pledges for children under 12 years (Kraak et al., 2019). The Global Policy was updated in August 2021 and applies to products that meet common nutrition criteria advertised through many media platforms (IFBA, 2021).

Voluntary industry codes of conduct are applied only to children under 13 years (International Food & Beverage Alliance, 2021; World Federation of Advertisers, 2021); fail to protect children aged 13–17 years, as recommended by the International Chamber of Commerce (2018), or children up to 18 years, as recommended by the WHO Europe (2016) and UNICEF (Garde et al., 2018); and have failed to adopt uniform nutrient-profiling standards to guide all IMC strategies targeted at young people (Kraak et al., 2019). Evaluations reveal that governments have often permitted industry to set their own targets through industry-funded programmes, firms have exploited loopholes and existing programmes lack adequate accountability and enforcement mechanisms for industry non-participation or when firms underperform and do not meet established targets. Over 15 years (2005–2020), no company or industry sector has set targets that adhere to the UN and WHO best-practice guidelines to protect children and adolescents from the marketing practices of industry actors that encourage predominantly unhealthy HFSS food and beverage products.

The UN Secretary General and WHO Director General should use legal approaches to enable states to take actions against commercial influences that undermine young people's diet. The 2020 WHO-UNICEF-Lancet Commission on the Future for the World's Children acknowledged the limitations of industry self-regulatory programmes and recommended that the UN develop an Optional Protocol to the Convention on the Rights of the Child for states to ratify to protect children from the marketing of unhealthy products (Clark et al., 2020). The WHO Director General should use Article 19 of the WHO Constitution to develop a legally binding Framework Convention to Protect and Promote Healthy and Sustainable Food Systems similar to the WHO Framework Convention on Tobacco Control. All food system actors should support the principles of healthy and sustainable food systems and be held accountable for policies that promote a commercial foodscape to protect and promote healthy dietary patterns. Table 14.4 summarizes recommended actions for UN System agencies, national governments, industry actors, civil society organizations and private foundations to create healthy food environments for young people globally.

**TABLE 14.4**
**Recommended Actions for Institutional Actors to Leverage Marketing Practices and Resources to Create Healthy Food Environments for Young People Globally Using Information from Kraak et al. (2020), free to Use under UN Permissions**

| Actor | Actions |
|---|---|
| United Nations agencies | The WHO, UN Global Compact and UN Committee on the Rights of the Child should convene actors to clarify common guidelines and standards for food and beverage marketing to children and adolescents from birth up to 18 years. |
| | WHO should provide technical assistance to national governments to develop comprehensive and cost-effective policies that restrict young people's exposure to the digital marketing of HFSS food and beverage products, and protect children's rights to adequate food and nutrition, health and privacy from marketing practices. |
| | WHO and its six regional offices should ensure that digital marketing is included in existing guidelines and standards to restrict HFSS food and beverage marketing to children and adolescents up to 18 years of age. |
| | WHO should assist states to monitor the implementation of commitments and evaluate the impact of actions to achieve targets. |
| | The WHO Director General should use Article 19 of the WHO Constitution to develop a legally binding Framework Convention to Protect and Promote Healthy Diets. |
| | The UN Secretary General should develop an optional protocol for the Convention on the Rights of the Child to protect children from the marketing of HFSS food and beverage products, social media, and the inappropriate use of their personal data. |
| States or national governments | Prioritize food marketing to children on the national agenda to restrict unhealthy HFSS food and beverage marketing policies that will also protect young people's digital privacy rights. |
| | Develop comprehensive national legislation, laws and regulations to cover all forms of digital marketing aimed at children and adolescents to align them with recommended best practices. |
| | Collaborate with international and regional bodies to develop cross-border policies to regulate transnational food and beverage marketing to young people. |
| | Monitor and evaluate how transnational companies are using marketing practices and digital media platforms including social media, and strengthen accountability for their practices in all countries where they operate. |
| | Appoint and empower independent bodies and regulatory institutions to require transparency and full disclosures to ensure accountability for industry actors. |
| | Support the WHO Director General to develop a legally binding Framework Convention to Protect and Promote Healthy and Sustainable Diets. |
| | Ratify international treaties and translate the principles and guidelines into national laws to protect children worldwide from the marketing of unhealthy food and beverage products. |
| | Prohibit businesses from collecting data from children and adolescents through digital marketing, including mobile applications. |
| | Ensure that international trade and investment agreements do not limit the ability of national governments to restrict and regulate HFSS food and beverage marketing to young people through digital marketing and media. |

*(Continued)*

**TABLE 14.4 (*Continued*)**
**Recommended Actions for Institutional Actors to Leverage Marketing Practices and Resources to Create Healthy Food Environments for Young People Globally Using Information from Kraak et al. (2020), free to Use under UN Permissions**

| Actor | Actions |
|---|---|
| Technology firms | Develop policies that protect the digital privacy rights of young people and enforce standards for digital platforms that support responsible food and beverage marketing to children and adolescents, aligning them with national, regional and international laws and recommended best practices. |
| | Ensure that digital marketing and privacy policies for children and adolescents are posted on firms' public websites in countries where they operate. |
| Food, beverage, restaurant and retailer firms | IFBA firms should amend their Global Policy on Marketing Communications to Children and apply the WHO-recommended nutrient profile standards for food and beverage marketing to young people on all social media platforms and digital and mobile devices. |
| | IFBA firms should ensure that children's rights are explicitly addressed in the amended Global Policy and identify processes for mitigating the adverse impacts of digital marketing and media on children's diet, health and well-being. |
| | All firms should update and harmonize the company policies on responsible food and beverage marketing to children with the policies of national, regional and international bodies and ensure that digital marketing and media policies are posted on companies' external websites in countries where they operate. |
| Civil society organizations | Advocate and mobilize populations to demand strong government policies to protect young people' digital privacy. |
| | Monitor and evaluate the effectiveness of voluntary commitments on digital marketing and media used to promote food and beverage brands and products to children and adolescents, as well as the impact of healthy and sustainable lifestyle programmes that use digital marketing and media to encourage healthy and responsible consumption behaviour. |
| | Hold national governments to account and encourage transnational firms to implement best-practice recommendations and voluntary codes of conduct that protect children from unhealthy food and beverage marketing practices. |
| Private foundations | Access to Nutrition Foundation, Gates Foundation, Clinton Foundation and Bloomberg Philanthropies could fund research and evaluations conducted by governments and civil society organizations that use common frameworks, tools and metrics to assess the impact of policies over time. |
| | Private foundations could fund and help to widely disseminate research through diverse communication channels including social media, to inform future policies and business practices. |

## 14.7 CONCLUSIONS

Two decades of evidence shows that the marketing practices used by industry actors have created unhealthy food environments that have influenced the attitudes, preferences, choices and eating behaviours and health risks for children, adolescents and their adult parents. The result has been to create a food environment where highly processed, branded HFSS food and beverage products are tasty, convenient, accessible and affordable compared with minimally processed foods such as fruits and vegetables, whole grains and plant-based proteins recommended by governments.

Evaluations of transnational industry actors' voluntary commitments and self-regulatory programmes compared with best-practice recommendations have revealed inherent inadequacies, and also that national governments have failed to adequately protect children from the consequences of marketing on young people's diets and health. States must implement strong accountability structures to protect children's diet and health. National governments that allow industry to make modest or no changes and continue "business as usual" are complicit in unethical and unconscionable actions. Many institutional actors must commit to using marketing that align with principles of healthy and sustainable food systems and restrict the marketing of unhealthy products to children and adolescents to meet the UN targets to ensure healthy lives for all.

## REFERENCES

Advertising Standards Authority. (2019). ASA monitoring report on online HFSS ads. Advertising Standards Authority. https://www.asa.org.uk/uploads/assets/uploaded/14be798d-bd30-49d6-bcfbc9ed7e66e565.pdf.

Advertising Standards Authority. (2020). Protecting children online: building a zero-tolerance culture to age-restricted ads in children's media. ASA, August 26. https://www.asa.org.uk/news/protecting-children-online.html.

American Marketing Association. (2020). Branding. https://www.ama.org/topics/branding/.

Boyland, E.J., Nolan, S., Kelly, B. et al. (2016). Advertising as a cue to consume: a systematic review and meta-analysis of the effects of acute exposure to unhealthy food and nonalcoholic beverage advertising on intake in children and adults. Am J Clin Nutr, 103:519–533. doi: 10.3945/ajcn.115.120022.

Cairns, G. (2019). A critical review of evidence on the sociocultural impacts of food marketing and policy implications. *Appetite*. 136:193–207. doi: 10.1016/j.appet.2019.02.002.

Clark, H., Coll-Seck, A.M., Banerjee, A., Peterson, S., Dalgleish, S.L., Ameratunga, S. et al. (2020). A future for the world's children? A WHO-UNICEF-lancet commission. *Lancet,* 395(10224):605–668. doi: 10.1016/S0140-6736(19)32540-1.

Committee of Advertising Practice (2016). CAP consultation: food and soft drink advertising to children. Regulatory statement. 8 December. https://www.asa.org.uk/asset/98337008-FA03-481B-92392CB3487720A8/.

Cornwell, T.B., McAlister, A.R., Polmear-Swendris, N. (2014). Children's knowledge of packaged and fast food brands and their BMI. Why the relationship matters for policy makers. *Appetite,* 81:277–283 doi: 10.1016/j.appet.2014.06.017.

Crone, E.A., Bullens, L., van der Plas, E.A.A., Kijkuit, E.J., Zelazo, P.D. (2008). Developmental changes and individual differences in risk and perspective taking in adolescence. *Dev Psychopathol,* 20(4):1213–1229. doi: 10.1017/S0954579408000588.

De Veirman, M., Hudders, L., Nelson, M.R. (2019). What is influencer marketing and how does it target children? A review and direction for future research. *Front Psych,* 10:2685. doi: 10.3389/fpsyg.2019.02685.

Dixon, H., Niven, P., Scully, M., Wakefield, M. (2017). Food marketing with movie character toys: effects on young children's preferences for unhealthy and healthier fast food meals. *Appetite*, 117:342–350. doi: 10.1016/j.appet.2017.07.014.

Dixon, H., Lee, A., Scully, M. (2019). Sports sponsorship as a cause of obesity. *Curr Obes Rep,* 8:480–494. doi: 10.1007/s13679-019-00363-z.

Elliott, C., Truman, E. (2020). The power of packaging: a scoping review and assessment of child-targeted food packaging. *Nutrients,* 12(4):958. doi: 10.3390/nu12040958.

Garde, A., Byrne, S., Gokani, N., Murphy, B. (2018). A child rights-based approach to food marketing: A guide for policymakers. United Nations Children's Fund (UNICEF), New York. https://www.unicef.org/csr/files/A_Child_Rights-Based_Approach_to_Food_Marketing_Report.pdf.

Gearhardt, A.N., Yokum, S., Harris, J.L., Epstein, L.H., Lumeng, J.C. (2020). Neural response to fast food commercials in adolescents predicts intake. *Am J Clin Nutr,* 11(3):493–502. doi: 10.1093/ajcn/nqz305.

Harris, J.L., Pomeranz, J.L. (2020). Infant formula and toddler milk marketing: opportunities to address harmful practices and improve young children's diets. *Nutr Rev,* 78(10):866–883. doi: 10.1093/nutrit/nuz095.

Hastings, G., Stead, M., McDermott, L., Forsyth, A., MacKintosh, A.M., Rayner, M., Godfrey, C., Caraher, M., Angus, K. (2003). Review of research on the effects of food promotion to children. Final Report, prepared for the Food Standards Agency. Glasgow, Scotland: University of Strathclyde Centre for Social Marketing. https://www.researchgate.net/publication/242490173_Review_Of_Research_On_The_Effects_Of_Food_Promotion_To_Children.

House of Commons Health Committee (2015). Childhood obesity – brave and bold action. 30 November. https://publications.parliament.uk/pa/cm 201516/cmselect/cmhealth/465/465.pdf.

International Chamber of Commerce (ICC). 2018. ICC advertising and marketing communication code, Paris, France. https://cms.iccwbo.org/content/uploads/sites/3/2018/09/icc-advertising-and-marketing-communications-code-int.pdf.

International Food & Beverage Alliance. (2021). IFBA Global Responsible Marketing Policy. https://ifballiance.org/publications/responsible-marketing-commitments/.

Kraak, V.I., Story, M. (2015). Influence of food companies' brand mascots and entertainment companies' cartoon media characters on children's diet and health: a systematic review and research needs. *Obes Rev,* 16(2):107–126. doi: 10.1111/obr.12237.

Kraak, V.I., Rincón-Gallardo Patiño, S., Sacks, G. (2019). Accountability evaluation for the International Food & Beverage Alliance's Global Policy on Marketing Communications to Children to reduce obesity: a narrative review to inform policy. *Obesity Rev,* 20(S2):90–106. doi: 10.1111/obr.12859.

Kraak, V.I., Zhou, M., Rincón-Gallardo Patiño, S. (2020). Digital marketing to young people: consequences for the health and diets of future generations. *UNSCN Nutr*, 45:9–24 https://www.unscn.org/uploads/web/news/UNSCN-Nutrition-45-WEB.pdf.

Labonté, M.È., Poon, T., Mulligan, C., Bernstein, J.T, Franco-Arellano, B., L'Abbé, M.R. (2017). Comparison of global nutrient profiling systems for restricting the commercial marketing of foods and beverages of low nutritional quality to children in Canada. *Am J Clin Nutr,* 106(6):1471–1481. doi: 10.3945/ajcn.117.161356.

Livingstone, S. (2006). Does TV advertising make children fat? What the evidence tells us. *Public Policy Res*, 13(1), 54–61. http://eprints.lse.ac.uk/1026.

Lobstein, T., Jackson-Leach, R., Moodie, M.L., Hall, K.D., Gortmaker, S.I., Swinburn, B.A., James, W.P.T., Wang, Y., McPherson, K. (2015). Child and adolescent obesity: part of a bigger picture. *Lancet,* 385(9986):2510–2520. doi: 10.1016/S0140-6736(14)61746-3.

Lycett, K., Juonala, M., Magnussen, C.G., et al. (2020). Body mass index from early to late childhood and cardiometabolic measurements at 11 to 12 years. *Pediatrics,* 146(2):e20193666. doi: 10.1542/peds.2019-3666.

Mennella, J.A. (2014) Ontogeny of taste preferences: basic biology and implications for health. *Am J Clin Nutr,* 99(3):704S–711S. doi: 10.3945/ajcn.113.067694.
Mytton, O.T., Boyland, E., Adams, J., et al. (2020). The potential health impact of restricting less-healthy food and beverage advertising on UK television between 05.30 and 21.00 hours: a modelling study. *PLoS Med,* 17(10):e1003212. doi: 10.1371/journal.pmed.1003212.
Office of Communication (Ofcom). (2007). Television advertising of food and drink products to children: final statement. Ofcom: London, UK. https://www.ofcom.org.uk/__data/assets/pdf_file/0028/47746/Television-Advertising-of-Food-and-Drink-Products-to-Children-Final-statement-.pdf.
Ofcom. (2008). Changes in the nature and balance of television food advertising to children: a review of HFSS advertising restrictions. 17 December, Ofcom: London, UK. https://www.ofcom.org.uk/__data/assets/pdf_file/0028/23977/hfssdec08.pdf.
Ofcom. (2010). HFSS advertising restrictions: final review. 26 July, Ofcom: London, UK. https://www.ofcom.org.uk/__data/assets/pdf_file/0024/31857/hfss-review-final.pdf.
Roberto, C.A., Swinburn, B., Hawkes, C., Huang T.T.K, Costa, S.A., Ashe, M., Zwicker, L., Cawley, J.H., Brownell, K.D. (2015). Patchy progress on obesity prevention: emerging examples, entrenched barriers, and new thinking. *Lancet,* 385(9985):2400–2409. doi: 10.1016/S0140-6736(14)61744-X.
Shekar, M., Popkin, B., eds. (2019). *Obesity Health and Economic Consequences of an Impending Global Challenge.* The World Bank Group. https://openknowledge.worldbank.org/bitstream/handle/10986/32383/211491ov.pdf?sequence=4&isAllowed=y.
Smith, R., Kelly, B., Yeatman, H., Boyland, E. (2019). Food marketing influences children's attitudes, preferences and consumption: a systematic critical review. *Nutrients,* 11(4):875. doi: 10.3390/nu11040875.
Tatlow-Golden, M., Parker, D. (2020). The devil is in the detail: challenging the UK Department of Health's 2019 impact assessment of the extent of online marketing of unhealthy foods to children. *Int J Environ Res Public Health,* 17(19):7231. doi: 10.3390/ijerph17197231.
Truman, E., Elliott C. (2019). Identifying food marketing to teenagers: a scoping review. *Int J Behav Nutr Phys Activity,* 16(1):67. doi: 10.1186/s12966-019-0833-2.
UK Government (2016). Childhood obesity: a plan for action. Updated 20 January 2017. https://www.gov.uk/government/publications/childhood-obesity-a-plan-for-action/childhood-obesity-a-plan-for-action.
UK Government (2019). Advancing our health: prevention in the 2020s, 1 July. https://assets.publishing.service.gov.uk/government/uploads/system/uploads/attachment_data/file/819766/advancing-our-health-prevention-in-the-2020s-accessible.pdf.
UK Government (2021). Consultation outcome. Introducing further advertising restrictions on TV and online for products high in fat, salt and sugar: government response. Updated 24 June 2021. https://www.gov.uk/government/consultations/further-advertising-restrictions-for-products-high-in-fat-salt-and-sugar/outcome/introducing-further-advertising-restrictions-on-tv-and-online-for-products-high-in-fat-salt-and-sugar-government-response.
UK Government, Department of Health (2004). Choosing health: making healthy choices easier. 16 November. https://webarchive.nationalarchives.gov.uk, http://www.dh.gov.uk/en/Publicationsandstatistics/Publications/PublicationsPolicyAndGuidance/DH_4094550.
UK Government, Department of Health and Social Care (2018). Childhood obesity: a plan for action, chapter 2, 25 June. https://www.gov.uk/government/publications/childhood-obesity-a-plan-for-action-chapter-2.
UK Government, Department of Health and Social Care. (2020). New obesity strategy unveiled as country urged to lose weight to beat coronavirus (COVID-19) and protect the NHS, 27 July [press release]. https://www.gov.uk/government/news/new-obesity-strategy-unveiled-as-country-urged-to-lose-weight-to-beat-coronavirus-covid-19-and-protect-the-nhs.

World Federation of Advertisers. (2021). Responsible advertising to children.
https://wfanet.org/services/connect-to-your-peers/responsible-advertising-and-children/detail.
WHO Europe. (2016). Tackling food marketing to children in a digital world: trans-disciplinary perspectives children's rights, evidence of impact, methodological challenges, regulatory options and policy implications for the WHO European Region. Copenhagen, Denmark. http://www.euro.who.int/__data/assets/pdf_file/0017/322226/Tackling-food-marketing-children-digital-world-trans-disciplinary-perspectives-en.pdf?ua=1.
WHO. (2010). Set of recommendations on the marketing of foods and non-alcoholic beverages to children. Geneva, Switzerland. http://whqlibdoc.who.int/publications/2010/9789241500210_eng.pdf.
WHO. (2012). A framework for implementing the set of recommendations on the marketing of foods and non-alcoholic beverages to children. Geneva, Switzerland. http://www.who.int/dietphysicalactivity/MarketingFramework2012.pdf.
WHO. (2020). Assessing national capacity for the prevention and control of noncommunicable diseases: report of the 2019 global survey. 23 March. https://www.who.int/publications/i/item/ncd-ccs-2019.
WHO Europe. (2018). Evaluating implementation of the WHO set of recommendations on the marketing of foods and non-alcoholic beverages to children: Progress, challenges and guidance for next steps in the WHO European Region. Copenhagen, Denmark. https://www.euro.who.int/__data/assets/pdf_file/0003/384015/food-marketing-kids-eng.pdf.
Wootan, M.G., Almay, J., Ugalde, M., Kaminski, M. (2019). How do nutrition guidelines compare for industry to market food and beverage products to children? World Health Organization nutrient profile standards versus the US Children's Food and Beverage Advertising Initiative. *Childhood Obesity,* 15(3):194–199. doi: 10.1089/chi.2018.0256.
World Cancer Research Fund International. (2020). Building momentum: lessons on implementing robust restrictions of food and non-alcoholic beverage marketing to children. https://www.wcrf.org/sites/default/files/PPA-Building-Momentum-3-WEB-3.pdf.
World Obesity Federation (2019). Atlas of childhood obesity. London, United Kingdom. https://www.worldobesity.org/nlsegmentation/global-atlas-on-childhood-obesity.
Zhou, M., Rajamohan, S., Hedrick, V., Rincón-Gallardo Patiño, S., Abidi, F., Polys, N., Kraak, V. (2019). Mapping the celebrity endorsement of branded food and beverage products and marketing campaigns in the United States, 1990–2017. *Int J Environ Res Public Health,* 16:3743. doi: 10.3390/ijerph16193743.

# 15 Portion and Serving Size of Energy- and Nutrient-Dense Foods

*Holly L. Rippin, Marion M. Hetherington, and Charlotte E.L. Evans*
University of Leeds

## CONTENTS



## 15.1 INTRODUCTION

Large portion sizes of energy dense foods have been identified as increasing risk of unhealthy weight gain. Portion sizes of many foods have increased over the last few decades, particularly in the US (Ledikwe et al., 2005). In the UK, portion sizes have increased in foods high in fats, sugars and salt (HFSS) in the last few decades, albeit to a lesser degree than in the US. For example, a UK review (British Heart Foundation, 2013) reported that since 1993 'American muffins' had increased in size by 81%, pies by 40% and a single serve packet of crisps by 50%. On the other hand, intakes of fruits and vegetables are too low in most populations, both in terms of frequency of consumption and portion sizes. Analysis of the UK National Diet and Nutrition Survey (NDNS), a large, repeated cross-sectional survey that measures food and nutrient consumption and food behaviours in a nationally representative sample, revealed that the average portion size of vegetables for children is 40 g and median intake is only once per day (Chawner et al., 2021).

DOI: 10.1201/9781003043720-15

Much of the research to date focusses on the impact on diet and health of *increasing* intakes of large portions of energy-dense foods. However, less is known about the impact on health and diet quality of *reducing* portions of energy-dense foods. This research is warranted as most recommendations and policies are based on reducing portion sizes of energy-dense foods. However, to increase diet quality, the aim is to simultaneously increase the portion size of nutrient-dense foods and reduce intake of high energy density, low nutrient-dense foods.

This chapter reviews the evidence for the effects of portion size of energy-dense foods and fruits and vegetables on diet quality in different age groups. It also investigates different strategies, and relevant factors, for optimising portion size of packaged and unpackaged foods.

## 15.2 PORTION SIZE OF ENERGY-DENSE FOODS

There is reliable, robust evidence that a 'portion size effect' exists, where large portion sizes encourage increased energy intake. Over time, large portions could result in weight gain, although few studies have examined the causal links between increased portion size and obesity. This is mainly due to the challenges of assessing manipulations of portion size and resulting effects of this on weight change in the long term. However, it is clear that portion sizes are important in terms of diet quality and health. Consequently, the effects of habitual exposure to large portion sizes of energy-dense foods and drinks are crucial to investigate.

Most studies linking portion size to increased energy intakes have been conducted in the US. These laboratory-based experiments mainly suggest that consumption increases when individuals are exposed to large portions (Rolls et al., 2002). Well-controlled, albeit short-term, laboratory-based studies have repeatedly demonstrated that large portion sizes of energy-dense food increase energy intake over a period of days, in both adults and children (Rolls et al., 2007, Smethers et al., 2019). These studies also show that both adults and children fail to adjust intake with the resulting cumulative effect of increased intake over time.

These studies indicate that not only is the portion size effect reliably demonstrated in adults and children but that when participants are served bigger portions, of macaroni cheese for example, half do not notice any difference and that people adjust their level of satiety to accommodate greater energy intakes (Rolls et al., 2002). The 'portion size effect', where energy intake and portion size are positively associated, is also shown when the food served is a discrete unit, for example a sandwich (Rolls et al., 2004).

Hollands et al. (2015) conducted a systematic review on portion and package size which concluded that individuals consistently ate more when offered larger portion sizes. The meta-analysis conducted on the effect of portion and package size estimated that a 67% increase in portion size increased energy intake by about 16%. If this increase was sustained over time, it would be sufficient to promote weight gain. Figure 15.1 presents drivers of the portion size effect and some downsizing strategies (Hetherington et al., 2018).

Strategies to reduce portion size effects of energy-dense foods can mainly focus on individuals or on the food environment. Individual approaches include increasing

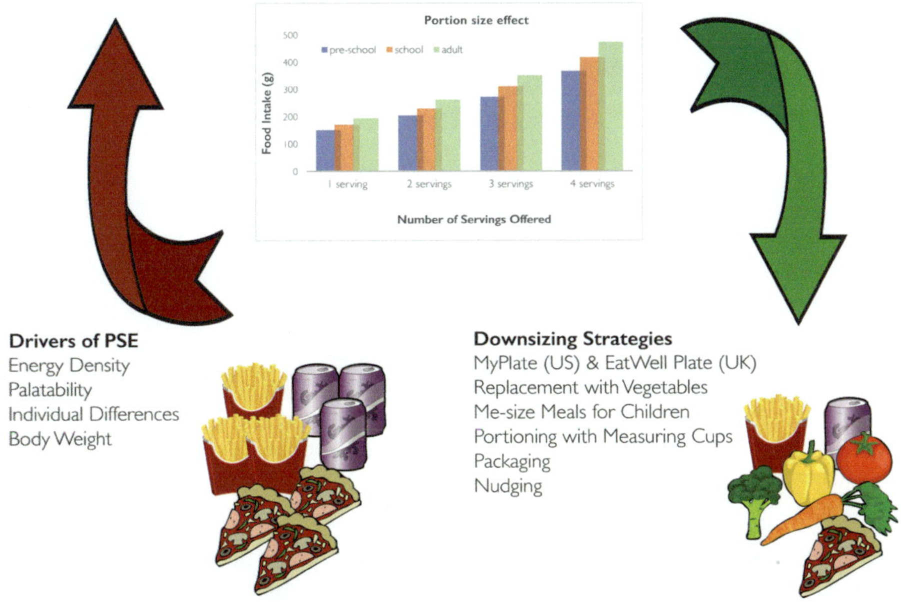


**FIGURE 15.1** Potential drivers of the portion size effect and potential strategies to counteract the portion size effect reprinted under licence CC 4.0. (From Hetherington et al. (2018).)

awareness of appropriate portion sizes for children at home which when coupled with increased availability of appropriate sized children's meals out of the home have the potential to change social norms. Acceptability of smaller portions by consumers is important in terms of effectiveness in reducing portions and price is also key. If the price per portion remains the same while portions decrease, this represents worse value for money for consumers. Suggested environmental methods for reducing average portion sizes without reducing consumer acceptability include offering a range of portions and changing the default portion size and restricting super-size portions (Marteau et al., 2015). An example is provided in Figure 15.2 which depicts bowls of rice in four sizes sold in a Japanese university canteen. Changing the default portion size offered is a form of nudging (see Chapter 16).

Another approach, to reduce portion sizes of energy-dense foods, is to reduce the use of non-proportional pricing whereby larger portion sizes are cheaper per gram than smaller portions (Marteau et al., 2015). This is common practice in food outlets and is demonstrated in Figure 15.3 where a menu informs customers that four doughnuts cost £3.00 whilst six doughnuts cost £3.50, only 50 p extra for 50% more doughnuts. This desire for value for money is also related to price (see Chapter 17).

An updated review of the effects of portion size (Almiron-Roig et al., 2020) provided further information on food environment and individual-level strategies both on reducing and increasing portion size of energy-dense foods. This review concluded that modifying portion size (in either direction) leads to a small to medium effect on consumption. Strategies such as modifying glass, bottle, bowl or plate size or shape also appeared to be effective, but there was a great deal of heterogeneity

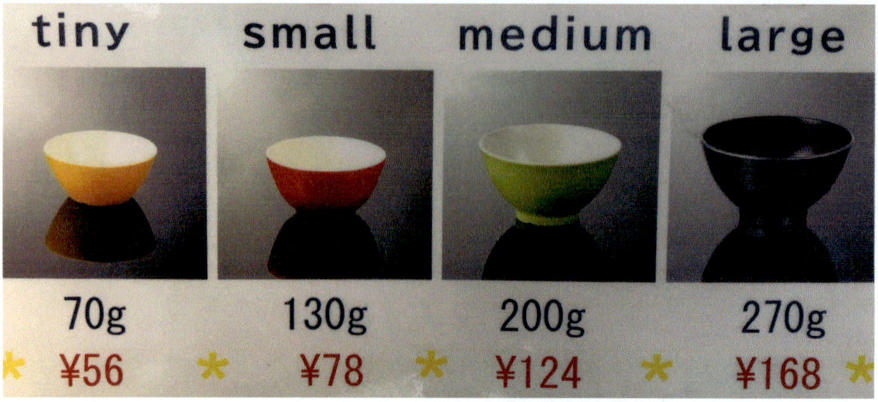


**FIGURE 15.2** Four different sized bowls of rice offered for purchase in a Japanese university canteen.

(variation) between studies. Furthermore, it should be noted that, whilst experimental studies usually provide evidence of a 'portion size effect', this association is not necessarily linear. In one review and meta-analysis, energy intake increased by 35% when the offered serving size was doubled but was not uniform across all population groups (Zlatevska et al., 2014).

Whatever the research study design used, there are challenges. Lab-based studies conducted in controlled environments, by definition, do not represent a real-world situation. Consumption patterns observed under experimental conditions may not be replicated by individuals in a natural setting such as in a restaurant or at home. A further limitation of experimental studies is that they typically have small sample sizes and do not shed light on the mechanisms behind any 'portion size effect'. Although potential mechanisms have been discussed by researchers (Steenhuis and Poelman, 2017), there is limited research into the mechanisms of portion size interventions and measures of portion control. It is unclear as to what type of interventions work best, for whom and in what context and more well-evaluated experimental studies are needed.

Observational studies on larger groups of participants have their own limitations. These studies are able to analyse relationships in different groups but are not as strong a study design for determining causal factors. In terms of observational research, studies looking at the cross-sectional relationships between portion size and health outcomes are more biased than longitudinal studies where participants are followed up over time; but this type of observational study has nevertheless provided some useful additional information from larger samples of free-living participants. Analysis of the UK NDNS has added to the research literature on portion sizes in different population groups. For example, a positive cross-sectional association was seen between BMI and the portion size of biscuits and cakes in UK adolescents aged 11–18 years (Albar et al., 2014). Another study investigating French and UK adults found that BMI was positively associated with portion size of certain energy-dense foods (Rippin et al., 2019a).

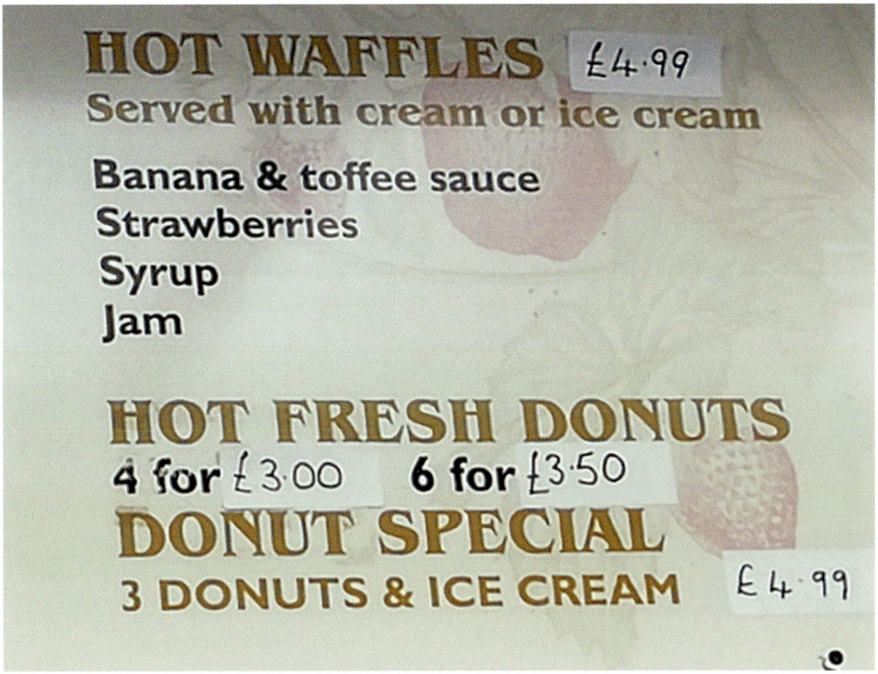
HOT WAFFLES £4.99
Served with cream or ice cream
Banana & toffee sauce
Strawberries
Syrup
Jam
HOT FRESH DONUTS
4 for £3.00 6 for £3.50
DONUT SPECIAL
3 DONUTS & ICE CREAM £4.99

**FIGURE 15.3** An example of non-proportional pricing at a waffle and doughnut concession stall in the UK.

One of the additional issues in larger observational studies is the validity of the method used to estimate portion sizes of foods and drinks. Whilst lab-based experimental studies can closely control the measurement of portion sizes, observational studies often provide less-accurate estimates to minimise participant burden. For example, the UK NDNS estimates portion size using a combination of household measures, photographs and food packaging labels. Although this is a comprehensive approach, it is susceptible to errors in portion size estimates, which should be taken into consideration when interpreting results and comparing with other studies. In addition, not all studies account for under-reporting, so observations drawn from the results may be less accurate (Murakami and Livingstone, 2014).

As well as reviews by university-based researchers, a McKinsey report was published in 2014 (Dobbs et al., 2014) that took into consideration the opinions of experts involved in research in this area. The review identified interventions to reduce portion sizes as a higher-impact intervention than other strategies such as information alone and concluded that they could help make healthier choices easier for individuals by changing the food environment rather than requiring conscious action from individuals. The report also concluded that the evidence base was 'sufficient for behaviour change' and identified portion size as the most impactful intervention type. The authors estimated that reducing portion sizes of both pre-packaged and out–of-home products could potentially save 2,000,000 disability-adjusted life years (DALYS) over a lifetime and 4% of the disease burden attributable to overweight and obesity

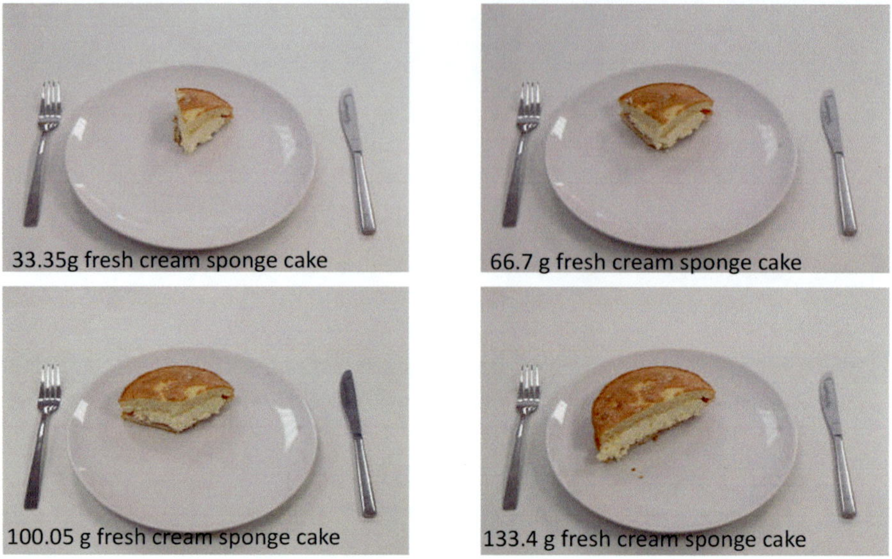
33.35g fresh cream sponge cake
66.7 g fresh cream sponge cake
100.05 g fresh cream sponge cake
133.4 g fresh cream sponge cake

**FIGURE 15.4** Four different portions of cake ranging from 33 to 133 g.

(Dobbs et al., 2014). This is partly due to the ubiquitous nature of large portion sizes which many of us are exposed to on a near-daily basis. Figure 15.4 depicts four possible portion sizes of cake from half the recommended to double the recommended size, but unless these are presented together, it is hard for consumers to select the recommended (66.7 g) portion size. Policies to reduce portion sizes of energy-dense foods are cost-effective, as they have a low average cost at $400 per DALY (Dobbs et al., 2014); however, the challenge is successfully changing social norms to enable customers to accept the smaller portion as normal, when most consumers are seeking value for money (i.e. larger portion at lower unit cost).

Successful reductions in portion size could be achieved through a number of different approaches such as reducing packaging sizes of individual, energy-dense packaged products including confectionery, as well as reducing the portion size of energy-dense meals such as meals typically served at fast food restaurants.

## 15.3 EFFECTS OF FOOD PACKAGING

It is important to distinguish between consumed portion sizes and on-pack serving sizes. The former is the quantity a person eats on one occasion and the latter is the quantity suggested to be eaten on one occasion (Almiron-Roig et al., 2020). This is typically indicated on the pack in pre-packed foods. Reducing the on-pack serving size of energy-dense foods forms part of the UK's calorie reduction drive and is one of the objectives in Public Health England's (PHE) calorie and sugar reduction strategy in the UK (Public Health England, 2018a).

Whilst on-pack serving sizes are not standardised but set individually by manufacturers in the UK and Europe (Kirwan et al., 2016), the US Reference Amounts

Customarily Consumed (RACCs), which inform American portion sizes, are based on typically consumed portion sizes from the National Health and Nutrition Examination Survey (NHANES) national dietary survey (US Food and Drug Administration (FDA), 2019). These standardised RACCs were updated in 2014 and 2016, increasing on-pack serving sizes to better reflect typical consumed portion sizes (Dallas et al., 2015).

On-pack serving sizes that better reflect consumed portion sizes may enable people to more accurately judge their energy intake and therefore avoid over-consumption. Yet Dallas et al. (2015) found that consumers erroneously believed that on-pack serving sizes referred to the quantity to be consumed for a healthy diet rather than a typically consumed portion size. In addition, when exposed to the new higher RACCs, American participants ate 41% more cookies, which suggests that the higher on-pack serving sizes could result in increased consumption in certain food categories. However, European evidence suggests that increasing serving sizes may condition individuals to believe that larger portion sizes are normal (World Health Organization (WHO), 2014).

A systematic review of the impact of food packaging on food intake identified 40 relevant studies that either aimed to reduce the portion size of energy-dense food or increase the portion size of nutrient-rich foods such as vegetables (Chu et al., 2021). The authors concluded that altering food packaging in a variety of ways had the potential to reduce consumed portion size of energy-dense foods. The most common method was through different types of visual cues such as pictures of the recommended portion size on the packaging, where pictures of fewer units of energy-dense foods resulted in lower intakes. Physically smaller packet sizes (physical visual cues) and partitioning were also effective at reducing intakes as was the ability to reseal packaging in some, although not all, consumers.

These interventions related to packaging overlap with approaches covered in other chapters such as the inclusion of written information on packaging which is discussed in the food labelling chapter (Chapter 13), advertising and food marketing covered in Chapter 14 and nudging in Chapter 16.

## 15.4 RECOMMENDATIONS FOR REDUCING PORTION SIZE OF ENERGY DENSE FOODS

Portion size guidance is not regularly updated and the information on which UK guidelines are based has not been updated since 1993 (Ministry of Agriculture Fisheries & Food, 1994). The British Nutrition Foundation has more recently released adult portion size guidance based on the UK Eatwell Guide (British Nutrition Foundation (BNF), 2019) shown in Chapter 1. Although this represents a combination of what individuals actually consume and previous government guidance, these are not official government recommendations, creating uncertainty for both the food industry and consumers.

Evidence suggests that in the UK on-pack serving-sizes have increased in some energy-dense food categories (British Heart Foundation, 2013) and therefore more action is needed. In addition, a study comparing UK on-pack serving-sizes with consumed portion sizes of popular energy-dense foods found that consumed portion sizes were significantly higher than on-pack serving size in all main food groups and most subgroups (Rippin et al., 2019b). For example, portion size of cakes, biscuits, chocolate and savoury snacks were 16%, 27%, 26% and 44% higher than the packet serving size, respectively. For popcorn (a product within the savoury snacks category), it was 151% higher. This suggests that updated guidance is needed as merely reducing on-pack serving sizes of energy-dense foods is unlikely to reduce energy intake and therefore weight change at a population level. Interventions to reduce portion sizes are included in the WHO Best Buys to reduce NCD risk (World Health Organization (WHO), 2017). However, policy action should be carefully considered, as even if on-pack serving sizes or pack sizes are decreased, it is not clear exactly what impact this would have on consumption and whether impact varies by demographic factors. Individuals may consume multiples of the smaller portions, thus maintaining or potentially increasing energy intake. Gradual reductions in portion size may enable new social norms to develop. Consequently, although outdated government guidelines may no longer reflect currently consumed portion sizes in the UK and Europe, careful consideration is needed in future policy development.

## 15.5 PORTION SIZE OF FRUIT AND VEGETABLES

In addition to understanding portion sizes of energy-dense foods, it is important to define and clearly communicate recommended portion sizes of nutrient-dense foods such as fruits and vegetables. To maintain and improve population health, WHO currently recommends the daily consumption of 400 g of fruit and vegetables, which equates to five 80 g portions (World Health Organization (WHO), 2004). However, guidance on fruit and vegetable consumption is not standardised across different countries. For example, the US Department of Agriculture (USDA) recommends that American adults consume two cups of fruit and 2.5 cups of vegetables per day. In Germany, adults are advised to eat two portions of fruit and three of vegetables, whilst Australian guidelines encourage the consumption of two portions of fruit and five portions of vegetables daily (including potatoes).

The UK national guidance for fruit and vegetable consumption follows WHO guidance with its widely communicated '5-a-day' message, which does not split out fruit and vegetable intake. This is detailed in the Eatwell Guide (Public Health England, 2016) (also see Chapter 1), which includes suggestions of what foods are included. For example, fresh, tinned and frozen fruit and vegetables are all included, whereas dried fruit (30 g) and pure fruit juices and smoothies (150 mL) can only count for one portion per day. Pulses can count for one portion, but potatoes do not count, as they are classed as a starchy carbohydrate.

According to UK NDNS data, people do not consume enough fruits and vegetables with mean daily intakes of 4.2 portions of fruit and vegetables for adults and only 31% meeting the 5-a-day guidelines (Public Health England (PHE), 2019). Worryingly, only 8% of children aged 11–18 years consume the recommended five portions each day, with this age group consuming an average of 2.7 portions daily (Public Health England, 2018b). This undesirable situation is not new – changes in fruit and vegetable consumption over the 9-year NDNS rolling programme have been minimal due to both a lack of frequency as well as smaller than optimal portion sizes of fruits and vegetables. Effective communication of the 5-a-day message in terms of frequency as well as portion size is therefore vital to safeguard and improve population health, particularly in lower-income groups where health literacy (see Chapter 13 on food labelling) may be lacking.

Interventions have been carried out to increase fruit and vegetable intakes in children in particular as higher intakes of fruits and vegetables early in life track into adulthood (Nekitsing et al., 2018) but have focused more on frequency than portion size. In pre-school children aged 2–5 years (Nekitsing et al., 2018), a review of interventions found repeated exposure to vegetables to be the most effective strategy to encourage their consumption. One study reported that offering a variety of vegetables to young children increased total portion size of vegetables consumed at lunchtime when compared with offering one vegetable, from 30–37 g (Carstairs et al., 2018); however, more research is needed in this area to identify the most successful strategies to increase portions of fruits and vegetables in different age groups.

## 15.6 DIFFERENCES IN PORTION SIZES BETWEEN HOME SETTINGS AND THE OUT-OF-HOME SECTOR

Portion sizes, particularly of processed, often energy-dense foods, may differ depending on the setting. Food and beverage products in the out-of-home sector often have portion sizes that are larger than their supermarket equivalents. Even within supermarkets, the portion size of, for example, American-style muffins may be larger in an in-store bakery than in the pre-packed aisle. As the suggested on-pack serving sizes are currently set by manufacturers and retailers rather than being based on (often outdated) government guidelines, these have consequently changed at different rates across manufacturers, product varieties and settings. This has led to the wide range of on-pack serving sizes seen in commercially available foods (Kirwan et al., 2016). This may create confusion in consumers and lead to inappropriate consumed portion sizes, over-consumption and an exacerbation of obesity-related health problems. In addition, the proportion of eating occasions that take place in the out-of-home sector has increased. One (non-representative) survey of ten European countries found that every fifth meal was consumed outside of the home, and 80% of these were from commercial outlets (IRI, 2020). As portion sizes in the out-of-home sector are larger than their retail counterparts, this creates even more scope for over-consumption, obesity and related NCD-risk. The out-of-home sector is therefore one of a range of stakeholders from whom coordinated action is needed if the obesity crisis is to be abated (Dobbs et al., 2014).

The mismatch between out-of-home and retail portion sizes, and lack of standardised, updated, evidence-based guidelines, means that voluntary measures by manufacturers to limit the availability of large serving sizes may not effectively reduce the consumed portion size in individuals. Portion-size reductions have been made in chocolate bars in the UK, but these measures have not been rigorously evaluated (Marteau et al., 2015); indeed, the recent evaluation of the sugar reduction plan in the UK concluded that sugar from chocolate confectionery bought outside the home has increased in the last 3 years and not decreased (Public Health England (PHE), 2020). It is possible that consumed portion size could actually increase if individuals consume multiple units when individual packaged portion sizes are perceived as too small. More research is needed to determine whether this is because portion sizes have not reduced in the out-of-home sector as in retail, or whether different consumer behaviours operate in different contexts.

## 15.7 INEQUALITIES, PORTION SIZE AND HEALTH

In addition, socioeconomic inequities should be considered in any set of recommendations or policy response. Energy-dense foods are disproportionately consumed by lower income groups (Food Standards Agency (FSA), 2007). There is currently little published work on the differential impact of portion size interventions on lower income groups either in the UK or across Europe. Some studies included in the recent review on food packaging noted that some interventions only influenced consumption when attention was paid to the packaging, and it is likely that the amount of attention varies by demographic (Chu et al., 2021). The same review also found that participants were more likely to respond to the intervention if they were not cognitively occupied and this, again, may vary with different groups of customers. More research on how to introduce policy guidance that is not inadvertently regressive and widens inequalities is needed in this area. Evidence is also missing on the effect of socioeconomic inequities on actions to optimise portion sizes in the out-of-home sector such as in takeaway restaurants. One small-scale study of a deprived UK locality found larger portions of energy-dense foods in fast-food outlets, higher than those reported in the literature for the US and elsewhere (Saunders et al., 2015). The authors described the community as both a 'food desert' and 'fat swamp', with regulation and interventions urgently required, including portion size reduction.

## 15.8 CONCLUSIONS

In summary, the increase in portion sizes of energy-dense foods and snacks has implications for increased energy intake and reduced diet quality and is likely to be cost effective to address (in health economic terms). Increasing portions of nutrient-rich foods such as fruits and vegetables also has the potential to improve diet quality. Guidance or stronger regulations may be needed. A holistic approach that takes into account the findings from a range of different types of research with different study designs while acknowledging the known limitations has the best chance of success. However, portion size on its own is not enough to improve health and additional strategies such as changes in marketing and economic strategies will also be needed.

## REFERENCES

Albar, S. A., Alwan, N. A., Evans, C. E. & Cade, J. E. 2014. Is there an association between food portion size and BMI among British adolescents? *Br J Nutr,* 112, 841–51.

Almiron-Roig, E., Forde, C. G., Hollands, G. J., Vargas, M. A. & Brunstrom, J. M. 2020. A review of evidence supporting current strategies, challenges, and opportunities to reduce portion sizes. *Nutr Rev,* 78, 91–114.

British Heart Foundation. 2013. Portion distortion. https://www.bhf.org.uk/what-we-do/news-from-the-bhf/news-archive/2013/october/portion-distortion

British Nutrition Foundation (BNF). 2019. Find your balance: get portion wise! https://www.nutrition.org.uk/media/csapwcse/457881-2.pdf

Carstairs, S. A., Caton, S. J., Blundell-Birtill, P., Rolls, B. J., Hetherington, M. M. & Cecil, J. E. 2018. Can reduced intake associated with downsizing a high energy dense meal item be offset by increased vegetable variety in 3-5-year-old children? *Nutrients,* 10, 1879.

Chawner, L. R., Blundell-Birtill, P. & Hetherington, M. M. 2021. Predictors of vegetable consumption in children and adolescents: analyses of the UK National Diet and Nutrition Survey (2008–2017). *Br J Nutr,* 126, 295–306.

Chu, R., Tang, T. & Hetherington, M. M. 2021. The impact of food packaging on measured food intake: a systematic review of experimental, field and naturalistic studies. *Appetite,* 166, 105579.

Dallas, S. K., Liu, P. J. & Ubel, P. A. 2015. Potential problems with increasing serving sizes on the Nutrition Facts label. *Appetite,* 95, 577–84.

Dobbs, R., Sawers, C., Thompson, F., Manyika, J., Woetzel, J., Child, P., Mckenna, S. And Spatharou, A. 2014. Overcoming obesity: an initial economic analysis.

Food Standards Agency (FSA). 2007. Low income diet and nutrition survey.

Hetherington, M. M., Blundell-Birtill, P., Caton, S. J., Cecil, J. E., Evans, C. E., Rolls, B. J. & Tang, T. 2018. Understanding the science of portion control and the art of downsizing. *Proc Nutr Soc*, 77, 347–55.

Hollands, G. J., Shemilt, I., Marteau, T. M., Jebb, S. A., Lewis, H. B., Wei, Y., Higgins, J. P. T. & Ogilvie, D. Portion, package or tableware size for changing selection and consumption of food, alcohol and tobacco. *Cochrane Database Syst Rev,* Issue 9. Art. No.: CD011045.

IRI. 2020. 1 in 5 meals eaten out of home as European consumers favour service over home cooking.

Kirwan, L., Walsh, M. C., Brennan, L., Gibney, E. R., Drevon, C. A., Daniel, H., Lovegrove, J. A., Manios, Y., Martinez, J. A., Saris, W. H., Traczyk, I., Mathers, J. C. & Gibney, M. 2016. Comparison of the portion size and frequency of consumption of 156 foods across seven European countries: insights from the Food4me study. *Eur J Clin Nutr,* 70, 642–4.

Ledikwe, J. H., Ello-Martin, J. A. & Rolls, B. J. 2005. Portion sizes and the obesity epidemic. *J Nutr,* 135, 905–9.

Marteau, T. M., Hollands, G. J., Shemilt, I. & Jebb, S. A. 2015. Downsizing: policy options to reduce portion sizes to help tackle obesity. *BMJ,* 351, h5863.

Ministry of Agriculture Fisheries & Food 1994. Food portion sizes, London.

Murakami, K. & Livingstone, M. B. 2014. Eating frequency in relation to body mass index and waist circumference in British adults. *Int J Obes (Lond),* 38, 1200–6.

Nekitsing, C., Blundell-Birtill, P., Cockroft, J. E. & Hetherington, M. M. 2018. Systematic review and meta-analysis of strategies to increase vegetable consumption in preschool children aged 2–5 years. *Appetite,* 127, 138–154.

Public Health England (PHE). 2019. NDNS: time trend and income analyses for years 1 to 9. https://www.gov.uk/government/statistics/ndns-time-trend-and-income-analyses-for-years-1-to-9

Public Health England (PHE). 2020. Sugar reduction. Report on progress between 2015 and 2019, London. https://assets.publishing.service.gov.uk/government/uploads/system/uploads/attachment_data/file/984282/Sugar_reduction_progress_report_2015_to_2019-1.pdf

Public Health England. 2016. The Eatwell Guide. https://www.gov.uk/government/publications/the-eatwell-guide

Public Health England. 2018a. Calorie reduction: the scope and ambition for action. https://www.gov.uk/government/publications/calorie-reduction-the-scope-and-ambition-for-action

Public Health England. 2018b. National diet and nutrition survey: results from years 7 and 8 (combined) of the rolling programme (2014/2015 to 2015/2016). https://www.gov.uk/government/statistics/ndns-results-from-years-7-and-8-combined

Rippin, H. L., Hutchinson, J., Jewell, J., Breda, J. J. & Cade, J. E. 2019a. Portion size of energy-dense foods among French and UK adults by BMI status. *Nutrients,* 11(1), 12.

Rippin, H. L., Hutchinson, J., Jewell, J., Breda, J. J. & Cade, J. E. 2019b. Comparison of consumed portion sizes and on-pack serving sizes of UK energy dense foods. *Appetite,* 134, 193–203.

Rolls, B. J., Morris, E. L. & Roe, L. S. 2002. Portion size of food affects energy intake in normal-weight and overweight men and women. *Am J Clin Nutr,* 76, 1207–13.

Rolls, B. J., Roe, L. S., Meengs, J. S. & Wall, D. E. 2004. Increasing the portion size of a sandwich increases energy intake. *J Am Diet Assoc,* 104, 367–72.

Rolls, B. J., Roe, L. S. & Meengs, J. S. 2007. The effect of large portion sizes on energy intake is sustained for 11 days. *Obesity (Silver Spring),* 15, 1535–43.

Saunders, P., Saunders, A. & Middleton, J. 2015. Living in a 'fat swamp': exposure to multiple sources of accessible, cheap, energy-dense fast foods in a deprived community. *Br J Nutr,* 113, 1828–34.

Smethers, A. D., Roe, L. S., Sanchez, C. E., Zuraikat, F. M., Keller, K. L., Kling, S. M. R. & Rolls, B. J. 2019. Portion size has sustained effects over 5 days in preschool children: a randomized trial. *Am J Clin Nutr,* 109, 1361–72.

Steenhuis, I. & Poelman, M. 2017. Portion size: latest developments and interventions. *Curr Obes Rep,* 6, 10–17.

US Food and Drug Administration (FDA). 2019. Guidance for Industry: Serving Sizes of Foods That Can Reasonably Be Consumed At One Eating Occasion, Reference Amounts Customarily Consumed, Serving Size-Related Issues, Dual-Column Labeling, and Miscellaneous Topics, Washington, DC. https://www.fda.gov/regulatory-information/search-fda-guidance-documents/guidance-industry-serving-sizes-foods-can-reasonably-be-consumed-one-eating-occasion-reference

World Health Organization (WHO). 2004. Global strategy on diet, physical activity and health. Diet and physical activity: a public health priority. https://www.who.int/dietphysicalactivity/strategy/eb11344/strategy_english_web.pdf

World Health Organization (WHO). 2014. Limiting portion sizes to reduce the risk of childhood overweight and obesity. https://www.who.int/elena/titles/portion_childhood_obesity/en/

World Health Organization (WHO). 2017. Tackling NCDS: best buys. https://apps.who.int/iris/handle/10665/259232

Zlatevska, N., Dubelaar, C. & Holden, S. S. 2014. Sizing up the effect of portion size on consumption: a meta-analytic review. *J Mark,* 78, 140–54.

# 16 Choice Architecture and Nudging for Better Food Choice

*Hannah Ensaff*
University of Leeds

*Naoki Kondo*
Kyoto University

**CONTENTS**



## 16.1 INTRODUCTION

Our daily food choice is largely automatic, heavily reliant on non-cognitive processing (Cohen & Babey, 2012). To help make quick decisions, we often use heuristics (rules of thumb) and biases. This means that our food choice can be susceptible to influence, and in this way, environmental cues can direct food choice. As a result, there is merit in purposefully changing the environment to steer food choice in a particular direction – and this is what nudging is about. In the last decade, there has been a growing interest in understanding and incorporating nudge strategies to promote better food choice. Related to this, choice architecture has become an area of immense international interest and activity.

DOI: 10.1201/9781003043720-16

## 16.2 CHOICE ARCHITECTURE

Nudging is rooted in behavioural economics, the irrationality and automaticity of behaviour (Kahneman, 2003, 2011; Tversky & Kahneman, 1974) and choice architecture (Thaler & Sunstein, 2008). First coined in 2008, choice architecture (Thaler & Sunstein, 2008) relates to the context in which we make choices and the influence of this on the decisions that we make. Food choice architecture relates specifically to food decisions and encompasses all aspects of how a food option is framed, and how this then affects our food selections (Ensaff et al., 2015). For instance, relevant aspects include the presentation, accessibility and availability of food options. These influence food choice – either encouraging or discouraging certain food options – and can be in place through purposeful design or incidentally. Nudging relates to the former, i.e. where the choice architecture is manipulated to steer food selection, either towards or away from specific food options.

Nudge strategies themselves are changes to the features of the choice architecture. They are small and inconspicuous adjustments to the social and physical environment. These can be changes to the placement (Broers, De Breucker, Van den Broucke, & Luminet, 2017), availability (Hollands et al., 2019) (e.g. number/proportion) and presentation (Thorndike, Sonnenberg, Riis, Barraclough, & Levy, 2012; Van Kleef, Otten, & Van Trijp, 2012) of food options, and the use of point of purchase prompts (Schwartz, 2007).

As well as making changes to the food options themselves (or their packaging or labelling), nudge strategies have also been implemented on menus (Feldman, Mahadevan, Su, Brusca, & Ruzsilla, 2011; Feldman, Su, Mahadevan, Brusca, & Hartwell, 2014; Sinclair, Cooper, & Mansfield, 2014), e.g. changes to the position of options on a menu and how the options are described or labelled.

Libertarian paternalism (Thaler & Sunstein, 2003, 2008) is another term relevant to nudging; this refers to safeguarding a consumer's freedom of choice, whilst steering in a direction beneficial to society and the consumer themselves. Therefore, food options are not restricted (Marteau, Ogilvie, Roland, Suhrcke, & Kelly, 2011; Thaler & Sunstein, 2003, 2008). Likewise, significantly changing economic incentives are excluded (Thaler & Sunstein, 2008) (see Chapter 17).

A recent review provided an overview of different nudge strategies for changing food choice, and the changes that these entail (Ensaff, 2021), as shown in Figure 16.1. Nudge strategies to change food choice can include: repositioning food to eye level or first in a buffet line; changing the availability of options; contrasting food with surroundings, e.g. boxing on a menu; providing food as grab-and-go; adding icons or symbols, e.g. smiley face; providing written or verbal prompts, e.g. "Would you like to add a salad to your order?"; describing food in an attractive way, e.g. creamy mushroom stroganoff; changing the default, e.g. adjusting standard food options.

Empirical evidence on the effectiveness of nudge strategies is growing, and various interventions have targeted foods such as fresh fruit (Vermote et al., 2020), vegetables (Mistura, Fetterly, Rhodes, Tomlin, & Naylor, 2019), leafy greens (Spence, 2020), plant-based foods (Ensaff et al., 2015), wholegrain pasta (Sogari et al., 2019) and vegetarian options (Bacon & Krpan, 2018). Several systematic reviews (Bucher et al., 2016; Lycett et al., 2017; Marcano-Olivier, Horne, Viktor, & Erjavec, 2020;

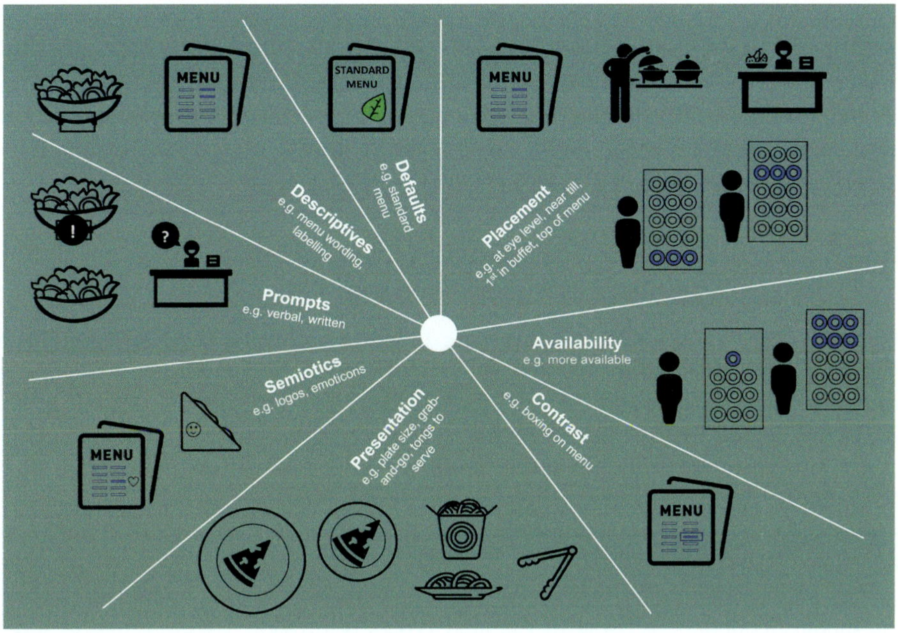


**FIGURE 16.1** Nudge strategies to change food choice. (Reprinted from Ensaff (2021) under license CC BY 4.0, https://creativecommons.org/licenses/by/4.0/.)

Nørnberg, Houlby, Skov, & Peréz-Cueto, 2016; Wright & Bragge, 2018) and meta-analyses (Arno & Thomas, 2016; Broers et al., 2017; Cadario & Chandon, 2020) have summarised findings, and highlighted, for instance, the success of changing availability and positioning (Hollands et al., 2019), and placement (Broers et al., 2017) on food choice. Interestingly, one meta-analysis indicated that the most effective nudge strategies may be behaviourally oriented, where changes aim to affect behaviour without changing knowledge or feelings (Cadario & Chandon, 2020). This work also outlined how the best nudge scenario increases effectiveness six-fold from the typical nudge-based intervention (Cadario & Chandon, 2020).

The mechanisms underpinning the effects observed with nudge strategies are still under investigation – and in determining effective nudge strategies, several aspects seem to be relevant. Changes can look to reduce overall effort and cognitive load for the individual, enhance the salience and tastiness of the food option being promoted and emphasise social norms (Ensaff, 2021).

## 16.3 CASE STUDIES OF NUDGE-BASED INTERVENTIONS IN REAL-WORLD SETTINGS

Nudge-based interventions to change food choice behaviour straddle multiple disciplines, including behavioural economics, nutrition, sociology and psychology. Drawing on theory, and practice across these, we can develop nudge-based interventions to steer food choice. To illustrate the application of nudge strategies in interventions to change food choice, we present three real-world case studies, across different countries, settings and nudges. Below, we describe the nudge strategies implemented, the foods promoted and the results observed. The first takes place in a secondary school setting in the United Kingdom, the second describes action that has been instigated in the wider eating out-of-home environment in Japan, and the third relates to a hospital workplace cafeteria in the United States.

### 16.3.1 Shifting Adolescents' Food Choice in a School Setting: A Case Study from Yorkshire, UK

Time-pressured food choice can be more liable to automatic food decisions, and therefore more disposed to nudging. An example of such an environment is a secondary school canteen, and this was the setting for an intervention (Ensaff et al., 2015) that aimed to shift the food choice of students (11–18 years) towards plant-based foods (whole fruit, vegetarian daily specials, sandwiches with salad, fruit pots). Interestingly, the cashless system used in the canteen automatically captured students' food choice; previous studies had demonstrated the power and utility of such data (Ensaff et al., 2013).

The intervention comprised nudge strategies targeting specific items already on the menu. Secondary schools in England typically provide a wide range of meal options, e.g. freshly prepared meals (such as vegetarian curry, beef lasagne), pizza, sandwiches, jacket potatoes, salad boxes. Foods with high plant-based content (evaluated through menus and recipes) and with designated codes on the cashless system (so that changes in the foods could be registered) were selected as the target foods.

The nudge strategies included changes to the placement, labelling and presentation as well as availability. These were determined by reviews of previous real-world nudge-based interventions, observation visits and consultation with catering and school leadership. In keeping with nudge theory, the intervention did not comprise any changes to the content of foods on offer. The strategies are depicted in Figure 16.2.

The intervention was implemented for 6 weeks, with a post-intervention period of 3 weeks (when the choice architecture reverted to its baseline condition). Results showed that overall selection was significantly different during the intervention compared to the rest of the year and also to the same time from the previous year. Compared to baseline, the selection of target foods during the intervention and post-intervention increased significantly (1.4% at baseline; 3.0% during the intervention; 2.2% post-intervention). Students were 2.5 times as likely to choose the plant-based food items nudged during the intervention, compared to baseline, controlling for age, socioeconomic status, day of the week and price. Interestingly, a spillover effect was observed for salads; there was an increase in selection despite it not having been a target food and not a focus for any nudge strategy. Overall, students were three times as likely during the intervention to select a fruit, vegetable or salad item, compared to baseline.

In considering the study's findings, it is important to acknowledge the context of the population sample, e.g. a higher-than-national average profile for Free School Meals (the national programme to provide a free school meal to students coming

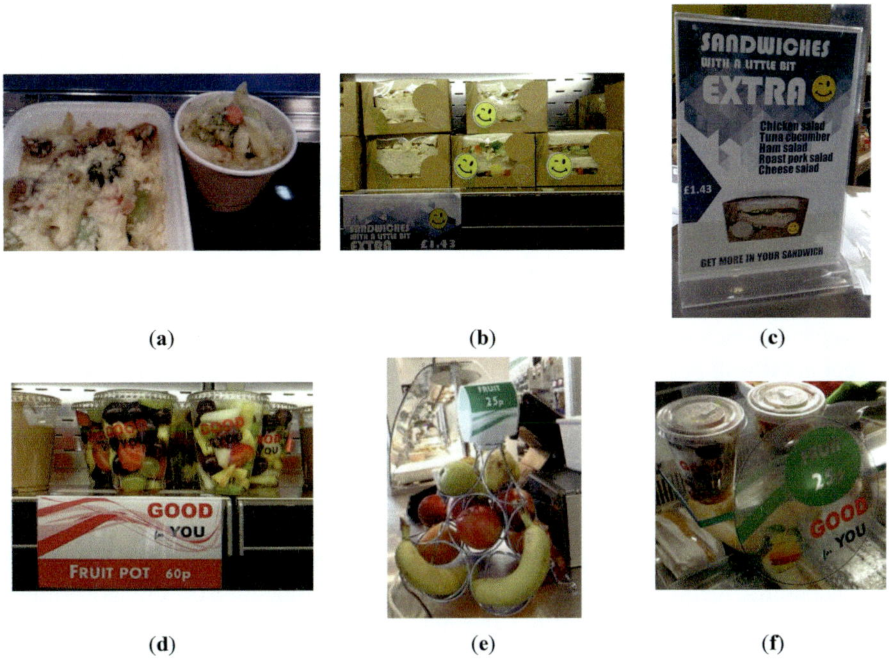


**FIGURE 16.2** Nudge strategies implemented for (a) *vegetarian daily specials* – convenient grab-and-go pots displayed prefilled and ready for selection; (b) *sandwiches containing salad* – emoticon smiley face sticker on packaging; (c) *sandwiches containing salad* – poster with written prompt "Get more in your sandwich"; (d) *fruit pots* – written prompt "GOOD for YOU" used on end-of-shelf label and stickers on containers; (e) *whole fruit* – displayed on pyramid stand and repositioned near till; (f) *whole fruit* – window sticker on display unit. (Adapted from Ensaff et al. (2015) licensed under CC BY 4.0, https://creativecommons.org/licenses/by/4.0/.)

from families with low income); and the food choice data in the study, that relied on canteen staff inputting student selections at the till.

The findings from this study point to the relevance of nudge-based interventions within schools and their potential in changing the food choice of adolescents.

### 16.3.2 Nudging for Better Food Choice in an Out-of-Home Food Setting, a Case Study from Adachi City, Japan

In 2019, the Organisation for Economic Co-operation and Development (OECD) highlighted health-promoting activities taking place in Adachi City (in Tokyo's metropolitan area) as best practice (OECD, 2019). The city had also achieved the sixth Healthy Longevity Award by the Ministry of Health, Labour and Welfare. One of the key features was the close partnerships that the city had developed with local restaurants. These partnerships aimed to build a community environment in which people had more opportunities to eat vegetables daily.

The average vegetable intake in Adachi was ~100 g less than Nagano – an area in Japan known for its longevity. The health promotion division in Adachi redesigned their strategy towards having more focus on vegetable intake and started a new programme called "Adachi veji-tabe-raifu" (meaning eating vegetables daily in Adachi). The goal was to increase access to *tasty* vegetable meals, thereby making it *easy* for people to make healthy choices in daily life.

Many of the activities related to nudging, targeting our behavioural traits, based on our cognitive characteristics, e.g. loss aversion bias (Kahneman & Tversky, 1979) – where we favour avoiding loss compared to gaining the equal amount; i.e. the amount of happiness gained by acquiring £20 for some reason is less than the amount of happiness lost by dropping a £20 note in the street. Under the city's government–restaurant partnerships, the partner restaurants served vegetable meals (i.e. vegetable-rich meals containing at least 120 g or more of vegetables per serving (except potatoes)) or prepared set meals with a vegetable dish served first. This government certification scheme increased the proportion of restaurants serving larger portions of vegetables with a main dish. Restaurants were encouraged to not only increase the quantity of vegetables but also ensure high-quality vegetable dishes, encourage their selection by customers and increase sales of these.

One challenge was that in most restaurants the certified vegetable meals were more expensive than regular meals, which could potentially lead to widening of socioeconomic inequality in vegetable intake. To overcome this, the city government implemented a campaign in 2016, offering a 1-week limited-time offer of a small discount of 50 yen (equivalent to £0.33/$0.44/€0.38) for the vegetable-rich meals. The discount was too small to make most of the vegetable-rich meals comparable in price to the regular meals (in the same restaurant); however, the limited-time offer could promote the vegetable-rich meals, given people's inherent loss aversion bias. Evaluation of this intervention found that orders of vegetable-rich meals increased by 1.5 times, with daily sales 1.77 times higher (even when accounting for the cost of cash-back payments) (Nagatomo, Saito, & Kondo, 2019). Researchers evaluated customers' socioeconomic status during the campaign by asking about their average cost for eating out for lunch, as a proxy measure of their income or financial leeway. Before the campaign, those with a lower socioeconomic position (lowest average payments for lunch) and categorised as non-regular workers were the least likely to order a vegetable-rich meal. However, during the campaign, the ordering rate increased the most among this group of customers (Nagatomo et al., 2019).

Overall, the campaign was successful in improving access to vegetables, offering more opportunities for local residents to order and consume vegetables while eating outside the home. Furthermore, the campaign contributed to increased sales in local restaurants and a positive reputation potentially for partner restaurants. The following year, the campaign was repeated with more restaurants, despite there being no subsidy compensating for the costs of the 50 yen discount. Findings from this experience could inform similar campaigns to improve vegetable intake in other cities.

### 16.3.3 Changing Employees' Food Purchases in a Workplace Hospital Cafeteria: A Case Study from Boston, USA

Our third case study is based in a workplace hospital cafeteria in Boston (Massachusetts, US), the setting of a longitudinal cohort study evaluating a choice architecture programme (Thorndike, Gelsomin, McCurley, & Levy, 2019). Workplace cafeterias are an important setting (see Chapter 4) where large sectors of the population acquire food regularly, and furthermore foods typically obtained are high in fat, added sugar or sodium (Onufrak et al., 2019). The overall aim was to test whether this programme was associated with reduced energy content of the foods and beverages bought by employees. The study tracked the food and beverage purchases of more than 5,000 employees for more than 2 years. Using employees' ID cards to log purchases, these were converted to energy content. In this way, researchers were able to examine the mean energy content per transaction across the duration, and critically the changes assessed were in-person differences.

The choice architecture programme comprised placement changes as well as 'traffic light' labels for all items. All items were assigned a red, yellow or green label to indicate healthy, less healthy and least healthy items, respectively. Red/yellow/green labels were allocated based on a number of positive (e.g. fruit or vegetable, wholegrain) and negative criteria (e.g. saturated fat content). Once assigned, foods and beverages were labelled accordingly, e.g. on food packaging, on menu boards or on shelf labels. Placement nudge strategies were then introduced (3 months after the labelling had been instigated) and included the promotion of the healthiest choices by placing these at eye level and/or near food stations for convenience. Once implemented, the choice architecture programme was in place for the duration of the study.

Study findings revealed a significant reduction in the energy content of transactions, and at year 2, a reduction of 35 kcal (146.4 kJ) per transaction was observed, a 6.2% reduction from baseline. The changes in energy did not differ by age or sex, but did by ethnicity, job type and part-time job status. Interestingly, red-labelled items provided the largest reduction, i.e. a 42 kcal (175.7 kJ) reduction per transaction at year 2 (a 23.0% drop), and the reduction in energy content of purchases for frequent cafeteria users (at least 36 transactions per quarter) was of the order of 4,275 kcal/quarter (17.9 MJ).

Integrating choice architecture programmes into workplace health and well-being provides a valuable opportunity for potential gains, particularly for employers with large numbers of employees.

## 16.4 SUSTAINABLE PARTNERSHIPS AND COMMUNITY ORGANISING: ESSENTIALS FOR NUDGE-BASED INTERVENTIONS

Nudge strategies provide useful tools to design physical and social environments to support people to make better choices with reduced cognitive burden. The development of nudge-based interventions is contingent on meaningful engagement with relevant stakeholders within organisations, such as key decision makers and those implementing change, for example catering staff. Early discussion and involvement are key to ensuring changes are feasible and practical. This supports not only better design of nudge-based interventions but also their successful implementation as intended.

In public health, creating organisational partnerships or community organising as it is sometimes called is "the process by which community groups are helped to identify common problems or goals, mobilise resources and develop and implement strategies to reach goals they have set collectively" (Minkler, 2012). According to the final report of the Commission for Social Determinants of Health, community organising is especially important in achieving equity in health promoting actions as organisational partnerships are critical to "tackle the inequitable distribution of power, money, and resources" (Commission on Social Determinants of Health, 2008). Providing resources for community organising is essential to make nudge-based interventions effective. These make it possible to not just employ public health professionals but also staff involved in public relations in the government, as well as marketing, advertising, product development and services in businesses.

There is another reason why community organising is important. The effect of a nudge for an individual person is relatively small. A single nudge may change only one food choice for an individual; however, the potential impact over an extended period with multiple choices is considerable. The lasting effects of nudges are also unclear. Therefore, to continuously improve people's dietary behaviour, we need a series of nudge interventions that are implemented in a long-lasting programme involving a range of relevant stakeholders. In this way, a variety of nudge strategies can be created together, across many channels and settings.

Nudge interventions can reduce the cognitive burden by approaching people's heuristics and affects, but we need to identify the triggers that make people take specific actions. Nudge as used in dietary behaviour change does not provide direct messages for their needs (healthy choice) but for their wants (interesting/attractive choice). In marketing, such triggers, or the relevant realities that people actually want, are called insights. Moreover, because individual interests may vary across subpopulations (e.g. based on characteristics such as age, gender, employment, culture), a nudge intervention may be effective in one subpopulation but not another. Hence, identifying the primary target of the intervention (targeting) and the "marketing mix" (product, its price, place where they can use the service and the ways to promote the services or communicate with the targets) are important in the design of interventions.

For example, in Adachi, the government's 10-year plan had many goals across different areas including diet and disease prevention. Towards the end of the last planning period, the city's health promotion division reviewed the achievements and realised that their activities might focus too much on the individual rather than the shared environment and that might not attract those most affected but instead participants who were highly motivated and relatively healthy. The health promotion division redesigned their strategy with a focus on vegetable intake and started the new programme called "Adachi veji-tabe-raifu". The programme involved a wide range of public and private organisations including major department stores located at the central train stations, supermarkets, local restaurants, leading convenience store companies, schools, childcare facilities and university researchers. The city obtained more than 900 partner restaurants consisting of 15% of all restaurants in the city. This multisector partnership provided the platform for co-designing effective interventions, including the 50 yen cashback campaign. They also had various interventions including vegetable cooking classes at public elementary and junior high schools and preschools (with a specific goal: all Adachi junior high school children can cook steamed rice, miso-soup and fried egg by themselves, by graduation) and offering small and low-price vegetable carry-out meals at local supermarkets.

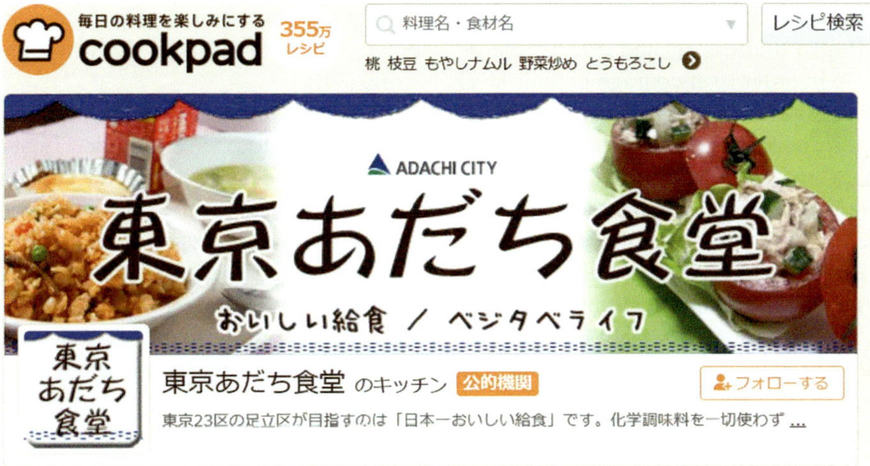


**FIGURE 16.3** Cookpad recipes from the Adachi ward government website (https://cookpad.com/kitchen/13386555).

As a branding strategy of their high-quality school lunches, the city of Adachi also launched a special website "Tokyo Adachi cafeteria" in Cookpad (a popular recipe website in Japan) and published a recipe book *The school kitchens in Adachi: nutrition-balanced meals for your daily lunch*, covering easy-to-cook nutritious dishes served in the public schools in the city (Figure 16.3).

In summary, strong community partnerships are necessary to improve a variety of community food environments through nudging. This necessarily entails support for engagement and strong leadership and networking.

## 16.5 CONCLUSIONS AND FUTURE DIRECTIONS

We are beginning to appreciate and understand the implication of choice architecture on food choice. Further, there is a growing body of literature attesting to the effect of nudge strategies. There is much still to be done, particularly with respect to study design and reporting (Broers et al., 2017), research in different settings (Arno & Thomas, 2016; Hollands et al., 2019), with different foods and for longer durations (Hollands et al., 2019) and also with populations of different sociodemographic characteristics. Given the promising evidence to date, and the typical low cost associated with such interventions, further work is recommended. This includes the extent of the effects of multiple nudge strategies and potential unintended consequences (Vermeer, Steenhuis, Leeuwis, Heymans, & Seidell, 2011; Wisdom, Downs, & Loewenstein, 2010). There is also a need to understand if consumers' awareness of being nudged influences the effects observed; indications are that it may not (Bruns, Kantorowicz-Reznichenko, Klement, Luistro Jonsson, & Rahali, 2018; Cheung et al., 2019; Kroese, Marchiori, & De Ridder, 2016). Work to explore public approval of nudging (Junghans, Cheung, & De Ridder, 2015; Evers, Marchiori, Junghans, Cremers, & De Ridder, 2018; Reisch, Sunstein, & Gwozdz, 2017) will determine if behaviour change interventions based on nudging are acceptable to the public and will also address related ethical considerations (Blumenthal-Barby & Burroughs, 2012) in order to encourage greater levels of transparency.

This is particularly relevant to the recent rapid emergence of digital technologies of information, communication and machine learning. These have provided further opportunities to design novel ways to nudge behaviour. Indeed, digital interface cues can act as nudge strategies to influence food decisions (Hou, 2017), which can be useful, for example, in the use of food-related apps. Such settings are particularly valuable as they contrast with physical nudge strategies and provide further opportunities for future interventions. The digital interface can also be modified frequently, at low cost and in a timely fashion. This enables interventions to be tailor-made to the individual's characteristics and interests. This is pertinent given that nutrition interventions that are personalised may be more effective in behaviour change (Celis-Morales, Lara, & Mathers, 2015) and are often considered cost-effective compared to a conventional approach (Galekop, Uyl-de Groot, & Ken Redekop, 2021). Nudging algorithms can be updated based on app user data to make the owner's experience easier and more enjoyable, for example while improving their diet. Ethical aspects of such endeavours are an important consideration (Hou, 2017) as well as the safe use of data in the digital food environment.

The potential of nudge-based interventions is substantial, particularly when considered across multiple settings (including those showcased in our three case studies) and in combination with other approaches such as financial incentives addressed in the next chapter. Integrating appropriate choice architecture across food settings in the future, provides the opportunity to radically change food choice and address the ongoing associated challenges that we face.

## REFERENCES

Arno, A., & Thomas, S. (2016). The efficacy of nudge theory strategies in influencing adult dietary behaviour: A systematic review and meta-analysis. *BMC Public Health*, *16*(1), 676. doi: 10.1186/s12889-016-3272-x.

Bacon, L., & Krpan, D. (2018). (Not) Eating for the environment: The impact of restaurant menu design on vegetarian food choice. *Appetite*, *125*, 190–200. doi: 10.1016/j.appet.2018.02.006.

Blumenthal-Barby, J. S., & Burroughs, H. (2012). Seeking better health care outcomes: the ethics of using the "Nudge." *The American Journal of Bioethics*, *12*(2), 1–10. doi: 10.1080/15265161.2011.634481.

Broers, V. J. V., De Breucker, C., Van den Broucke, S., & Luminet, O. (2017). A systematic review and meta-analysis of the effectiveness of nudging to increase fruit and vegetable choice. *European Journal of Public Health*, *27*(5), 912–920. doi: 10.1093/eurpub/ckx085.

Bruns, H., Kantorowicz-Reznichenko, E., Klement, K., Luistro Jonsson, M., & Rahali, B. (2018). Can nudges be transparent and yet effective? *Journal of Economic Psychology*, *65*, 41–59. doi: 10.1016/j.joep.2018.02.002.

Bucher, T., Collins, C., Rollo, M. E., McCaffrey, T. A., De Vlieger, N., Van Der Bend, D., … Perez-Cueto, F. J. A. (2016). Nudging consumers towards healthier choices: A systematic review of positional influences on food choice. *British Journal of Nutrition*, *115*(12), 2252–2263. doi: 10.1017/S0007114516001653.

Cadario, R., & Chandon, P. (2020). Which healthy eating nudges work best? A meta-analysis of field experiments. *Marketing Science*, *39*(3), 465–486. doi: 10.1287/mksc.2018.1128.

Celis-Morales, C., Lara, J., & Mathers, J. C. (2015). Personalising nutritional guidance for more effective behaviour change. *Proceedings of the Nutrition Society*, *74*(2), 130–138. doi: 10.1017/S0029665114001633.

Cheung, T. T. L., Gillebaart, M., Kroese, F. M., Marchiori, D., Fennis, B. M., & De Ridder, D. T. D. (2019). Cueing healthier alternatives for take-away: A field experiment on the effects of (disclosing) three nudges on food choices. *BMC Public Health*, *19*(1), 974. doi: 10.1186/s12889-019-7323-y.

Cohen, D. A., & Babey, S. H. (2012). Contextual influences on eating behaviours: Heuristic processing and dietary choices. *Obesity Reviews*, *13*(9), 766–779. doi: 10.1111/j.1467-789X.2012.01001.x.

Commission on Social Determinants of Health. (2008). Closing the gap in a generation: Health equity through action on the social determinants of health. Final Report of the Commission on Social Determinants of Health. Geneva, Switzerland: World Health Organization.

Ensaff, H. (2021). A nudge in the right direction: The role of food choice architecture in changing populations' diets. *Proceedings of the Nutrition Society*, *80*, 195–206.

Ensaff, H., Russell, J., & Barker, M. E. (2013). Meeting school food standards: Students food choice and free school meals. *Public Health Nutrition*. doi: 10.1017/S1368980012005575.

Ensaff, H., Homer, M., Sahota, P., Braybrook, D., Coan, S., & McLeod, H. (2015). Food choice architecture: An intervention in a secondary school and its impact on students' plant-based food choices. *Nutrients*, *7*(6), 4426–4437.

Evers, C., Marchiori, D. R., Junghans, A. F., Cremers, J., & De Ridder, D. T. D. (2018). Citizen approval of nudging interventions promoting healthy eating: The role of intrusiveness and trustworthiness. *BMC Public Health*, *18*(1), 1182. doi: 10.1186/s12889-018-6097-y.

Feldman, C., Mahadevan, M., Su, H., Brusca, J., & Ruzsilla, J. (2011). Menu engineering: A strategy for seniors to select healthier meals. *Perspectives in Public Health*, *131*(6), 267–274. doi: 10.1177/1757913911419897.

Feldman, C., Su, H., Mahadevan, M., Brusca, J., & Hartwell, H. (2014). Menu psychology to encourage healthy menu selections at a New Jersey University. *Journal of Culinary Science & Technology*, *12*(1), 1–21. doi: 10.1080/15428052.2013.798605.

Galekop, M. M. J., Uyl-de Groot, C. A., & Ken Redekop, W. (2021). A systematic review of cost-effectiveness studies of interventions with a personalized nutrition component in adults. *Value in Health*, *24*(3), 325–335. doi: 10.1016/j.jval.2020.12.006.

Hollands, G. J., Carter, P., Anwer, S., King, S. E., Jebb, S. A., Ogilvie, D., … Marteau, T. M. (2019). Altering the availability or proximity of food, alcohol, and tobacco products to change their selection and consumption. *Cochrane Database of Systematic Reviews*. doi: 10.1002/14651858.CD012573.pub3.

Hou, J. (2017). Can interface cues nudge modeling of food consumption? Experiments on a food-ordering website. *Journal of Computer-Mediated Communication*, *22*(4), 196–214. doi: 10.1111/jcc4.12190.

Junghans, A. F., Cheung, T. T., & De Ridder, D. D. (2015). Under consumers' scrutiny: An investigation into consumers' attitudes and concerns about nudging in the realm of health behavior health policies, systems and management. *BMC Public Health*, *15*(1), 1–13. doi: 10.1186/s12889-015-1691-8.

Kahneman, D. (2003). Maps of bounded rationality: Psychology for behavioral economics. *American Economic Review*, *93*(5), 1449–1475. doi: 10.1257/000282803322655392.

Kahneman, D. (2011). *Thinking, Fast and Slow*. London, UK: Penguin.

Kahneman, D., & Tversky, A. (1979). Prospect theory: An analysis of decision under risk. *Econometrica*. doi: 10.1111/j.1536-7150.2011.00774.x.

Kroese, F. M., Marchiori, D. R., & De Ridder, D. T. D. (2016). Nudging healthy food choices: A field experiment at the train station. *Journal of Public Health (Oxford), 38*(2), e133–e137. doi: 10.1093/pubmed/fdv096.

Lycett, K., Miller, A., Knox, A., Dunn, S., Kerr, J. A., Sung, V., & Wake, M. (2017). 'Nudge' interventions for improving children's dietary behaviors in the home: A systematic review. *Obesity Medicine, 7*, 21–33. doi: 10.1016/j.obmed.2017.06.001.

Marcano-Olivier, M. I., Horne, P. J., Viktor, S., & Erjavec, M. (2020). Using nudges to promote healthy food choices in the school dining room: A systematic review of previous investigations. *Journal of School Health, 90*(2), 143–157. doi: 10.1111/josh.12861.

Marteau, T. M., Ogilvie, D., Roland, M., Suhrcke, M., & Kelly, M. P. (2011). Judging nudging: Can nudging improve population health? *British Medical Journal, 342*, d228.

Minkler, M. (2012). *Community Organizing and Community Building for Health and Welfare*. Ithaca, NY: Rutgers University Press. doi: 10.36019/9780813553146.

Mistura, M., Fetterly, N., Rhodes, R. E., Tomlin, D., & Naylor, P. J. (2019). Examining the efficacy of a 'Feasible' nudge intervention to increase the purchase of vegetables by first year university students (17–19 years of age) in British Columbia: A pilot study. *Nutrients, 11*(8). doi: 10.3390/nu11081786.

Nagatomo, W., Saito, J., & Kondo, N. (2019). Effectiveness of a low-value financial-incentive program for increasing vegetable-rich restaurant meal selection and reducing socioeconomic inequality: A cluster crossover trial. *International Journal of Behavioral Nutrition and Physical Activity, 16*(1), 1–10. doi: 10.1186/s12966-019-0830-5.

Nørnberg, T. R., Houlby, L., Skov, L. R., & Peréz-Cueto, F. J. A. (2016). Choice architecture interventions for increased vegetable intake and behaviour change in a school setting: A systematic review. *Perspectives in Public Health, 136*(3), 132–142. doi: 10.1177/1757913915596017.

OECD. (2019). *OECD Reviews of Public Health: Japan: A Healthier Tomorrow*. Paris, France: OECD Publishing. Retrieved from doi: 10.1787/9789264311602-en.

Onufrak, S. J., Zaganjor, H., Pan, L., Lee-Kwan, S. H., Park, S., & Harris, D. M. (2019). Foods and beverages obtained at worksites in the United States. *Journal of the Academy of Nutrition and Dietetics, 119*(6), 999–1008. doi: 10.1016/j.jand.2018.11.011.

Reisch, L. A., Sunstein, C. R., & Gwozdz, W. (2017). Beyond carrots and sticks: Europeans support health nudges. *Food Policy, 69*, 1–10. doi: 10.1016/j.foodpol.2017.01.007.

Schwartz, M. B. (2007). The influence of a verbal prompt on school lunch fruit consumption : A pilot study. *The International Journal of Behavioral Nutrition and Physical Activity, 4*(1), 3–7. doi: 10.1186/1479-Received.

Sinclair, S. E., Cooper, M., & Mansfield, E. D. (2014). The influence of menu labeling on calories selected or consumed: A systematic review and meta-analysis. *Journal of the Academy of Nutrition and Dietetics, 114*(9), 1375–1388.e15. doi: 10.1016/j.jand.2014.05.014.

Sogari, G., Li, J., Lefebvre, M., Menozzi, D., Pellegrini, N., Cirelli, M., … Mora, C. (2019). The influence of health messages in nudging consumption of whole grain pasta. *Nutrients, 11*(12), 2993. doi: 10.3390/nu11122993.

Spence, C. (2020). Gastrophysics: Nudging consumers toward eating more leafy (salad) greens. *Food Quality and Preference, 80*, 103800.

Thaler, R. H., & Sunstein, C. R. (2003). Libertarian paternalism. *American Economic Review, 93*(2), 175–179. doi: 10.1257/000282803321947001.

Thaler, R. H., & Sunstein, C. R. (2008). *Nudge: Improving Decisions about Health, Wealth, and Happiness*. New Haven, CT: Yale University Press.

Thorndike, A. N., Sonnenberg, L., Riis, J., Barraclough, S., & Levy, D. E. (2012). A 2-phase labeling and choice architecture intervention to improve healthy food and beverage choices. *American Journal of Public Health, 102*(3), 527–533. doi: 10.2105/AJPH.2011.300391.

Thorndike, A. N., Gelsomin, E. D., McCurley, J. L., & Levy, D. E. (2019). Calories purchased by hospital employees after implementation of a cafeteria traffic light-labeling and choice architecture program. *JAMA Network Open*, *2*(7), 1–12. doi: 10.1001/jamanetworkopen.2019.6789.

Tversky, A., & Kahneman, D. (1974). Judgment under uncertainty: Heuristics and biases. *Science*, *185*(4157), 1124–1131.

Van Kleef, E., Otten, K., & Van Trijp, H. C. M. M. (2012). Healthy snacks at the checkout counter: A lab and field study on the impact of shelf arrangement and assortment structure on consumer choices. *BMC Public Health*, *12*(1), 1072. doi: 10.1186/1471-2458-12-1072.

Vermeer, W. M., Steenhuis, I. H. M., Leeuwis, F. H., Heymans, M. W., & Seidell, J. C. (2011). Small portion sizes in worksite cafeterias: Do they help consumers to reduce their food intake. *International Journal of Obesity*, *35*(9), 1200–1207. doi: 10.1038/ijo.2010.271.

Vermote, M., Nys, J., Versele, V., D'Hondt, E., Deforche, B., Clarys, P., & Deliens, T. (2020). The effect of nudges aligned with the renewed Flemish Food Triangle on the purchase of fresh fruits: An on-campus restaurant experiment. *Appetite*, *144*, 104479. doi: 10.1016/j.appet.2019.104479.

Wisdom, J., Downs, J. S., & Loewenstein, G. (2010). Promoting healthy choices: Information versus convenience. *American Economic Journal: Applied Economics*, *2*, 164–178. doi: 10.1257/app.2.2.164.

Wright, B., & Bragge, P. (2018). Interventions to promote healthy eating choices when dining out: A systematic review of reviews. *British Journal of Health Psychology*, *23*(2), 278–295. doi: 10.1111/bjhp.12285.

# 17 Financial Incentives to Promote Healthier Diets

*Adam Martin*
University of Leeds

*Elisa J. Vargas-Garcia*
Universidad Iberoamericana León

## CONTENTS



## 17.1 INTRODUCTION

Dietary financial incentives are interventions that alter the prices people pay for selected foods or drinks and are typically instigated by policy makers to encourage better diets and health. Examples include recent interest in subsidising sales of fruits or vegetables and in taxing saturated fat or added sugar, including through levies on manufacturers of sugar-sweetened beverages (SSBs; Finkelstein et al., 2013) (see case study 17.2.3.). Other examples include the more established practice of providing free fruit and vegetables for low-income families and free school meals for disadvantaged children.

These incentives can be implemented nationwide, (Smed et al., 2016) in certain localities, or in particular settings such as primary schools or selected restaurants (Cornelsen et al., 2017); they can be imposed on consumers, retailers or manufacturers; and may target broadly defined food types or very specific nutrient content. Those that lead to price increases, or *negative financial incentives,* may penalise or discourage unhealthy food choices whilst those that lead to price reductions, or

DOI: 10.1201/9781003043720-17

*positive financial incentives*, are typically designed to encourage healthier food choices or address food insecurity (see Chapter 11).

One argument supporting the use of financial incentives is based on the ideas of an early 20th-century British economist, Arthur Pigou. It is that the prices people pay should reflect not only the costs incurred directly by the producers and suppliers of products, but also any hidden costs or benefits that are experienced by other people or society.

Examples of negative financial incentives being used to try and account for hidden costs, or *negative externalities*, include car fuel duty which partially reflects the environmental harm posed to others by greenhouse gas (GHG) emissions (Martin et al., 2012; Don Fullerton et al., 2010), and tobacco duty, which may be justified by the harm caused by passive smoking. The externalities in these two cases also extend to healthcare costs (arising from physical inactivity or smoking-induced illnesses) that are typically paid for by the public at large through collectively funded healthcare systems. Given the high cost of treating and managing obesity-related non-communicable diseases (NCDs) (Biener et al., 2020; Dixon et al., 2019; Cawley and Meyerhoefer, 2012), including heart disease, cancer and type 2 diabetes, a similar case can be made for taxing unhealthy foods and drinks.

Examples of benefits that are accrued by others but not reflected in retail prices may include improved classroom behaviour and educational outcomes associated with eating healthy meals during childhood, the value of which extends beyond a single child to their classmates and the wider economy. The use of positive financial incentives, including subsidies, to account for these *positive externalities* may be favoured by policy makers because they do not restrict individual choices, particularly among those on lower incomes, in the way that negative financial incentives may. For this reason, the Nuffield Council on Bioethics' Interventions Ladder (see Chapter 1) lists "Guiding choice through disincentives" above "Guiding choice through incentives", indicating that negative financial incentives are more intrusive and that more robust evidence would be needed before they can be implemented. On the other hand, some policy makers may oppose positive financial incentives because they require Government funding, whereas negative financial incentives are revenue generating. A potentially neat idea lies in the so-called "double dividend" (Don Fullerton et al., 2010) (as proposed by some advocates of GHG emission taxes) whereby carefully designed food or drink taxes might discourage unhealthy diets whilst simultaneously generating revenue to fund subsidies of healthier alternatives.

Other more contested arguments supporting the use of financial incentives include the problem of *internalities*. These are hidden costs or benefits that accrue to consumers themselves which might be overlooked when making purchasing decisions (Allcott et al., 2019). This could include long-term health consequences that result from the strong habitual properties of some unhealthy food products. People may also be time inconsistent in that they plan to consume less in the future but, when the time comes, they choose not to (see Chapter 16). Although prices could be adjusted to better reflect people's own best interests, policy makers may be reluctant to act for fear of being too paternalistic. On the other hand, the public may support financial incentives that enable people to have more self-control over their dietary choices (Crawford et al., 2010; Gruber, 2010).

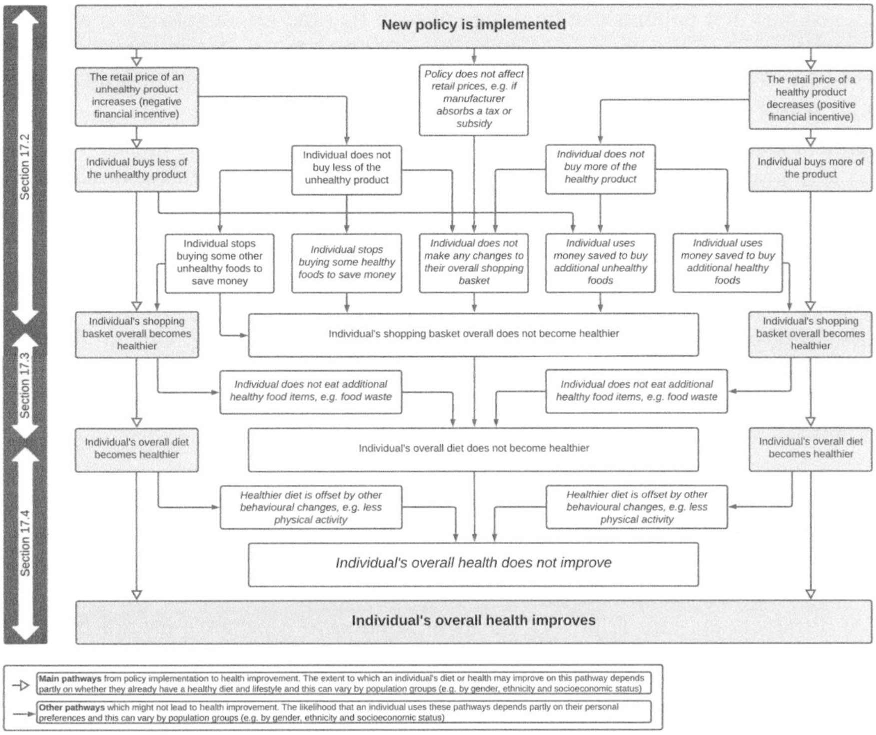


**FIGURE 17.1** Pathways linking dietary financial incentives with health improvement.

With reference to Figure 17.1, which shows the possible effects of dietary financial incentives on an individual's health behaviours, the remainder of this chapter examines the potential impact of dietary financial incentives on purchasing behaviour, diet and, finally, health.

## 17.2 DO FOOD AND DRINK PRICE CHANGES AFFECT HOW MUCH WE BUY?

### 17.2.1 Price Elasticities of Demand

A measure of the degree to which demand for a particular product changes when its price changes is the *price elasticity of demand* (PED). It is calculated by dividing observed percentage increases (or decreases) in the demand for a product by observed percentage decreases (or increases) in its price. The higher the value of the PED, the more 'elastic' the demand for a product is in terms of its responsiveness to price changes.

On the face of it, higher values of PED could be desirable from a policy-making perspective. This is because the total cost of subsidising healthy products would be lower for a given increase in sales and because only relatively modest tax measures would be necessary for a given decrease in sales of unhealthy products. However, this assumes that policies can be designed such that the tax or subsidy is passed on to consumers through retail price changes, rather than being absorbed by retailers or producers. This is least likely to happen when taxes are imposed on products with a higher PED, or subsidies are imposed on products with a lower PED, due to those suppliers fearing lost sales and revenue. Another consideration is that taxing products with lower PED values could be beneficial from the point of view of generating tax revenue because relatively few people will stop buying the product, despite an increased retail price, and thus will incur the tax.

Published price elasticity of demand estimates typically vary at the general population level between 0.2 and 0.8 for different types of food and drink (Andreyeva et al., 2010; Green et al., 2013). This indicates that a 10% price increase (or decrease) may be associated with a relatively small 2%–8% reduction (or increase) in purchases of those products (see Table 17.1). These values vary by product type for several reasons:

- Products that are considered necessities (e.g. staple foods) tend to be less price elastic than those that are considered luxuries (e.g. restaurant meals) because people are more likely to need similar quantities of them after a price change.
- Products that are relatively cheap in relation to a person's overall budget (e.g. a loaf of bread that lasts several days) tend to be less price elastic than more expensive items (e.g. a single portion of red meat). This also suggests that people with smaller budgets might be more sensitive to price changes than their wealthier counterparts (Pechey et al., 2013), particularly if they suffer from financial insecurity (see Chapter 11), and that PED would be higher in low- and middle-income countries (indicating that policy changes would have a larger impact on consumption in those countries) (Green et al., 2013).
- Broadly defined product types (e.g. 'vegetables' or 'soft drinks') tend to be less price elastic than narrowly defined product types (e.g. "organic broccoli" or "cloudy apple juice") because there are fewer close substitute products that people can buy instead.

Other relevant determinants of PED include:

- The size and direction of the price change (Schmacker and Smed, 2020). In some instances, small changes may not be noticed. In others they can have a disproportionately large impact – some people enjoy snapping up special offers, for example, while others begrudge even the smallest price increases.
- The rationale for the price change. People might be more responsive to financial incentives imposed by policy makers in the public interest than those promoted by retailers. An example of the former may be the large fall in demand for plastic shopping bags in response to the relatively small, nominal charges that are now imposed for environmental reasons. Similarly, a dietary financial incentive might provide a signal that 'nudges' people

**TABLE 17.1**
**Elasticities of demand**

| Definition | Interpretation | Example | Other published estimates |
|---|---|---|---|
| Price elasticity of demand (PED) $\frac{\%\text{ change in demand for a product}}{\%\text{ change in price of a product}}$ | If \|PED\| > 1 then demand is price elastic<br>If \|PED\| < 1 then demand is price inelastic<br>Absolute values of PED are used | The PED of eggs is estimated to be 0.27, indicating that if the price increased by 10%, demand would decrease by 2.7% [1] | Food not at home: 0.81<br>Soft drinks: 0.79<br>Beef: 0.75<br>Fruit: 0.70<br>Cereals: 0.60<br>Vegetables: 0.58<br>Fish: 0.50<br>Dairy: 0.65<br>Fats/oils: 0.48<br>Sweets/sugars: 0.34 [1] |
| Cross price elasticity of demand (XPED) $\frac{\%\text{ change in demand for product A}}{\%\text{ change in price of product B}}$ | If XPED > 0 then the two products may be substitutes<br>If XPED < 0 then the two products may be complements<br>Larger absolute values of XPED indicate a stronger relationship between the two products | The XPED of dairy products in relation to the price of cereals is estimated to be +0.06, indicating that these are weak substitute products where a 10% increase in cereal prices could be associated with a 0.6% increase in demand for dairy products [2] | XPED in relation to a change in the price of cereals:<br>Dairy: +0.06<br>Fruit and vegetables: +0.01<br>Meat: +0.01<br>XPED in relation to a change in the price of fish:<br>Dairy: −0.09<br>Fruit and vegetables: −0.08<br>Meat: −0.07 [2] |
| Income elasticity of demand (YED) $\frac{\%\text{ change in demand for a product}}{\%\text{ change in personal income}}$ | If YED is between 0 and 1 then the product may be considered a necessity<br>If YED > 1 then the product may be considered a luxury<br>YED is rarely negative | The YED for fruit and vegetables is estimated to be 0.62, indicating that if incomes increase by 10%, demand would increase by 6.2% [3] | Soft drinks: 1.24<br>Dairy: 0.81<br>Meat, fish and eggs: 0.79<br>Fruits and vegetables: 0.62<br>Fat and oil: 0.58<br>Root vegetables: 0.42<br>Cereals: 0.4<br>Legumes and nuts: 0.4 [3] |

[1] Based on U.S. data collected between 1938 and 2007 (Andreyeva et al., 2010)
[2] Based on 2008 estimates for middle-income countries (Cornelsen et al., 2015b)
[3] Based on data from 48 African countries collected between 1991 and 2015 (Colen et al., 2018)

towards healthier diets, independent of the price change itself. In some cases, this signal may be the dominant factor in driving behaviour change. Alternatively, people may be less responsive if they resent Government interference.

- The type of actions needed by consumers. People may be less responsive to incentives if they are cumbersome or inconvenient to claim and redeem. This might include means-tested healthy food vouchers (Griffith et al., 2018) and free school meals, which can also be unattractive due to social stigma. People might be more responsive to universal in-store food price changes, for instance, since little effort is required to change the quantity or type of products in their shopping baskets.
- The time period. People may respond to price changes in the short term but then switch back to old habits once they've got used to them. Alternatively, it may only be in the longer term that people change their habits, after learning different cooking skills or gaining knowledge of alternative products, for example. Manufacturers would also have more time to develop better alternative products (e.g. meat- or sugar-free versions of people's preferred foods and drinks), which has been one stated objective of SSB levies (see case study 17.2.3). However, other factors also influence decisions to switch production to healthier products. These include how the cost of making changes to production processes compare with the cost in terms of lost sales and revenue that would arise from passing the levy onto consumers through higher retail prices (or the cost in terms of absorbing it themselves).

### 17.2.2 Not Everyone's the Same

Differences in the PED between the general population and the intended target population have rarely been studied in relation to food or drink but would affect how dietary financial incentives work. Ideally, people who already typically buy healthier products would be less responsive to price changes than people whose diets typically include a larger proportion of less healthy products. Otherwise the policy may achieve little more than reduce the shopping bills of people who already have healthier diets and potentially widen diet inequalities. In the case of taxes on unhealthy products (e.g. SSBs), reductions in diet inequalities would probably require behaviour change among those disproportionately impacted by their consumption (e.g. younger people and those with lower socio-economic status).

It is likely that PED also depends on people's current habitual level of consumption. For example, those who have never purchased a product or who already buy ample amounts of it may be less responsive to price reductions because they may not consider buying more. On the other hand, they at least have more potential scope for making relatively large changes in the quantity they purchase.

There are also differences in how much spare time people have. For many people, time is money, and if that's the main reason why they choose fast-food over healthier meals cooked at home then they might not be so reactive to food price changes.

### 17.2.3 Case Study: Levies on Sugar-Sweetened Beverages (SSBs)

Recent evidence shows promising effects of price changes on purchasing behaviours and sales of non-essential foods high in energy and sugars (Pfinder et al., 2020).

A systematic review of real-world evaluations of SSB taxes reported declines of 10% (95% CI –5% to –15%) in purchases of taxed beverages with the equivalent of a 10% SSB tax (Teng et al., 2019). The largest effects were seen amongst lowest socioeconomic status (SES) groups, indicating its potential to narrow diet inequalities. A review of virtual or experimental scenarios showed that intention to purchase decreased more when combined with other financial incentive or educational schemes (i.e. healthier food subsidies or improved labelling) (Redondo et al., 2018).

Chile and the UK have implemented a tax or levy on SSBs based on thresholds of sugar content in terms of grams of sugar per 100 mL. In Chile, which has the highest SSB sales per capita in Latin America (188 kcals per capita per day) (Popkin and Hawkes, 2016), tax rates on SSBs exceeding 6.3 g/100 mL were increased from 13% to 18% in 2014, whilst tax rates on SSBs with lower or no sugar content were decreased from 13% to 10%. A controlled before-after study showed that household purchases of SSBs above the lower sugar tier declined in volume by 3.4% and in calories by 4.0%. Analyses revealed larger reductions in purchases of SSBs with higher sugar content amongst higher SES groups when compared to lower SES groups (–6.4% vs –1.6%) (Caro et al., 2018) possibly due to the tax not being fully passed onto consumers and lower responsiveness to price increases amongst low SES households (Cuadrado et al., 2020).

In April 2018, the UK government implemented the Soft Drinks Industry Levy where SSBs exceeding 8g/100 mL were charged £0.24 per litre and those ranging from 5 to <8 g/100 mL were charged £0.18 per litre. This levy, aimed at drinks companies, successfully encouraged product reformulation. In 2019, the purchased volume of drinks above the higher (>8 g/100 mL) and lower (5 to <8 g/100 mL) sugar thresholds had decreased by 44% and 86%, respectively (Pell et al., 2021). Prices of lower tier drinks (5 to <8 g/100 mL), in particular, reduced by £0.17 per litre and the proportion of low-sugar beverages (<5 g/100 mL) as a proportion of market share increased from 16% to 28% (Scarborough et al., 2020) indicating the impact of the levy was due to reduced availability of sugary drinks as well as differences in price. Total added sugars purchased also fell by around one-third in all SES groups (Niblett et al., 2019).

Evidence of the effectiveness of taxation of SSBs on beverage (and thus added sugar) consumption rather than purchasing is more complex and still emerging (Pfinder et al., 2020; Madsen et al., 2019). In North America, two studies assessing the City of Berkeley's tax over the first 3 years of its implementation found reductions of up to 52% in self-reported SSB consumption across all SES groups (Falbe et al., 2016; Lee et al., 2019). A similar analysis from the city of Philadelphia indicated a decrease of 26% in intakes in the short term, albeit offset by increased purchases across nearby cities without the tax (Roberto et al., 2019). In the UK, the National Diet and Nutrition Survey shows that intakes of SSBs and added sugars are overall significantly lower compared with previous years before the implementation of the levy in most age groups (Public Health England and Food Standards Agency, 2020).

## 17.3 CAN DIETARY FINANCIAL INCENTIVES LEAD TO HEALTHIER DIETS?

### 17.3.1 What Else Is in Your Shopping Basket?

Dietary financial incentives can affect diet directly if they lead to changes in how much people buy of the particular healthy or unhealthy product that is the target of a price change. But those price changes can also affect diet indirectly if they lead to changes in other food or drink purchases:

- People who decide to buy less of an unhealthy product in response to a price increase may spend the money they have saved on other products instead. Similarly, those who buy more of a healthy product in response to its price going down may need to save money elsewhere in their budget by spending less on other food or drinks. These are examples of a *substitution effect.*
- If people's reaction to financial incentives is limited, then price increases on the targeted unhealthy products may lead to fewer purchases of other food or drinks. Similarly, price reductions on selected healthy products may lead to more purchases of other food or drinks. These are examples of an *income effect.*

A measure of how changing the price of one product could affect the demand for another product is the *cross-price elasticity of demand* (*XPED*). It is calculated by dividing the percentage change in demand for another food or drink product by the percentage change in price of the product that is subjected to the dietary financial incentive (Table 17.1). The higher the value of the XPED, the more 'elastic' the demand for another product is in response to a change in price of the targeted product. Like PED, the XPED is likely to vary between the target population and the general population and between the short and long term.

From a policy-making perspective, it could be desirable if, in relation to the product that is the target of a dietary financial incentive, the XPED for other healthy food or drink products was much higher than the XPED for other unhealthy products. If the substitution effects were dominant, then this would imply that in response to a new tax on unhealthy products (such as fast food takeaways or SSBs), people would spend the money they save from buying less of it on more healthy products (such as vegetables, fruit or sugar free drinks) relative to unhealthy products (such as processed ready meals or savoury or sweet snacks). Alternatively, if the income effects were dominant, then this would imply that people who want to continue buying the taxed product but don't want to spend more on food or drink overall would reduce purchases of other healthier products (e.g. fruit) at a slower rate than they reduce purchases of other unhealthy products (e.g. SSBs).

A key determinant of XPED is the degree to which the two products are considered complements (e.g. fast food and SSBs may be complements, so a tax on one could reduce demand for both) or substitutes (e.g. fruit may be a weak substitute and biscuits a strong substitute for chocolate bars, so a chocolate tax might increase demand for biscuits more than it would for fruit). Compared with PED, fewer studies have examined XPED in relation to the products that would be the target of dietary financial incentives. Some evaluations of SSB taxes have looked at substitution effects, but commercially sensitive estimates of both PED and XPED may not be publicly available, such as the impact of end-of-aisle or other in-shop price promotions designed using consumer data from supermarket loyalty cards (Cornelsen et al., 2015a; Finkelstein et al., 2013; Miao et al., 2013; Schroeter et al., 2008; Dharmasena and Capps Jr, 2012; Cornelsen et al., 2015b).

### 17.3.2 Who Eats What?

An important feature of dietary financial incentives is that the targeted products are unlikely to be universally good or bad for us. When compared with the example of tobacco duty noted earlier (Section 17.1), where each additional cigarette is somewhat harmful to people who smoke, most foods benefit the undernourished and are unlikely to cause harm when consumed in moderation as part of a healthy balanced diet. Ideally those who have most to gain from changing their diet would be the most responsive to financial incentives, but often this may not be the case. Therefore, it is necessary to consider and investigate how different groups of people respond to financial incentives before they are introduced.

Another consideration is how food purchases translate into food consumption. For example, the purchase of large amounts of heavily processed foods for consumption by one person in a short space of time is likely to be more harmful than one household storing their purchases for consumption over a longer period. It is also necessary to examine how the consumption of food that is bought at the household level, perhaps by a parent, is shared between different household members (Griffith et al., 2018). Finally, not all food gets eaten, and there are reasons to presume this applies most to healthier, less processed and fresh foods that are more perishable (Yu and Jaenicke, 2020).

### 17.3.3 Other Things Are Happening

Not all dietary financial incentives are designed with health improvement in mind. Examples involving positive financial incentives include the UK Government's £849 million 'Eat Out to Help Out' subsidy for restaurant meals in August 2020 and product price promotions used by food retailers (Watt et al., 2020), sometimes to offset policies designed to increase the price of unhealthy foods (Cornelsen et al., 2015a). They are also used in many countries to support agricultural product markets, including sugar, (Bonnet and Requillart, 2011) and ostensibly to maintain reasonable prices for people's basic food needs (Walls et al., 2016). Examples involving negative financial incentives include proposed environmental taxes on meat and dairy produce to account for the high levels of GHG emissions generated in their production, which (on some measures at least) cause similar damage globally as those generated by the entire transport sector where environmental taxes are much more common. Food prices are also affected by more established sales taxes which are frequently applied to selected foods with little apparent consideration of their nutritional content – in the UK, bakery shoppers pay 0% value-added tax (VAT) on hot Cornish pasties and 20% on cakes, whilst supermarket shoppers pay 0% on ice cream and 20% on red meat (Gruber, 2010).

People's demand for particular products is also dependent on their food purchasing power, which tends to increase over time due to technological change (Lakdawalla and Philipson, 2009) and their income. In general, people buy more when incomes rise and less if incomes fall. This relationship can be measured by the *income elasticity of demand* (Table 17.1), which can help predict how sales of particular foods or drinks may change when people's financial circumstances change (e.g. after losing a job) or when the economy experiences an economic recession or upturn.

Since all these factors could have large incidental effects on the balance of healthy and unhealthy food and drinks in our diets, health policy makers need to consider the degree to which they may reinforce or undermine the effects of their own (potentially more modest) dietary financial incentives. Evidence from recent decades also indicates that the price of healthy foods has increased faster than the price of unhealthy foods in many countries including the UK (Jones et al., 2014), suggesting that more stringent policies to encourage healthier diets may be needed to weaken these underlying market trends.

## 17.4 DO DIETARY FINANCIAL INCENTIVES IMPROVE HEALTH?

In addition to the complex relationships between food and drink prices and healthier diets, assessing the success of dietary financial incentives is complicated by further potential avenues for unpredictable consequences to emerge on the pathway between healthier diets and health-related outcomes (see Figure 17.1) (Lakdawalla and Philipson, 2009). For example, even if product price changes did lead to better diets, these price changes may affect other health-related behaviours. Since some people would have to spend more time in the kitchen and doing shopping, one study suggests that a fast food tax might lead to weight gain if people end up having less time for exercise (Yaniv et al., 2009). More encouragingly, another study suggests healthy food subsidies can boost the chances that children attend routine check-ups with their doctor, because their parents are experiencing less financial stress (Bronchetti et al., 2019).

A further complicating factor in assessing the success of dietary financial incentives arises if there is ambiguity about the health policy objective; for instance, if obesity is poorly defined (e.g. whether the aim is to reduce population average BMI or the proportion of people who are obese) or if there are multiple objectives (e.g. related to health inequalities or food insecurity). This might not matter, but it is unlikely that all objectives can be met with the same policy. Expecting that a policy can tackle hunger among some people, for instance, whilst addressing over-eating among others is potentially unrealistic.

In terms of the empirical evidence, there is a shortage of studies that have examined the impact of specific financial incentive policies on health outcomes, due partly to the long time period that effects would be expected to materialise and methodological challenges in attributing cause to effects. Studies that have examined the relationship between general food price fluctuations and health outcomes nevertheless provide policy makers some hope. For example, several studies show that higher fast food prices are associated with lower weight outcomes, especially among younger people, and that lower fruit and vegetable prices are associated with lower body weight, including among low-income groups (Powell et al., 2013).

## 17.5 FURTHER CONSIDERATIONS AND CONCLUSION

Dietary financial incentives are more popular with policy makers than regulations that restrict choice and may be better at changing behaviour than nudging. They may also help to reduce inequalities in diet. But designing them is challenging. Optimal results may require combining financial incentives with additional policies, such as educational interventions (Afshin et al., 2017). Furthermore, because of the long and complex pathways between price changes and better health (Figure 17.1), unintended consequences may occur. For example, some people will adopt worse diets and others will be unfairly penalised.

Compared to the example of car fuel duty, which leads more directly and unequivocally to the goal of reduced GHG emissions, opportunities for a shorter, less complex pathway are limited – taxing people with obesity or subsidising healthy weight (Bhattacharya and Bundorf, 2009; Gruber, 2010; The Economist, 2009) would be wholly unpalatable and likely impractical. Another (more feasible) policy would make greater use of the tax or social security systems to tackle financial insecurity in order to free people experiencing deprivation from the heavily skewed economic incentives that arise from constant uncertainty about their future income and lead many to rely on food banks. Such financial insecurity may be a root cause of poor outcomes and inequalities in relation to diet, (as indicated by the lower consumption of fruit and vegetables in more deprived households (Public Health England and Food Standards Agency, 2020)), as well as in relation to other important determinants of health including housing and education (Marmot, 2020). Other than that, policy makers may conclude that the risk of unintended consequences means the scope for using economic incentives to improve diets is limited to subsidising the purchase of products that are universally good by people who otherwise wouldn't buy them (e.g. means-tested healthy food vouchers) or taxing a small range of products that are considered universally bad (e.g. SSBs). Danish politicians apparently confirmed this when they withdrew a wide-ranging 'fat tax' encompassing meat, dairy produce and processed food when unintended consequences emerged shortly after its introduction in 2011. More recently, however, growing clamour for tougher action on GHG emissions from food production (e.g. meat and dairy) (Rippin et al., 2021) could lead to an increased political acceptability of multilateral food taxes that couldn't be justified solely by people's unhealthy food choices. If so, then policy interest in dietary financial incentives looks set to continue for many years to come.

In conclusion, whilst dietary financial incentives have an important role to play in promoting health, so far they have proved insufficient on their own to address the scale of the public health challenge.

## ACKNOWLEDGEMENTS

We are grateful to Laura Cornelson for her invaluable feedback on earlier manuscripts.

## REFERENCES


Afshin, A., Peñalvo, J. L., Del Gobbo, L., Silva, J., Michaelson, M., O'Flaherty, M, et al. 2017. The prospective impact of food pricing on improving dietary consumption: A systematic review and meta-analysis. *PLoS One* 12(3), e0172277.

Allcott H., Lockwood, B.B. & Taubinsky, D. 2019. Regressive sin taxes, with an application to the optimal soda tax. *Quarterly Journal of Economics*, 134 (3), 1557–1626. https://doi.org/10.1093/qje/qjz017

Andreyeva, T., Long, M. W. & Brownell, K. D. 2010. The impact of food prices on consumption: A systematic review of research on the price elasticity of demand for food. *American Journal of Public Health,* 100, 216–222.

Bhattacharya, J. & Bundorf, M. K. 2009. The incidence of the healthcare costs of obesity. *Journal of Health Economics,* 28, 649–658.

Biener, A. I., Cawley, J. & Meyerhoefer, C. 2020. The medical care costs of obesity and severe obesity in youth: An instrumental variables approach. *Health Economics,* 29, 624–639.

Bonnet, C. & Requillart, V. 2011. Does the EU sugar policy reform increase added sugar consumption? An empirical evidence on the soft drink market. *Health Economics,* 20, 1012–1024.

Bronchetti, E. T., Christensen, G. & Hoynes, H. W. 2019. Local food prices, SNAP purchasing power, and child health. *Journal of Health Economics,* 68, 102231.

Caro, J. C., Corvalán, C., Reyes, M., Silva, A., Popkin, B. & Taillie, L. S. 2018. Chile's 2014 sugar-sweetened beverage tax and changes in prices and purchases of sugar-sweetened beverages: An observational study in an urban environment. *PLoS Medicine,* 15, e1002597.

Cawley, J. & Meyerhoefer, C. 2012. The medical care costs of obesity: An instrumental variables approach. *Journal of Health Economics,* 31, 219–230.

Colen, L., Melo, P. C., Abdul-Salam, Y., Roberts, D., Mary, S. & Gomez, Y., Paloma, S. 2018. Income elasticities for food, calories and nutrients across Africa: A meta-analysis. *Food Policy,* 77, 116–132.

Cornelsen, L., Green, R., Dangour, A. & Smith, R. 2015a. Why fat taxes won't make us thin. *Journal of Public Health,* 37, 18–23.

Cornelsen, L., Green, R., Turner, R., Dangour, A. D., Shankar, B., Mazzocchi, M. & Smith, R. D. 2015b. What happens to patterns of food consumption when food prices change? Evidence from a systematic review and meta-analysis of food price elasticities globally. *Health Economics,* 24, 1548–1559.

Cornelsen, L., Mytton, O. T., Adams, J., Gasparrini, A., Iskander, D., Knai, C., Petticrew, M., Scott, C., Smith, R. & Thompson, C. 2017. Change in non-alcoholic beverage sales following a 10-pence levy on sugar-sweetened beverages within a national chain of restaurants in the UK: Interrupted time series analysis of a natural experiment. *Journal of Epidemiology Community Health,* 71, 1107–1112.

Crawford, I., Keen, M. & Smith, S. 2010. Value added tax and excises. In: S. Adam, T. Besley, R. Blundell, S. Bond, R. Chote, M. Gammie, P. Johnson, G. Myles & J. Poterba (eds.) *Dimensions of Tax Design: The Mirrlees Review.* Oxford: Oxford University Press.

Cuadrado, C., Dunstan, J., Silva-Illanes, N., Mirelman, A. J., Nakamura, R. & Suhrcke, M. 2020. Effects of a sugar-sweetened beverage tax on prices and affordability of soft drinks in Chile: A time series analysis. *Social Science & Medicine,* 245, 112708.

Dharmasena, S. & Capps, J. R. 2012. Intended and unintended consequences of a proposed national tax on sugar-sweetened beverages to combat the US obesity problem. *Health Economics*, 21, 669–694.

Dixon, P., Davey Smith, G. & Hollingworth, W. 2019. The association between adiposity and inpatient hospital costs in the UK Biobank Cohort. *Applied Health Economics and Health Policy,* 17, 359–370.

Falbe, J., Thompson, H. R., Becker, C. M., Rojas, N., Mcculloch, C. E. & Madsen, K. A. 2016. Impact of the Berkeley excise tax on sugar-sweetened beverage consumption. *American Journal of Public Health,* 106, 1865–1871.

Finkelstein, E. A., Zhen, C., Bilger, M., Nonnemaker, J., Farooqui, A. M. & Todd, J. E. 2013. Implications of a sugar-sweetened beverage (SSB) tax when substitutions to non-beverage items are considered. *Journal of Health Economics,* 32, 219–239.

Fullerton, D., Leicester, A. & Smith, S. 2010. Environmental taxes. In: S. Adam, T. Besley, R. Blundell, S. Bond, R. Chote, M. Gammie, P. Johnson, G. Myles & J. Poterba (eds.) *Dimensions of Tax Design: The Mirrlees Review.* Oxford: Oxford University Press.

Green, R., Cornelsen, L., Dangour, A. D., Turner, R., Shankar, B., Mazzocchi, M. & Smith, R. D. 2013. The effect of rising food prices on food consumption: Systematic review with meta-regression. *BMJ,* 346, f3703.

Griffith, R., Von Hinke, S. & Smith, S. 2018. Getting a healthy start: The effectiveness of targeted benefits for improving dietary choices. *Journal of Health Economics,* 58, 176–187.

Gruber, J. 2010. Commentary on 'value added tax and excises'. In: S. Adam, T. Besley, R. Blundell, S. Bond, R. Chote, M. Gammie, P. Johnson, G. Myles & J. Poterba (eds.) *Dimensions of Tax Design: The Mirrlees Review.* Oxford: Oxford University Press.

Jones, N. R., Conklin, A. I., Suhrcke, M. & Monsivais, P. 2014. The growing price gap between more and less healthy foods: Analysis of a novel longitudinal UK dataset. *PLoS One,* 9, e109343.

Lakdawalla, D. & Philipson, T. 2009. The growth of obesity and technological change. *Economics and Human Biology,* 7, 283–293.

Lee, M. M., Falbe, J., Schillinger, D., Basu, S., Mcculloch, C. E. & Madsen, K. A. 2019. Sugar-sweetened beverage consumption 3 years after the Berkeley, California, sugar-sweetened beverage tax. *American Journal of Public Health,* 109, 637–639.

Madsen, K. A., Krieger, J. & Morales, X. 2019. Sugar-sweetened beverage taxes: Emerging evidence on a new public health policy. *JAMA,* 321, 1777–1779.

Marmot, M., Allen, J., Boyce, T., Goldblatt, P. & Morrison, J.. 2020. *Health equity in England: The Marmot Review 10 years on.* London: Institute of Health Equity https://www.health.org.uk/publications/reports/the-marmot-review-10-years-on

Martin, A., Suhrcke, M. & Ogilvie, D. 2012. Financial Incentives to Promote Active Travel: An Evidence Review and Economic Framework. *American Journal of Preventive Medicine,* 43, e45–e57.

Miao, Z., Beghin, J. C. & Jensen, H. H. 2013. Accounting for product substitution in the analysis of food taxes targeting obesity. *Health Economics,* 22, 1318–1343.

Niblett, P., Coyle, N., Little, E. A., Beaton, C., Burton, J., Chisholm, C., Tedstone, A., Targett, V., Nicholas, J. & Montel, S. 2019. Sugar reduction: Report on progress between 2015 and 2018. London, Public Health England.

Pechey, R., Jebb, S. A., Kelly, M. P., Almiron-Roig, E., Conde, S., Nakamura, R., Shemilt, I., Suhrcke, M. & Marteau, T. M. 2013. Socioeconomic differences in purchases of more vs. less healthy foods and beverages: Analysis of over 25,000 British households in 2010. *Social Science & Medicine,* 92, 22–26.

Pell, D., Mytton, O., Penney, T. L., Briggs, A., Cummins, S., Penn-Jones, C., Rayner, M., Rutter, H., Scarborough, P., Sharp, S. J., Smith, R. D., White, M. & Adams, J. 2021. Changes in soft drinks purchased by British households associated with the UK soft drinks industry levy: Controlled interrupted time series analysis. *BMJ,* 372, n254.

Rippin, H. L., Cade, J. E., Berrang Ford, L., Benton, T. G., Hancock, N., & Greenwood, D. C. (2021). Variations in greenhouse gas emissions of individual diets: associations between the greenhouse gas emissions and nutrient intake in the United Kingdom. PLoS One, 16(11): e0259418.

Pfinder, M., Heise, T. L., Hilton Boon, M., Pega, F., Fenton, C., Griebler, U., Gartlehner, G., Sommer, I., Katikireddi, S. V. & Lhachimi, S. K. 2020. Taxation of unprocessed sugar or sugar-added foods for reducing their consumption and preventing obesity or other adverse health outcomes. *Cochrane Database of Systematic Reviews*, 2020(4): CD012333.

Popkin, B. M. & Hawkes, C. 2016. Sweetening of the global diet, particularly beverages: Patterns, trends, and policy responses. *The Lancet Diabetes & Endocrinology,* 4, 174–186.

Powell, L. M., Chriqui, J. F., Khan, T., Wada, R. & Chaloupka, F. J. 2013. Assessing the potential effectiveness of food and beverage taxes and subsidies for improving public health: A systematic review of prices, demand and body weight outcomes. *Obesity Reviews,* 14, 110–128.

Public Health England and Food Standards Agency. 2020. National diet and nutrition survey rolling programme years 9 to 11 (2016/2017 to 2018/2019).

Redondo, M., Hernández-Aguado, I. & Lumbreras, B. 2018. The impact of the tax on sweetened beverages: A systematic review. *The American Journal of Clinical Nutrition,* 108, 548–563.

Roberto, C. A., Lawman, H. G., Levasseur, M. T., Mitra, N., Peterhans, A., Herring, B. & Bleich, S. N. 2019. Association of a beverage tax on sugar-sweetened and artificially sweetened beverages with changes in beverage prices and sales at chain retailers in a large urban setting. *JAMA,* 321, 1799–1810.

Scarborough, P., Adhikari, V., Harrington, R. A., Elhussein, A., Briggs, A., Rayner, M., Adams, J., Cummins, S., Penney, T. & White, M. 2020. Impact of the announcement and implementation of the UK soft drinks industry levy on sugar content, price, product size and number of available soft drinks in the UK, 2015–19: A controlled interrupted time series analysis. *PLoS Medicine,* 17, e1003025.

Schmacker, R. & Smed, S. 2020. Do prices and purchases respond similarly to soft drink tax increases and cuts? *Economics & Human Biology,* 37, 100864.

Schroeter, C., Lusk, J. & Tyner, W. 2008. Determining the impact of food price and income changes on body weight. *Journal of Health Economics,* 27, 45–68.

Smed, S., Scarborough, P., Rayner, M. & Jensen, J. D. 2016. The effects of the Danish saturated fat tax on food and nutrient intake and modelled health outcomes: An econometric and comparative risk assessment evaluation. *European Journal of Clinical Nutrition,* 70, 681–686.

Teng, A. M., Jones, A. C., Mizdrak, A., Signal, L., Genç, M. & Wilson, N. 2019. Impact of sugar-sweetened beverage taxes on purchases and dietary intake: Systematic review and meta-analysis. *Obesity Reviews,* 20, 1187–1204.

The Economist. 2009. Waist banned: Does a tax on junk food make sense? *Finance and Economics Section*, August 1, 2009.

Walls, H. L., Cornelsen, L., Lock, K. & Smith, R. D. 2016. How much priority is given to nutrition and health in the EU Common Agricultural Policy? *Food Policy,* 59, 12–23.

Watt, T. L. S., Beckert, W., Smith, R. D. & Cornelsen, L. 2020. Reducing consumption of unhealthy foods and beverages through banning price promotions: What is the evidence and will it work? *Public Health Nutrition,* 23, 2228–2233.

Yaniv, G., Rosin, O. & Tobol, Y. 2009. Junk-food, home cooking, physical activity and obesity: The effect of the fat tax and the thin subsidy. *Journal of Public Economics,* 93, 823–830.

Yu, Y. & Jaenicke, E. C. 2020. Estimating food waste as household production inefficiency. *American Journal of Agricultural Economics,* 102, 525–547.

# 18 Importance of Sustainable Food Environments

*Christine L. Cleghorn*
University of Otago

*Christian J. Reynolds*
City, University of London

**CONTENTS**



## 18.1 INTRODUCTION

In the past decade, more countries have started to incorporate sustainability considerations into their food policies, dietary guidance, and consumer facing programmes (Reynolds et al., 2014). Such recommendations include – consuming a mostly plant-based diet, consuming seasonal and local foods, reducing food waste, consuming fish from sustainable stocks, and reducing consumption of red and processed meat, highly processed foods, and sugar-sweetened beverages. These actions may all seem to be quite distinct; however, due to the complex and multifaceted concepts involved, each of these recommendations contributes to a different (but interrelated) aspect of sustainability. This chapter will explore and introduce this multi-dimensional topic which will almost certainly influence the foods available in the food system and chosen by individuals in years to come.

In the broadest context, sustainable diets can be described as "food choices that support life and health within natural system limits into the foreseeable future"

DOI: 10.1201/9781003043720-18

(Gussow and Clancy, 1986). However, this definition misses the nuance and breadth of scope that the 2010 FAO definition provides:

> Those diets with low environmental impacts which contribute to food and nutrition security and to healthy life for present and future generations. Sustainable diets are protective and respectful of biodiversity and ecosystems, culturally acceptable, accessible, economically fair and affordable; nutritionally adequate, safe and healthy; while optimizing natural and human resources.
>
> *Burlingame and Dernini (2012)*

Yet to operationalize this definition in a practical nutrition setting is challenging. Few policy makers or practitioners have access to information or expertise to balance multiple nutrition, and environment, economic, and socio-cultural dimensions for each dietary recommendation, or policy choice; and so fall back upon the definition that sustainable diets are those that have a low impact on the environment. Until recently, this was often equated to mean that the production and consumption of this diet is associated with lower levels of greenhouse gas (GHG) emissions. Sustainable diets have become almost synonymous with GHG emissions for three reasons: (i) GHG emissions data was one of the first types of environmental impact data widely available for multiple types of food products and production systems. (ii) Climate change is one of the largest threats facing humanity and has knock on effects into other domains of sustainability. (iii) The embodied GHG emissions of different foods are correlated to other environmental impacts (including water use, energy use, biodiversity loss, and land use (Poore and Nemecek, 2018)).

Communicating what a sustainable diet is to consumers is also challenging. Currently there is limited consumer understanding of what is a sustainable dietary pattern (Van Loo et al., 2017), or which foods have a low environmental impact (Camilleri et al., 2019) – with these two topics becoming easily conflated. However, these again are two different concepts. Indeed, not all foods consumed within a sustainable diet have to be low impact. However, the diet as a whole needs to be within environmental bounds – as will be discussed here.

The act of food production generates environmental impacts at each stage of the food system; from farming and processing, transportation, transit packaging, consumer packaging, warehouse, and distribution, to refrigeration and storage at the supermarkets and shops, through to driving home, cooking, and waste disposal. As the food that we choose to eat drives food production, changing dietary patterns at a population level or widespread changes in food choice can impact on the environmental impact associated with food production. Additionally changes made across the supply chain of food production can change the environmental impact of specific foods and, if widespread enough, the whole food system.

## 18.2 PLANETARY BOUNDARIES EFFECTED BY FOOD PRODUCTION

The planet we live on has finite resources and limits to the amount of environmental damage it can suffer without system collapse. Rockström et al. (2009) outlined the

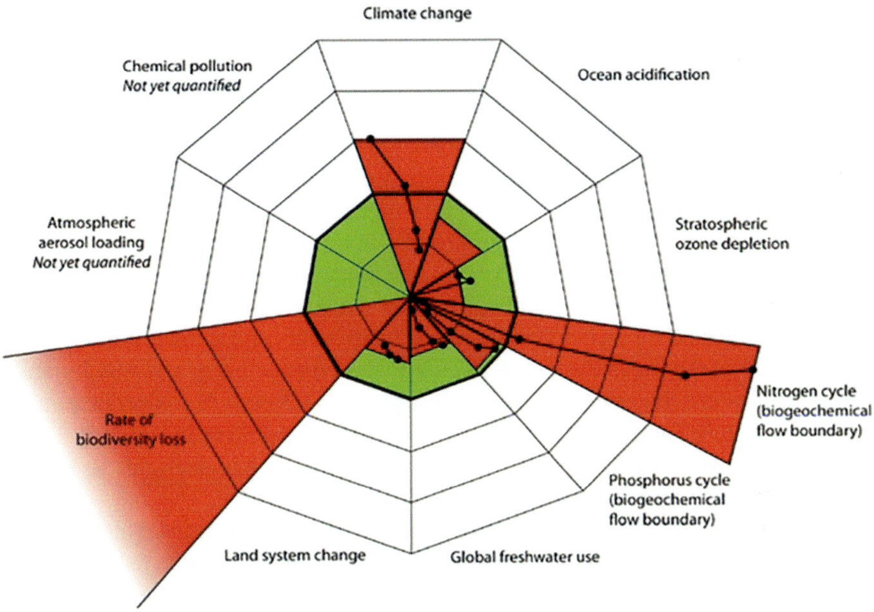


**FIGURE 18.1** Estimate of quantitative evolution of control variables for seven planetary boundaries from pre-industrial levels to the present. The inner (green) shaded area represents the safe operating space with proposed boundary levels at its outer contour. The wedges for each boundary show the estimate of current position of the control variable. (Reprinted under licence CC BY-NC 4.0 from Rockström et al. (2009), https://creativecommons.org/licenses/by-nc/4.0/.)

nine planetary boundary limits within which we expect that humanity can operate safely. These earth system processes are climate change; ocean acidification; stratospheric ozone depletion; atmospheric aerosol loading; biogeochemical flows – interference with phosphorus and nitrogen cycles; global freshwater use; land system change; rate of biodiversity loss; and chemical pollution (see Figure 18.1).

Five of these are greatly affected by food production and should be considered when discussing sustainable food production and therefore sustainable diets (climate change, interference with the global nitrogen and phosphorus cycles, freshwater use, land-system change, and biodiversity loss) with special attention given to the three that have already breached the safe operating limits (see Figure 18.1).

Climate change is the planetary boundary most often discussed as it poses an immense threat to global health alongside its impact to the physical environment and the world is now at a critical point for avoiding catastrophic climate change. The global food system is responsible for up to 29% of all anthropogenic GHG emissions (Costello et al., 2009). Changes to the global food system alongside changes to the foods we all eat are essential to reduce global GHG emissions to levels compatible with the Paris agreement.

Human modification of the Nitrogen cycle is particularly notable with more conversion from atmospheric $N_2$ to reactive forms due to human activities than all other terrestrial processes combined. The main purpose is to enhance food production through fertilisation but much is lost to the environment causing pollution of waterways and the atmosphere. Phosphorus is added in food production as fertilizer, and this increased inflow to oceans has been suggested as the main cause of ocean anoxic events causing widespread marine death.

Global manipulations of the freshwater cycle affect biodiversity and ecological functioning which have knock-on effects to food production and food and water security. This manifests through a loss of soil moisture, human water supply, and aquatic water needs as well as through impacts in climate regulation.

Land-system change is mainly driven by agricultural expansion and intensification, and there is much concern internationally about the conversion of biodiverse rainforests into grazing land for cattle. This threatens biodiversity and is undermining regulatory capacities of the Earth System through impacts on the climate and water systems.

Biodiversity loss is particularly serious, due to biodiversity's importance in sustaining ecosystem functioning. There is concern that non-linear and largely irreversible consequences are likely. Recent biodiversity loss has been due to land-use change, introduction of species and climate change.

One area of biodiversity that deserves further mention is the impact of overfishing on the health of oceans. The consumption of omega 3 fatty acids from fish reduces the risk of cardiovascular disease, and regular consumption of fish is therefore recommended widely. These nutrition recommendations do not consider the environmental impact of overfishing or the knock-on effects onto human health. Fish populations have been exploited for many years and regulation is almost impossible to enforce. The extinction of fish species used for food can have significant and catastrophic follow-on effects on other species and the ocean ecosystems which can then contribute to ocean dead zones (Jackson, 2008). With the alternative source of fish, aquaculture, having its own environmental impacts such as habitat destruction and overfishing for feed ingredients (Troell et al., 2014).

These planetary boundaries are interrelated with the degradation of one planetary boundary affecting others. Much of the research showing sustainable diets are high in unprocessed plant-based foods and low in animal-based foods focus on GHG emissions (Drew et al., 2020; Green et al., 2015) with less attention given to the other planetary boundaries (Willett et al., 2019). However, synergies between GHG emission impact of diets and impact on other planetary boundaries such as land use and water use have been shown (Clark et al., 2019; Gephart et al., 2016) and can be seen in Figure 18.2 from the EAT Lancet Commission (Willett et al., 2019). Research into the impact of dietary intake on 'sustainability' should continue to investigate impacts on all relevant planetary boundaries.

## 18.3 GHG EMISSIONS ASSOCIATED WITH FOOD PRODUCTION AND CONSUMPTION

Each type of food has different environmental impacts in different parts of the food system. This has most recently been illustrated by the meta-analysis conducted by Poore and Nemecek (2018), the results of which are presented in Figure 18.3. Overall, animal-based foods tend to be much higher in environmental impacts than plant-based foods. With the production of a kilogram of beef emitting 60 kg

| Food item | GHG emissions (10kg$CO_2$/serving) | Cropland use (10m$^2$/serving) | Water use (10m$^3$/serving) |
|---|---|---|---|
| wheat | 0.10 | 1.51 | 0.22 |
| rice | 0.53 | 1.58 | 0.48 |
| maize | 0.08 | 0.89 | 0.07 |
| other grains | 0.13 | 2.76 | 0.07 |
| roots | 0.08 | 0.76 | 0.05 |
| legumes | 0.08 | 3.86 | 0.33 |
| soybeans | 0.04 | 1.38 | 0.05 |
| nuts & seeds | 0.21 | 1.92 | 0.13 |
| vegetables | 0.05 | 0.41 | 0.07 |
| fruits (temperate) | 0.11 | 1.65 | 0.47 |
| fruits (tropical) | 0.13 | 1.32 | 0.45 |
| fruits (starchy) | 0.15 | 1.18 | 0.16 |
| sugar | 0.01 | 0.07 | 0.05 |
| palm oil | 0.26 | 0.43 | 0.00 |
| vegetable oil | 0.09 | 1.44 | 0.07 |
| beef | 35.74 | 4.64 | 0.24 |
| lamb | 36.33 | 6.86 | 0.54 |
| pork | 3.21 | 6.69 | 0.38 |
| poultry | 1.55 | 7.25 | 0.44 |
| eggs | 0.79 | 3.43 | 0.22 |
| milk | 2.93 | 3.21 | 0.19 |
| shellfish | 0.08 | 0.40 | 0.04 |
| fish (freshwater) | 0.33 | 1.66 | 0.11 |
| fish (demersal) | 0.02 | 0.14 | 0.01 |
| fish(pelagic) | 0.00 | 0.00 | 0.00 |

**FIGURE 18.2** Global average environmental impact per serving of major food groups from the EAT Lancet Commission (Willett et al., 2019). Colours indicate environmental impacts from low – green; medium – orange; high – red. The EAT Lancet diet is high in vegetables, legumes, whole grains, fruit, and plant sources of protein and low in animal sources of protein compared to many currently practiced dietary patterns (see Section 18.7). (Reprinted under fair use clause.)

of GHG ($CO_2$ equivalent), lamb and cheese emit more than 20 kg. Poultry and pork are slightly lower at 6 and 7 kg. For comparison, production of a kilogram of peas emits just 1 kg of GHG emissions. The finding that animal products are high impact compared to plant-based products holds regardless of the functional unit used (e.g. what the impact is measured against). Figure 18.4 shows this same relationship with the functional unit of "gram of Protein" rather than per kilogram of end product (Ranganathan, 2016).

For the majority of foods, most GHG emissions result from land use change and from processes at the farm stage (including application of fertilisers and methane from cattle). Combined, land use, and farm-stage emissions account for more than 80% of the footprint for most foods.

However, the method of production and where on the planet the food is produced can dramatically alter the environmental impacts of individual foods. This creates opportunities for targeted interventions. For example, for beef, the highest impact

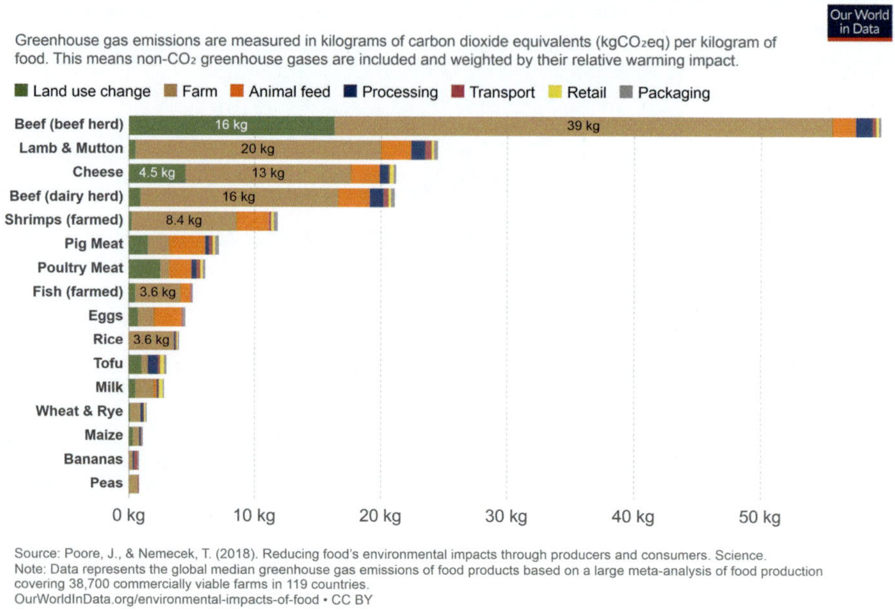


**FIGURE 18.3** Food-related greenhouse gas emissions across the supply chain. (Data from Poore and Nemecek (2018) published on OurWorldinData.org under licence CC BY 4.0, https://creativecommons.org/licenses/by/4.0/deed.en_US.)

25% of producers represent 56% of the beef's global GHG emissions (an estimated 1.3 billion metric tons of $CO_2$ equivalent). Across all products, 25% of producers contribute on average 53% of each food's environmental impact (Poore and Nemecek, 2018).

For many consumers, transport is (incorrectly) thought to be a large contributor to GHG emissions. However, transport is only a small contributor to total emissions. For most food products, transport accounts for <10% of total emissions, and it makes up a very small proportion for the largest GHG emitters. For example, in beef production, transport accounts for only 0.5% of total emissions. Indeed, all processes in the supply chain after the farm – processing, transport, retail, and packaging – mostly account for small shares of total emissions. The small contribution of transport emissions also holds for dietary patterns as well as individual products. In the EU, food transport was responsible for only 6% of emissions associated with dietary intake whilst production of dairy, meat, and eggs accounted for 83% of total emissions (Sandström et al., 2018). Notably post-retail transport emissions can be higher than pre-retail, due to the differences in efficiencies of scale. However, this is complicated and depends on the food product, amount purchased, and either the frequency and method of travel to and from the store (bike, car, on foot etc.) or the method of delivery by online shopping (Sonesson et al., 2005).

Food loss and waste is a large contributor to food-related GHG emissions. It is estimated that approximately 8% of all global GHG emissions caused by humans is related to food waste. This is equal to 24% of total global food emissions. Globally, two-thirds of food loss and waste is from losses in the supply chain, which are caused

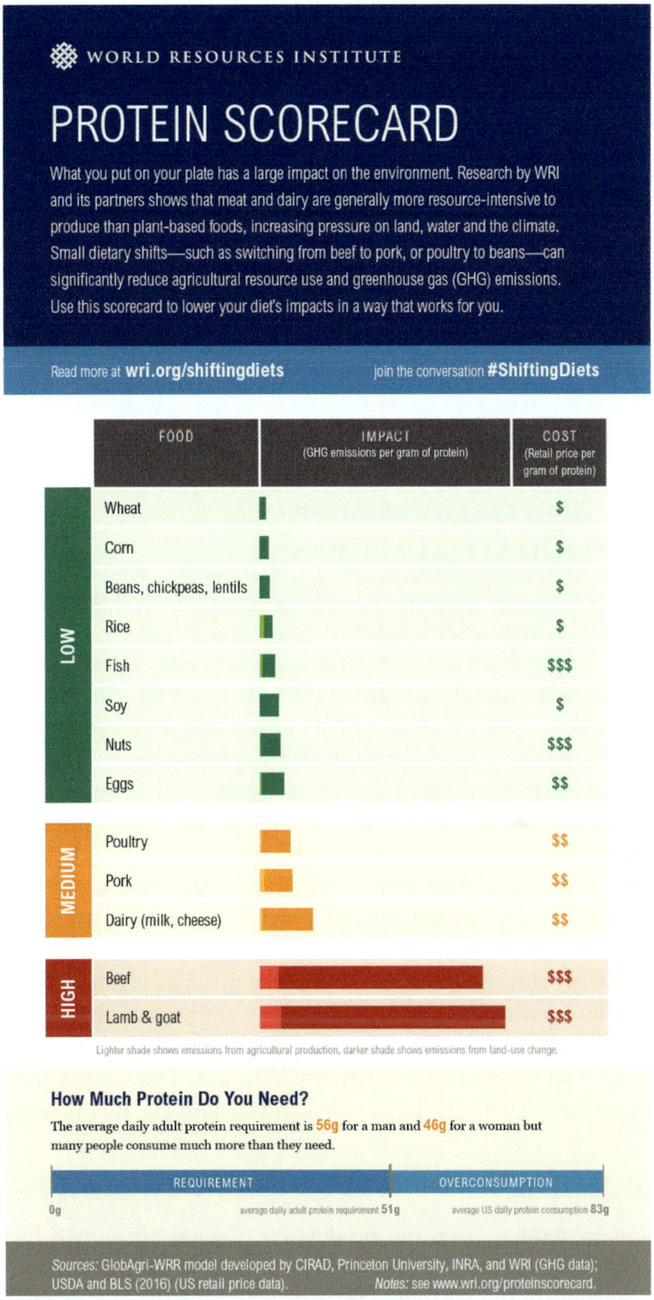


**FIGURE 18.4** Greenhouse gas emissions per gram of protein of a selection of low, medium, and high-emitting foods. (Reprinted under the open data commitment from Ranganathan (2016).)

by poor storage and handling techniques; lack of refrigeration; and spoilage in transport and processing. The other third comes from food thrown away by retailers and consumers (Poore and Nemecek, 2018). Food loss and waste can be reduced through changes to the supply chain, by giving consumers better food skills and through shifting diets to foods that are wasted less. The exact proportion of food loss vs food waste is different for each country, with industrialized food systems – such as the UK and USA – generating more food waste than food loss. In addition, the main food wasters in industrialised food systems are domestic households. For this reason, shifting consumer's food waste behaviours (including wasteful dietary patterns) is crucial for shifting towards sustainable diets. Changes to the food environment can reduce food waste. Successful interventions to reduce consumer food waste include changing the size of plate and serving ware, changing nutritional guidance, and information campaigns. Other less validated methods include cooking classes, fridge cameras, food sharing apps, advertising, and information sharing (Reynolds et al., 2019a).

## 18.4 REDUCTION OF GHG EMISSIONS FROM FOOD CONSUMPTION

Individuals can reduce the environmental impact from food production by choosing to eat foods with low associated environmental impact and through changing their dietary patterns to more sustainable overall diets (see Section 18.7). These decisions can be supported through changes in the food environment and food policy and through pricing mechanisms such as a GHG or red and processed meat tax, making the sustainable choice the easier and more affordable choice.

However, it has been highlighted that many types of sustainable (low GHG emission) diets are not culturally acceptable (Green et al., 2015) (being unpalatable, expensive, too far from what is currently eaten, etc.). Thus, it has been proposed that different dietary advice could be given to different sub-populations. One method to group subpopulations is by income. Studies from Australia (Reynolds et al., 2015), the Netherlands (van Dooren, 2018), Japan (Kanemoto et al., 2019) and the UK (Reynolds et al., 2019b) have all shown that different income groups consume different types of foods (and in differing quantities) with different environmental impacts. Due to these different consumption patterns, each income groups has different trade-offs and starting points on their pathways towards sustainable diets. The studies have shown that regardless of income, an affordable, healthy, and sustainable diet is possible.

## 18.5 GLOBAL VARIATION IN SUSTAINABILITY IMPACTS

GHG emissions generated from the production of food consumed in high-income countries are substantially higher that that from people in middle- and low-income countries. The responsibility for those emissions lies with those consuming diets associated with environmental degradation, putting aside where this food may have been produced. As low- and middle-income countries develop, there is a trend for dietary intake to move towards what is considered 'more western' diets, i.e. high in meat, dairy, and ultra-processed food. And with this trend comes the potential for substantial rises in global GHG emissions and impacts on the other planetary boundaries associated with food production. Due to this current and historical imbalance in responsibility, high-income countries have a responsibility to lead the way in sustainable food production and consumption. This variation in dietary pattern is also generational, with different generations (with distinct developmental food environments) leading to different dietary choices with their associated environmental impacts. For this reason, all ages of consumer must also shift towards a sustainable diet.

## 18.6 ENVIRONMENTAL HEALTH CO-BENEFITS OF SUSTAINABLE DIETS

There are likely to be significant health and environmental co-benefits of shifts in diet towards more sustainable foods. Foods with the highest associated GHG emission, red and processed meat (Drew et al., 2020), are also associated with increased risks of colorectal cancer (International Agency for Research on Cancer (World Health Organization), 2015), type 2 diabetes (Forouzanfar et al., 2015), and death from cardiovascular disease (CVD) (Abete et al., 2014). Substitutions for meat that have lower GHG emissions such as fruit, vegetables, nuts, seeds, and whole grains are associated with a reduction in CVD and some cancers (Forouzanfar et al., 2015).

A number of modelling studies have shown that more sustainable diets are lower in meat intake and higher in fruits, vegetables, and whole foods with the associated improvements in health. It has been estimated that global mortality could be reduced by 6%–10% and food-related GHG emissions by 29%–70% by 2050 with shifts towards more plant-based diets that are in line with dietary guidelines (Springmann et al., 2016). The EAT Lancet Commission estimated that changing global consumption to a healthy sustainable diet could avert 19%–24% of deaths per year (Willett et al., 2019). A systematic review found that dietary change could reduce GHG emissions and land-use demands by up to 50% compared to current diets (Hallström et al., 2015).

However, not all low emission or low environmental impact foods are healthier and shifts towards some low emission foods, such as sugary food and drink and ultra-processed foods (Drew et al., 2020; Willett et al., 2019) would not confer health benefits.

## 18.7 EXAMPLES OF SUSTAINABLE DIETS

There are a number of sustainable diets that have been proposed internationally that we can draw on. In all of these diets, there is the common element of increases in fruits, vegetables, and plant sources of protein and a decrease in meat intake. When this is taken to its full extent, you find the vegan diet which excludes all meat, fish, eggs, and dairy products and provides nutrition through plant sources. Modelled health benefits of dietary shifts towards sustainable diets are usually greatest for the vegan diet (Drew et al., 2020). A recent trend is also 'plant based diets' which are potentially less strict than vegan diets but follow the same principles. However, population diets do not need to shift to completely vegan diets to benefit the environment. Cultural shifts so plant-based meals are more normalised with small portions of meat viewed as optional additions would have a large impact on population health and sustainability. These cultural understandings are often more common in low- and middle-income countries than in high-income countries.

In 2011, the WWF-UK "LiveWell 2020" (https://www.wwf.org.uk/what-we-do/livewell) programme was created which aimed to develop diets in the UK, France, and Sweden that decreased GHG emissions by 25% from the current diet, cost no more, met national nutritional guidelines, and still resembled current diets sufficiently to be widely and easily accepted. In the UK, this reduction in emissions would be achieved by limiting the consumption of animal protein and increasing protein from legumes and nuts; in France by reducing consumption of meat and meat products and increasing consumption of legumes and cereals and in Sweden by reducing consumption of meat, dairy products, sugar, sweets, and fruit-based products and increasing consumption of vegetables, cereals, and nuts. In all countries, these modelled sustainable diets were cheaper than the current diets. These diets also implied health benefits due to reduced red and processed meat consumption and increases in the quantities of oily fish, vegetables, and nuts.

In 2019, the EAT Lancet Commission (Willett et al., 2019) proposed an internationally acceptable sustainable diet based on the six planetary boundaries (nitrogen and phosphorus were considered as separate planetary boundaries) that are greatly affected by food production (Rockström et al., 2009). The Commission proposed a 'Great Food Transformation' including a global reference diet to bring these six key earth system processes to within safe operating boundaries. The reference diet is high in vegetables, legumes, whole grains, fruit, and plant sources of protein and low in animal sources of protein. Modelling on shifting global consumption from current diets to the EAT Lancet reference diet showed substantial benefit to human health, averting about 10.8–11.6 million deaths per year, which is a reduction of 19%–24% (Willett et al., 2019).

## 18.8 MOVING TOWARDS SUSTAINABLE DIETS: CURRENT BEST PRACTICE

There are many tools and levers that have the potential to shift dietary consumption towards more sustainable foods. These range from education, through changing the food environment to fiscal measures and changes to legislation (Garnett, 2014).

First, those that are explicitly about sustainability. A number of countries have incorporated aspects of sustainability into their dietary guidelines; Brazil (Brazil, 2014) and Sweden (Sweden, 2015) provide two good examples. Other European countries have supporting documents to their guidelines on sustainable dietary intake (Fischer and Garnett, 2016). The Barilla double food pyramid was developed in 2010 and updated in 2016 by the Barilla centre for food and nutrition, a privately held, apolitical and non-profit think tank to show the close alignment between nutritional value and environmental impact (see Figure 18.5).

Food labels on the environmental impact of foods could help to educate the public on what food choices are the most environmentally friendly. Consumers could compare foods across and within food groups. Some have been proposed that include impacts onto GHG emissions, nitrogen, and water footprints (Leach et al., 2016), but these have not been evaluated. In 2008, the European Commission launched a project to create a European method of calculating the environmental impact of products, based on their life cycle and other environmental indicators. This has led to the development of the Product Environmental Footprint (PEF) which has been piloted and consulted on between 2013 and 2019.

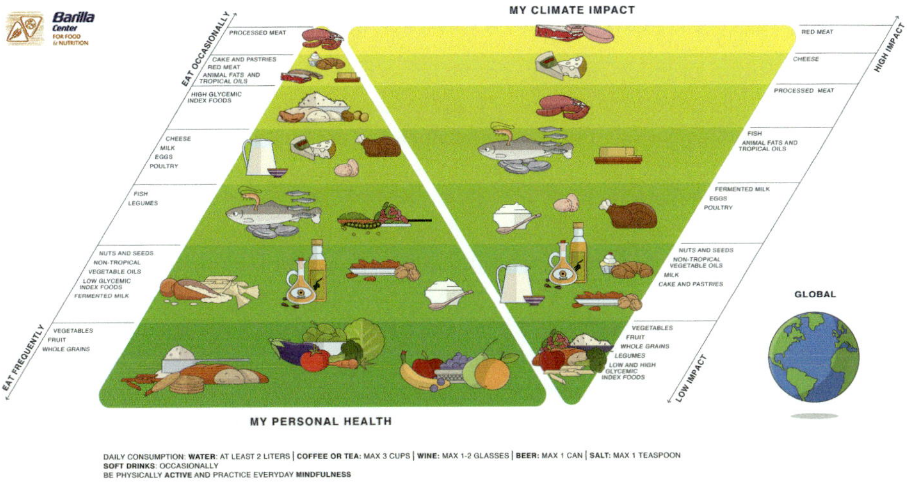


**FIGURE 18.5** The Barilla double food pyramid. (From Barilla Foundation (2021), The double food and environmental pyramid highlights the extremely close links between two aspects of every food: its nutritional value and the environmental impact it has through the stages of its production and consumption, https://www.barillacfn.com/en/dissemination/double_pyramid/.)

There have been a number of initiatives to promote more sustainable food choices that have evolved outside of the influence of government such as meat free Mondays and Veganuary. These could be capitalised on and expanded through support from government. Some institutions, such as the National Health Service in the UK, have a sustainability policy that extends to food provision (Department of Health, 2009).

High GHG emission foods could be taxed to discourage purchase and consumption. Modelling studies have shown that a tax on selected meat and dairy products would result in a 12% reduction in sector GHG emissions (Säll and Gren, 2012). The reduction in global deaths attributable to red and processed meat consumption decreased by 9% with a red and processed meat tax (Springmann et al., 2018).

But many interventions that aim to improve dietary intake for health would also have sustainability co-benefits as outlined above. Shifts towards following the dietary guidelines, taxes on unhealthy food, improvements to the food environment to encourage increased fruit and vegetable consumption and health warning labels on processed meat are likely to improve the sustainability of population dietary intake.

Changes to the food environment (Garnett et al., 2019) and food policy put in place by governments have the potential to make large impacts on both the environmental impact of food consumption and health, including legislation to change industry practices. Putting the responsibility onto individuals to changes their diets in order to decrease the impact of dietary GHG emissions and environmental degradation, although important, will not make the gains needed. A lot of the changes that need to be made are outside of the control of the public and require governments, international bodies and industry to act.

## 18.9 FUTURE CONSIDERATIONS AND CONCLUSIONS

It is now common practice in many countries to consider the sustainability of diets and food. Multiple government's dietary advice now include sustainability, alongside health and monetary costs. Future research needs to tackle a lack of understanding in how to implement sub-population-level sustainable diets and assist in shifting food environments (from local to global) towards making sustainable, healthy, low waste, and affordable options the default choice. One of the most difficult challenges is adapting this advice to multiple cultural contexts, with every country and gastronomic cuisine style needing its own advice. This knowledge gap is currently felt in low- and middle-income countries where there is limited evidence available.

There is a global imperative to change practice to reduce our impact on the environment with climate change being the most immediate focus. Food production, and by extension consumption, impacts on climate change, freshwater use, land-system use, biodiversity and interferes with the global nitrogen and phosphorus cycles. It is therefore imperative that changes are made to current consumption in order to reduce this impact. There are many changes that individuals can make to reduce their environmental food footprint but the largest and most necessary gains will come from regional, national, and global changes in the food production systems, food policy, and food environment.

## REFERENCES

Abete, I., Romaguera, D., Vieira, A. R., Lopez-de Munain, A. & Norat, T. 2014. Association between total, processed, red and white meat consumption and all-cause, CVD and IHD mortality: a meta-analysis of cohort studies. *British Journal of Nutrition,* 112, 762–775.

Brazil, M. 2014. Dietary guidelines for the Brazilian population. Brasília: Ministry of Health.

Burlingame, B. & Dernini, S. (2012). Sustainable diets and biodiversity: directions and solutions for policy, research and action. *International Scientific Symposium, Biodiversity and Sustainable Diets United Against Hunger,* FAO Headquarters, Rome, Italy, 3–5 November 2010.

Camilleri, A. R., Larrick, R. P., Hossain, S. & Patino-echeverri, D. 2019. Consumers underestimate the emissions associated with food but are aided by labels. *Nature Climate Change,* 9, 53–58.

Clark, M. A., Springmann, M., Hill, J. & Tilman, D. 2019. Multiple health and environmental impacts of foods. *Proceedings of the National Academy of Sciences,* 116, 23357–23362.

Costello, A., Abbas, M., Allen, A., Ball, S., Bell, S., Bellamy, R., Friel, S., Groce, N., Johnson, A. & Kett, M. 2009. Managing the health effects of climate change: lancet and University College London Institute for Global Health Commission. *The Lancet,* 373, 1693–1733.

Department of Health, NHS Purchasing and Supply Agency. 2009. Sustainable food. A guide for hospitals. UK: Department of Health.

Drew, J., Cleghorn, C., Macmillan, A. & Mizdrak, A. 2020. Healthy and climate-friendly eating patterns in the New Zealand Context. *Environmental Health Perspectives,* 128, 017007.

Fischer, C. G. & Garnett, T. 2016. Plates, pyramids, and planets: developments in national healthy and sustainable dietary guidelines: a state of play assessment, Food and Agriculture Organization of the United Nations.

Forouzanfar, M. H., Alexander, L., Anderson, H. R., Bachman, V. F., Biryukov, S., Brauer, M., Burnett, R., Casey, D., Coates, M. M. & Cohen, A. 2015. Global, regional, and national comparative risk assessment of 79 behavioural, environmental and occupational, and metabolic risks or clusters of risks in 188 countries, 1990–2013: a systematic analysis for the Global Burden of Disease Study 2013. *The Lancet,* 386, 2287–2323.

Garnett, T. 2014. Changing what we eat: a call for research & action on widespread adoption of sustainable healthy eating. Food Climate Research Network.

Garnett, E. E., Balmford, A., Sandbrook, C., Pilling, M. A. & Marteau, T. M. 2019. Impact of increasing vegetarian availability on meal selection and sales in cafeterias. *Proceedings of the National Academy of Sciences of the United States of America,* 116, 20923–20929.

Gephart, J. A., Davis, K. F., Emery, K. A., Leach, A. M., Galloway, J. N. & Pace, M. L. 2016. The environmental cost of subsistence: optimizing diets to minimize footprints. *Science of the Total Environment,* 553, 120–127.

Green, R., Milner, J., Dangour, A. D., Haines, A., Chalabi, Z., Markandya, A., Spadaro, J. & Wilkinson, P. 2015. The potential to reduce greenhouse gas emissions in the UK through healthy and realistic dietary change. *Climatic Change,* 129, 253–265.

Gussow, J. D. & Clancy, K. L. 1986. Dietary guidelines for sustainability. *Journal of Nutrition Education (USA),* 18, 1–5.

Hallström, E., Carlsson-Kanyama, A. & Börjesson, P. 2015. Environmental impact of dietary change: a systematic review. *Journal of Cleaner Production,* 91, 1–11.

International Agency for Research on Cancer (World Health Organisation). 2015. IARC monographs evaluate consumption of red meat and processed meat. No. 240, Lyon, France.

Jackson, J. B. 2008. Ecological extinction and evolution in the brave new ocean. *Proceedings of the National Academy of Sciences,* 105, 11458–11465.

Kanemoto, K., Moran, D., Shigetomi, Y., Reynolds, C. & Kondo, Y. 2019. Meat consumption does not explain differences in household food carbon footprints in Japan. *One Earth,* 1, 464–471.

Leach, A. M., Emery, K. A., Gephart, J., Davis, K. F., Erisman, J. W., Leip, A., Pace, M. L., D'odorico, P., Carr, J. & Noll, L. C. 2016. Environmental impact food labels combining carbon, nitrogen, and water footprints. *Food Policy,* 61, 213–223.

Poore, J. & Nemecek, T. 2018. Reducing food's environmental impacts through producers and consumers. *Science,* 360, 987–992.

Ranganathan, J. 2016. Protein scorecard [Online]. World Resources Institute. Available: https://www.wri.org/resources/data-visualizations/protein-scorecard [Accessed 2020].

Reynolds, C. J., Buckley, J. D., Weinstein, P. & Boland, J. 2014. Are the dietary guidelines for meat, fat, fruit and vegetable consumption appropriate for environmental sustainability? A review of the literature. *Nutrients,* 6, 2251–2265.

Reynolds, C. J., Piantadosi, J., Buckley, J. D., Weinstein, P. & Boland, J. 2015. Evaluation of the environmental impact of weekly food consumption in different socio-economic households in Australia using environmentally extended input–output analysis. *Ecological Economics,* 111, 58–64.

Reynolds, C., Goucher, L., Quested, T., Bromley, S., Gillick, S., Wells, V. K., Evans, D., Koh, L., Kanyama, A. C. & Katzeff, C. 2019a. Consumption-stage food waste reduction interventions: What works and how to design better interventions. Food Policy.

Reynolds, C. J., Horgan, G. W., Whybrow, S. & Macdiarmid, J. I. 2019b. Healthy and sustainable diets that meet greenhouse gas emission reduction targets and are affordable for different income groups in the UK. *Public Health Nutrition,* 22, 1503–1517.

Rockström, J., Steffen, W. L., Noone, K., Persson, Å., Chapin Iii, F. S., Lambin, E., Lenton, T. M., Scheffer, M., Folke, C. & Schellnhuber, H. J. 2009. Planetary boundaries: exploring the safe operating space for humanity. *Ecology and Society,* 14, 32.

Säll, S. & Gren, I.-M. 2012. Green consumption taxes on meat in Sweden.

Sandström, V., Valin, H., Krisztin, T., Havlík, P., Herrero, M. & Kastner, T. 2018. The role of trade in the greenhouse gas footprints of EU diets. *Global Food Security,* 19, 48–55.

Sonesson, U., Anteson, F., Davis, J. & Sjödén, P.-O. 2005. Home transport and wastage: environmentally relevant household activities in the life cycle of food. *AMBIO: A Journal of the Human Environment,* 34, 371–375.

Springmann, M., Godfray, H. C. J., Rayner, M. & Scarborough, P. 2016. Analysis and valuation of the health and climate change cobenefits of dietary change. *Proceedings of the National Academy of Sciences,* 113, 4146–4151.

Springmann, M., Mason-D'croz, D., Robinson, S., Wiebe, K., Godfray, H. C. J., Rayner, M. & Scarborough, P. 2018. Health-motivated taxes on red and processed meat: a modelling study on optimal tax levels and associated health impacts. *PLoS One,* 13(11): e0204139.

Sweden, N. F. A. 2015. Find your way to eat greener, not too much and be active. National Food Agency, Sweden.

Troell, M., Naylor, R. L., Metian, M., Beveridge, M., Tyedmers, P. H., Folke, C., Arrow, K. J., Barrett, S., Crépin, A.-S. & Ehrlich, P. R. 2014. Does aquaculture add resilience to the global food system? *Proceedings of the National Academy of Sciences,* 111, 13257–13263.

Van Dooren, C. 2018. Simultaneous optimisation of the nutritional quality and environmental sustainability of diets.

Van Loo, E. J., Hoefkens, C. & Verbeke, W. 2017. Healthy, sustainable and plant-based eating: perceived (mis) match and involvement-based consumer segments as targets for future policy. *Food Policy,* 69, 46–57.

Willett, W., Rockström, J., Loken, B., Springmann, M., Lang, T., Vermeulen, S., Garnett, T., Tilman, D., Declerck, F. & Wood, A. 2019. Food in the Anthropocene: the EAT–Lancet Commission on healthy diets from sustainable food systems. *The Lancet,* 393, 447–492.

# 19 Evaluation of Interventions, Programmes and Policies in Food Environments

*Charlotte F.L. Evans*
University of Leeds

*Atsushi Miyawaki*
The University of Tokyo

*Anja Mizdrak*
University of Otago

**CONTENTS**



## 19.1 INTRODUCTION

Evaluation of interventions and programmes is important for many reasons; the most important being to answer the question "Did it work?" Evaluation can be separated into different categories including process evaluation, outcome evaluation, and economic evaluation (Hughes and Margetts, 2012). Process evaluation examines to what extent the individual components of the intervention actually took place. Outcome evaluation examines how effective the intervention was in improving the main outcome of interest and economic evaluation examines the costs associated with achieving outcomes of interest – including whether it was cost effective.

DOI: 10.1201/9781003043720-19

This chapter covers outcome evaluation, evaluating effectiveness overall and in specific subgroups. We start with a description of measurement tools available before moving on to examining different evaluation methods such as randomised and non-randomised controlled trials that are suitable for measuring the effectiveness of programmes and policies targeting the food environment. Evaluating food systems rather than individual programmes is discussed further in the chapter on systems approaches (Chapter 20).

## 19.2 TOOLS TO MEASURE FOOD ENVIRONMENTS

Outcomes of interest include individual food components (e.g. fruit intake, sodium intake), summative assessments of the overall diet (e.g. diet quality indices), health outcomes (e.g. body mass index, prevalence of type 2 diabetes), and measures of the food environment itself (e.g. availability of healthy foods in a certain location). Often, programmes targeting multiple aspects of the food environment make it challenging to decide on the single most optimal outcome to measure. Outcomes that are diet behaviour rather than health related are suitable if there is substantial evidence that the diet behaviour of interest, for example fruit and vegetables consumption, is strongly related to health.

Few universally agreed upon validated methods or gold standards to measure effectiveness of policies targeting the food environment exist. Lytle and Sokol (2017) reviewed the tools that have been used to measure the food environment and identified measures for assessing accessibility, availability, affordability and quality of food environments. These tended to be mainly studies investigating stores selling food but also included restaurants and out-of-the-home eating environments. The authors found checklists to be the most common tool to be used (usually paper based) followed by questionnaires/interviews. A similar review by Glanz et al. (2016) found that tools were most likely to assess the availability of certain types of foods such as fruits and vegetables with many also assessing price and the quality of different food types. The Nutrition Environment Measures Survey for Stores (NEMS-S) was the most common tool to be used (http://nems-upenn.org/).

Traditionally, the most common method of analysis used in assessing environments has been geographical analysis (Lytle and Sokol, 2017). However, studies that use menu, food, nutrient, or sales analysis to determine the impact of the environmental programme or policy are becoming more common. Outcomes need to be measured as reliably as possible which may be more straightforward when analysing purchasing rather than individual or household dietary behaviour. Dietary outcomes are usually continuous such as grams of fruit and vegetables or in categories; for example four categories reporting how often families eat meals together (never, 1–2 times per week, 3–4 times per week, or most or every day). Table 19.1 provides information on different measures used in a range of food environments.

One of the limitations is that many of the tools available lack comprehensive validation. Criterion-related validity, comparison of the measure used with the gold standard for assessment of the measure, was only mentioned in 10% of the studies reviewed by Lytle and Sokol (2017). A good example of this is validation of a school healthfulness score with an inventory of school food (Hearst et al., 2009). However,

## TABLE 19.1
## Measures of the Food Environment

### Categories of the Food Environment

*Food Store Environment*: grocery stores, supermarkets, convenience stores, snack bars, specialty food stores, farmers' markets, bodegas, and food banks.

*Home Food Environment*: food available within the home.

*Macro Food Environment*: national and regional food supply.

*Public Facility Food Environment*: cafeterias, vending machines, and snack shops in recreation centres, health care facilities and other public venues.

*Restaurant Food Environment:* fast food and full-service restaurants.

*Food Environment:* cafeterias, vending machines and snack shops in daycare settings, schools, and/or colleges.

*Worksite Food Environment*: cafeterias, vending machines, and snack shops.

### Instruments

Instruments are standardised assessment tools, typically paper-based forms completed by subjects themselves or by trained observers.

*Checklist*: a pre-defined list of indicator foods which are selected based on pre-determined criteria, such as those foods that are identified by the researchers as aligning with current dietary guidance. A checklist may be used in food stores, restaurants, schools, or worksites.

*Interview/questionnaire*: a pre-determined list of questions that is administered by a trained interviewer or completed by the respondent via self-report. An interview/questionnaire may be used in food stores, restaurants, schools, or worksites.

*Inventory*: a form for recording all foods available in a given environment. An inventory may be used in food stores, restaurants, schools, or worksites.

*Market basket*: a pre-defined list of foods that represent a range of food choices across a total diet. These foods may be based on foods frequently consumed by the population or may reflect a standardised diet plan like the U.S. Department of Agriculture's Thrifty Food Plan. A market basket is usually used in food stores.

### Methodologies

Methodologies include geographic analysis, menu analysis, nutrient analysis, sales analysis, and food supply analysis.

*Food supply analysis*: uses macro-level data on food available for consumption at the national level.

*Geographic analysis*: draws data from specific geographic measures; this includes counts of the number of food stores or restaurants within a specific area; the nearest distance to food stores or restaurants; and/or the food type, price and quality available in food stores or at restaurants within a specific area.

*Menu analysis*: uses information on a menu as the basis for data collection and evaluation.

*Nutrient analysis*: uses nutrient data such as saturated fat, energy, and sodium to evaluate foods available for school lunches, as à la carte foods, and in vending machines.

*Receipt analysis*: uses annotated receipts to assess food purchasing and food supplies.

*Sales analysis*: uses data from sales, cashier receipts, and food service reporting forms to determine availability and patterns of purchase for certain foods (e.g., fruits and vegetables).

*Universal Product Code (UPC) Scanning*: uses barcode scanners to collect data on food products and food supplies.

*Source:* From Lytle and Sokol (2017), Used with permission from Elsevier.

there are currently few existing gold standards for researchers to use making it challenging to improve the criterion-related validity of these types of measurement tools. Construct validity, "the extent to which the measure is related to other constructs in an expected way, for example is food availability related to food purchases", is reported by even fewer studies (Lytle and Sokol, 2017). Furthermore, measurement tools need to be sufficiently sensitive (ability to identify true positives) and specific (ability to identify true negatives) to enable them to detect changes in the measure of interest. Validation can be context specific, and additional validation may be required if existing methods are refined and improved for use in different populations and contexts.

In the next sections, different types of evaluation approaches are briefly described. Further details can be found in the additional references provided and available text books (Lovegrove et al., 2015).

## 19.3 RANDOMISED CONTROLLED TRIALS

Randomised controlled trials (RCTs) are experimental studies where participants are randomly (in statistical terms) assigned to an intervention group that receives the programme or policy or a control (or usual practice) group. For example, an intervention group could be required to follow a high-fibre diet, while the control group is not required to change their diet. The groups are then followed up for a pre-specified period of time which could be weeks or months to determine whether the intervention group has performed better than the control group on the outcome of interest such as serum cholesterol. Data on the exposure (fibre for this example) and the health outcome (LDL cholesterol for this example) are collected at baseline at the beginning of the study and at the end of the time period. The time period, or duration of the study, must be long enough for the exposure to affect the outcome. Randomisation ensures that the intervention is the only difference between the intervention and the control group. This enables researchers to conclude that any difference between the intervention and control group is a direct cause of the intervention rather than any number of other actions that might be going on outside the study being conducted. It is a strong study design for looking at causality and is usually considered the gold standard in research methodology including in nutrition (Lovegrove et al., 2015). Figure 19.1 presents the flow of participants through a cluster RCT which aimed to improve diet quality in children (clustered within schools) in Guangzhou, a city in China (Li et al., 2019).

RCTs can also be used to assess changes in diet behaviour (not just health outcomes). Early good examples of these focussed on fruits and vegetables in children (Baranowski et al., 2000; Sahota et al., 2001). Analysis of RCTs is carried out using regression methods and the main measurement of interest is the difference between the outcome in the intervention and the control group at follow-up. The analysis needs to take account of clustering if participants are recruited in schools or other clusters as children within the same school may be more similar to each other than children in another school.

Although RCTs are considered high-quality evaluation methods, they are expensive and time-consuming. Furthermore, they may not be an accurate reflection of real-world behaviour, and different parts of the population may be less likely to be

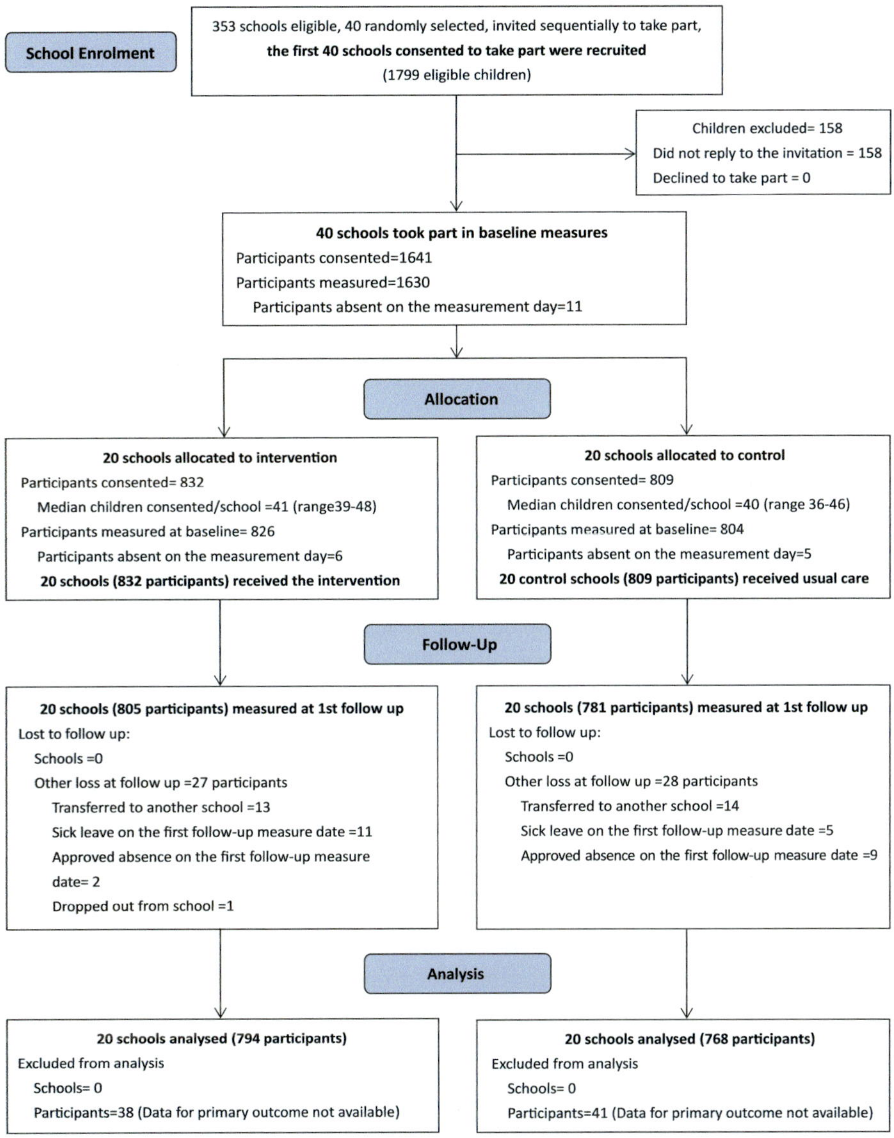


**FIGURE 19.1** Flow of participants (schools and children) through the Chirpy Dragon randomised controlled trial. (Reprinted from Li et al. (2019), under licence CC BY 4.0, http://creativecommons.org/licenses/by/4.0/.)

recruited into trials (leading to selection bias) or differences may result between groups in the number/types of people completing the trial (leading to attrition bias). Double-blind trials with food-based interventions where the participant and the researcher don't know which group they are in are also often impossible. Sometimes it is not ethical or feasible to have a control group or to randomise between the intervention and control group.

RCTs are also limited when behaviours occur in complex systems and childhood obesity is a good example of this (Brown et al., 2019). Evaluations of the food environment where a large number of relatively small individual changes need to be made to have an impact on long-term health are particularly challenging.

Overall, RCTs are a powerful method of evaluating the effectiveness of interventions. Systematic reviews of RCTs (both randomised and non-randomised) that synthesise the impact of different programmes in different populations are particularly useful to researchers and policy makers. Examples of these include reviews of school gardens on fruit and vegetable consumption in children (Robinson-O'Brien et al., 2009), school-based interventions to improve overall fruit and vegetable consumption (Evans et al., 2012) and financial incentives on health behaviours (Giles et al., 2014).

## 19.4 QUASI-EXPERIMENTAL TRIALS I: NON-RANDOMISED CONTROLLED TRIALS

Quasi-experimental trials offer an alternative approach when it isn't possible to successfully run an RCT. The most common quasi-experiment used in the social sciences is a non-randomised controlled trial, but there are others that are becoming more common such as interrupted time series (described in the next section). In non-randomised experiments, researchers compare those exposed to an intervention (the intervention group) with those that do not receive the intervention (the control group) on the outcome of interest, similar to RCTs. However, as individuals are not randomly allocated to the intervention and control group, there is a risk that observed differences between the two groups on the outcome of interest may be due to factors other than the intervention increasing risk of bias such as selection bias where the groups differ in key characteristics (Higgins and Green, 2020).

However, these types of studies are beneficial in terms of having a control group (compared with designs with no control group) and may be less prone to high rates of non-compliance and attrition (drop-out) rates than RCTs. With care, selection bias can be reduced, for example by ensuring both groups are similar to each other as possible – particularly in terms of factors that may impact on why participants select one group over another. An example of this type of approach is offering a school-based nutrition programme to a number of schools and each school decides whether to implement the intervention in the first or second round (academic year). The control group can serve as a waiting list group that will receive the intervention in the next round. A non-randomised design was used to evaluate the free school fruit and vegetable scheme in a region in England where 53 schools received free fruit as part of a pilot of a national scheme (the intervention) and 45 schools in a different region of England did not receive fruit (and served as the control) (Ransley et al., 2007). Fruit and vegetable intake was measured at the beginning and end of the intervention over one school year and analysed in a similar way to an RCT with the fruit and vegetable intakes of the two groups compared at follow up (adjusting for baseline values and relevant socio-economic factors). A further example is a study assessing an intervention encouraging families to eat dinner together to improve the home food environment (Gunther et al., 2019).

Non-randomised controlled trials are considered reasonably high-quality design and are often included in systematic reviews of trials. However, they are likely to have lower internal validity than randomised designs due to differences between the intervention and control groups. Risk of bias is reduced if participants are matched on key variables or a composite score (such as a propensity score) so that each participant in the intervention group is matched to a similar (within 0.2 standard deviations) participant/cluster in the control group. Another design that has been used in public health nutrition is the use of routinely collected data as the control group. Although it is possible that the participants in the intervention group are included in the routinely collected data, if the routinely collected data is large and includes mostly participants who aren't in the intervention, then this is a convenient (and potentially cheap) control group. An example of this is an Australian-based intervention to reduce risk of obesity in young children (Sanigorski et al., 2008). A stronger quasi-experimental design is the use of interrupted time series analysis which is covered in the next section.

## 19.5 QUASI-EXPERIMENTAL TRIALS II: INTERRUPTED TIME SERIES ANALYSIS

One of the most popular types of quasi-experimental design is the use of interrupted time series (ITS) analysis which involves collecting data over time, both before and after the introduction of a policy or programme. The actual results from after the policy are compared with the predicted results assuming continuation of the same trend and no new policy. Including a control group strengthens the design. As is the case for non-randomised controlled trials, it is used when evaluation using an RCT is challenging, either due to difficulties in recruiting or randomising without introducing considerable bias or because the intervention or policy is implemented in a large region so that a control group is likely to be very different from the intervention group.

This method builds on the use of a pre-post design, a weaker method of evaluation where data is collected at one time point at baseline before the introduction of the intervention and once at follow-up after completion of the intervention. ITS is well suited to the evaluation of programmes or policies over which researchers have little or no control (natural experiments) but could nonetheless have important impacts on diet or health outcomes (e.g. health-related food taxes and subsidies). The key limitation with a pre-post design is that any changes in the dietary behaviour of interest could be due to external factors unrelated to the intervention being evaluated that happen to occur at the same time as the intervention. For example, price increases following the introduction of a sugary drinks tax may be accompanied by mass media campaigns on the health impacts of sugary drinks. In this situation, it would be difficult to evaluate the effectiveness of the tax alone. However, ITS analysis uses data collected repeatedly, usually weekly or monthly, for a period before the intervention is introduced, and then again repeatedly for a period of time after the intervention or policy has been implemented. This enables any underlying trend or slope to be identified and adjusted for in the analysis. The observations before the

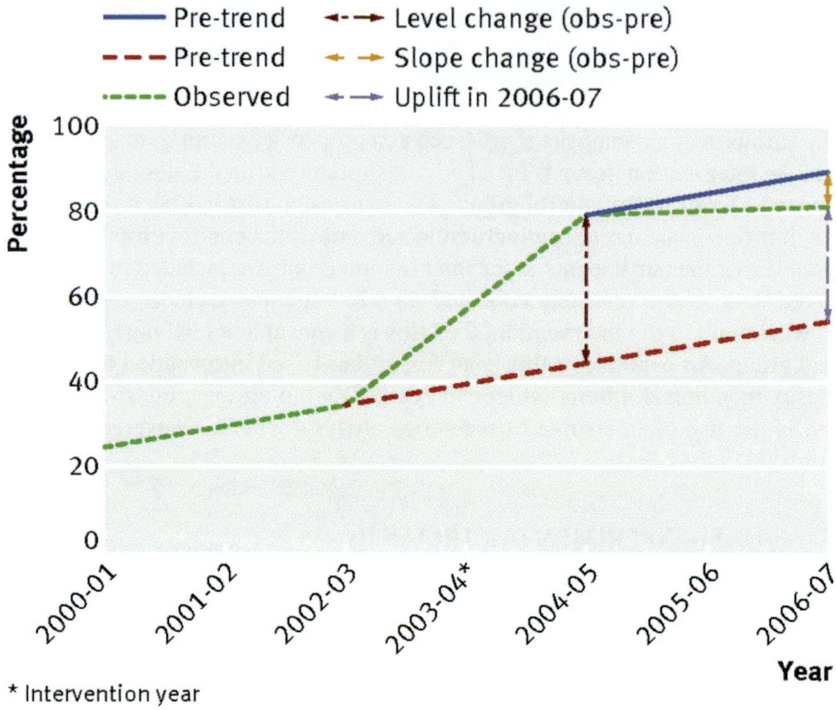


**FIGURE 19.2** The different components of interrupted time series analysis. (Reprinted from the *BMJ*, https://www.bmj.com/content/350/bmj.h2750.full, under licence CC BY 4.0, http://creativecommons.org/licenses/by/4.0/.)

intervention provide the counterfactual which is compared with observations after the intervention. The introduction of the intervention or policy could result in a dramatic increase in, for example, sales of fruit, which would indicate a change in level and/or a reduction in the slope compared with the projection of the counterfactual. See Figure 19.2 for an example of where a treatment or intervention effect produces a change in level and slope over time. As the analysis requires that data points are independent, further adjustments are usually needed for auto-correlation between the data points to provide robust results.

ITS is best suited to outcome measures that are collected routinely and automatically to reduce the burden of collecting data. A minimum of eight data points are needed both before and after the implementation of the policy (Reichardt, 2019). Controlled ITS analysis (CITS) has been used successfully to evaluate reductions in proportions of sugary drinks with free sugar levels higher than 5 g/100 mL in the UK after the announcement of the soft drinks industry levy in 2016 (see Figure 19.3) where the proportion reduced from 49% to 15% over 4 years (Scarborough et al., 2020). The control group used for comparison was drinks not subject to the levy (juices and milk based drinks). A further example is the analysis of a 10 p tax on sugary drinks at a chain of restaurants where the number of sugary drinks reduced by 9% over 6 months (Cornelsen et al., 2017).

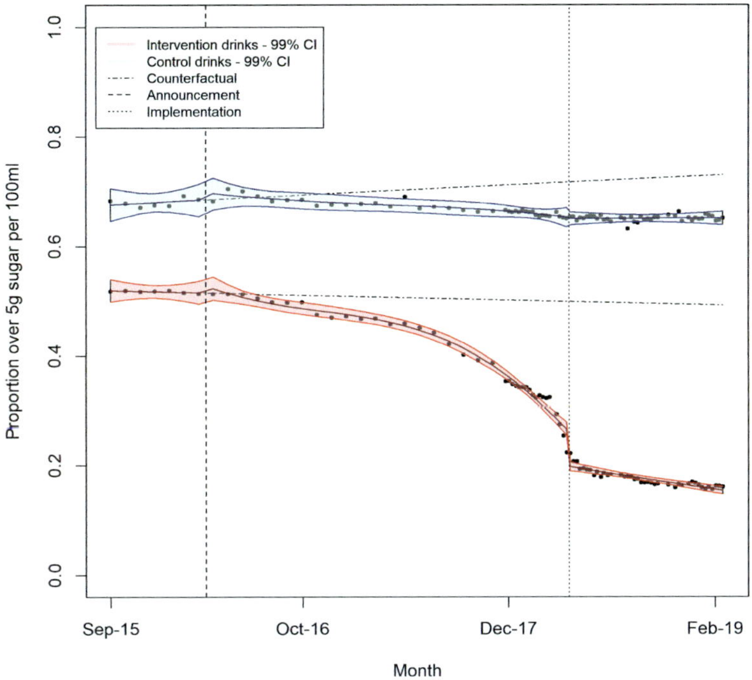


**FIGURE 19.3** Example of a controlled interrupted time series analysis (CITS) to evaluate the soft drinks industry levy in the UK. (Reprinted from Scarborough et al. (2020), doi: 10.1371/journal.pmed.1003025, under licence CC BY 4.0, http://creativecommons.org/licenses/by/4.0/.)

## 19.6 LONGITUDINAL STUDIES

In situations where it is not possible to use an experimental design, it may be necessary to rely on evidence from observational studies. There are different types of observational studies including longitudinal observational studies where the same participants are followed up over time. This is a stronger design than cross-sectional studies where data is collected only once (and which are not covered here). In prospective cohorts, the same participants may be followed up for years and the exposure, such as sugary drinks consumption, is measured before the health outcome, type 2 diabetes, for example. The data are analysed to determine whether participants with a lower exposure are less (or more) at risk. In the analysis of Australian data, where adults were recruited in 2006 and the same participants followed up for 3 years until 2009, the researchers investigated the relationship between the food environment (ratio of supermarkets to fast food outlets within pre-specified buffer zones) and weight gain (or change in weight from baseline to follow-up) (Feng et al., 2018). In practice, many cohort analyses use large established cohorts that have been followed up for many years, sometimes decades, and the exposure and outcome are usually measured at more than one time point. This leads to increasingly complex analysis and interpretation of the findings. A longitudinal study in the US using the National Longitudinal Survey of Youth recruited in 1979 investigated the impact of neighbourhood food environments on subsequent weight in adults (Gibson, 2011). Participants were recruited at age 14–22 years and followed up for more than 20 years when they were aged 33–48 years. Data were collected on the food environment and BMI every 2 years so the analysis focussed on the change in BMI in consecutive data collections and information on the food environment in the previous data collection. For example, the change in BMI between 1998 and 2000 was compared with the results for the food environment in 1998. Outcomes can also be measures of dietary behaviour; for example the Diet Quality Index (DQI) or fruit and vegetable consumption that are all associated with health outcomes can be used. An analysis of the well-known US CARDIA data (Boone-Heinonen et al., 2011) used follow-up data 7, 10 and 15 years after baseline to explore the impact of access to fast food restaurants on diet quality.

Repeated cross-sectional studies are sometimes used when prospective cohorts are not available or to explore new areas where there is little published information. These repeat data collections at different time points, but on different participants, are a slightly stronger study design than cross-sectional studies and have been used to evaluate novel policies with a small evidence base. For example, a study of the impact of policies at supermarket checkouts reported on the purchase of high fat, sugar or salt (HFSS) snacks (Ejlerskov et al., 2018), while another looked at the effect of advertising policies targeting children on exposure to advertising (Adams et al., 2012) over two time periods 1 year apart. A third study explored changes in children's packed lunches with two surveys 10 years apart (Evans et al., 2020).

## 19.7 ECOLOGICAL MODELS

Ecological studies collect indicators of exposure and disease for a group of people (e.g. a country or region) as a unit and look at their associations at the group level, rather than at the individual level. An example is a study looking at soy intake in 1980–1985 and cancer and heart disease mortality rates in 1995 in 47 provinces in Japan which found an inverse association for stomach cancer and heart disease death (Nagata, 2000). The data was aggregated at the regional (prefecture) level from the Japanese government's official statistics. An ecological approach often uses existing statistics and therefore has the advantages that it requires less money and less time than alternative individual-level studies. Another example is the evaluation of the school lunch programme in Japan where regions with high take up of the programme (and therefore lower proportions of children taking bento box style packed lunches to school) were associated with lower rates of childhood obesity (Miyawaki et al., 2019).

However, there are limitations to ecological studies, including the ecological fallacy. The ecological fallacy indicates that population-level associations do not necessarily coincide with individual-level associations, which is attributed to the lack of information on individual-level exposure and outcomes. For example, when observing individuals within the same province in the study of soy intake stated above, individuals with higher soy intake may not necessarily have lower rates of heart disease mortality than the individuals with lower soy intake. The negative association between province-level soy intake and heart disease mortality may be explained by other factors (such as demographic patterns, other dietary patterns and lifestyles or socio-economic factors). As such, one of the major causes of the ecological fallacy seems to be group-specific (observed or unobserved) characteristics. To partially solve this problem, we may remove the effect of the group characteristics by statistically controlling for these characteristics. Also, if we can observe the groups longitudinally, we may think about controlling for group-specific dummy variables to remove the effect of group-specific factors, regardless of the observed or unobserved factors (Li and Hashimoto, 2019; Miyawaki et al., 2019). Even if doing so, however, we should note that some factors would still confound the association.

This type of approach is most useful when there are macro-level exposures, such as policy and environmental/social factors by region, which are often difficult to measure at the individual level. Ecological approaches are well suited to forming hypotheses about the impact of different dietary behaviours or characteristics due to the food environment. Also, if the effect size and variations of the exposure of interest are large, and the effect of confounding factors is, at most, moderate, an ecological approach is likely to provide reasonable information on the direction of the association. With ecological studies such as these as a stepping stone, researchers can design future epidemiological studies with a stronger and more valid research design such as longitudinal observational studies or randomised or quasi-experimental trials. For example, based on the ecological studies of soy intake with cause-specific mortality (Nagata, 2000), researchers conducted longitudinal observational studies (prospective cohort studies) and reported the inverse association of soy intake and stomach cancer death (Nagata et al., 2002) as well as a lower risk of all-cause death and cardiovascular death with higher intakes of fermented soy products, represented by "natto" (Katagiri et al., 2020).

## 19.8 SIMULATION MODELLING

Simulation modelling can be used for both prospective and retrospective evaluation of interventions in the food environment. Models are simplified versions of reality that are used to estimate solutions to real-world problems by applying mathematical relationships between input and output variables (see chapter on modelling in public health (Regmi and Gee 2016)). There are a variety of modelling approaches that can be used in evaluations depending on the nature of the problem. Detail about specific modelling methodologies is beyond the scope of this chapter, instead we focus on some core principles that apply across a variety of modelling methodologies.

Simulation modelling has been widely used to evaluate interventions in the food environment and is particularly advantageous when real-world studies would be challenging or impossible to conduct. This includes evaluation of policy interventions that are difficult to accurately replicate in experimental studies such as food taxes and subsidies or reformulation (e.g. (Cobiac et al., 2017; Federici et al., 2019; Springmann et al., 2018a)). Simulation modelling can also be used to examine hypothetical scenarios such as overnight eradication of obesity (Blakely et al., 2020) and removal of specific dietary risks such as high sodium intake (GBD Obesity Collaborators, 2017). Modelling studies may combine evaluation of the health impacts of interventions with environmental or other outcomes (Springmann et al., 2018b). Whilst hypothetical scenarios are not evaluations of interventions per se, quantification of the maximum possible health gain that could be achieved by addressing particular features of the food environment is valuable to identify areas where intervention may positively impact health.

A strength of simulation modelling is that it can be used to evaluate impacts over long time horizons, including for the lifetime of a modelled population unlike experimental studies. The ability to assess long-term impacts of interventions in the food environment is particularly important as small changes in the environment may have large, cumulative health gains across the population – particularly when interventions result in long-term dietary change or change trajectories of behaviour.

Modelling studies combine evidence from a variety of data sources and other study designs. This may include combining dose–response relationships between dietary factors and diseases from cohort studies, with cross-sectional surveys of dietary patterns, and effect size estimates from meta-analyses. Simulation modelling is complementary to, but reliant on, evidence from other study designs. Robust calibration and validation of simulation models is needed to ensure that underlying assumptions are appropriate, with international frameworks providing some guidance about best practice (Caro et al., 2012). Analytic approaches such as sensitivity analyses and uncertainty analysis can be used to determine the extent to which changes in model assumptions alter the findings of simulation modelling studies. In addition to providing greater trust in modelled results, these approaches provide a guide as to the greatest areas of uncertainty and priorities for future empirical research.

Where comparable modelling methodologies are used to evaluate different interventions, simulation modelling can be a valuable tool to compare the impacts of different interventions. This includes the ability to evaluate interventions in the food environment against other public health interventions. For example, the Australia New Zealand Health Intervention League Table (University of Otago & University of Melbourne, 2019) has compiled hundreds of intervention evaluations, enabling users to compare the (modelled) health gains of interventions in the food environment with tobacco taxes, cancer screening and a variety of other public health interventions. Comparison of such a broad scope of interventions would not be possible without utilising simulation models that quantify the health impacts of these interventions onto a common metric.

## 19.9 CONCLUSIONS

Many great public health interventions are not properly evaluated (or the evaluation is not published) which is a problem for many reasons. Without high-quality evaluation, it is not possible to determine whether or how effective a programme or policy is and/or whether the programme is at least as effective in those that need it the most compared with those that don't and therefore does not widen inequalities.

The best evaluation design depends on the nature of the research question being addressed. RCTs provide robust evidence for individual-level interventions where researchers are able to control intervention implementation. Quasi-experimental trials such as non-randomised controlled trials are well suited to scenarios where randomisation is not possible, and where groups receiving and not receiving the intervention are similar. ITS analysis is well suited to evaluating interventions that researchers have little or no control over, occurring over broad areas such as national policies. For this type of analysis, care needs to be taken to adjust for background differences in time that are external to the intervention or policy being evaluated.

Currently, the majority of evaluations investigating the food environment are relatively weak as they are cross-sectional rather than longitudinal and typically without a control group. More robust evaluations are needed to strengthen the evidence on what works in this area. Traditionally, researchers have had input into the implementation of the intervention to be evaluated, as well as the evaluation itself. However, evaluation of natural experiments where researchers have no input into the intervention is becoming more common (Wrieden and Levy, 2016). It is hoped that nutrition policies introduced at national or local levels are properly evaluated more often going forward.

Those working to improve the food environment need to be aware that strong evidence means different things to different stakeholders and therefore, broadly speaking, a range of different techniques are recommended to evaluate interventions. Systematic reviews of RCTs and non-randomised controlled trials can also provide strong evidence for the effectiveness of different types of interventions, and these are routinely used in a number of countries including the UK (Scientific Advisory Committee on Nutrition (SACN), 2020). However, broad agreement and strong evidence that consensus has been reached on the effectiveness of a programme usually occurs when there is information from a variety of different types of studies and they converge to provide similar conclusions.

## REFERENCES

Adams, J., Tyrrell, R., Adamson, A. J. & White, M. 2012. Effect of restrictions on television food advertising to children on exposure to advertisements for 'less healthy' foods: repeat cross-sectional study. *PLoS One,* 7, e31578.

Baranowski, T., Davis, M., Resnicow, K., Baranowski, J., Doyle, C., Lin, L. S., Smith, M. & Wang, D. T. 2000. Gimme 5 fruit, juice, and vegetables for fun and health: outcome evaluation. *Health Educ Behav,* 27, 96–111.

Blakely, T., Cleghorn, C., Petrovic-Van Der Deen, F., Cobiac, L. J., Mizdrak, A., Mackenbach, J. P., Woodward, A., Van Baal, P. & Wilson, N. 2020. Prospective impact of tobacco eradication and overweight and obesity eradication on future morbidity and health-adjusted life expectancy: simulation study. *J Epidemiol Commun Health,* 74, 354–361.

Boone-Heinonen, J., Gordon-Larsen, P., Kiefe, C. I., Shikany, J. M., Lewis, C. E. & Popkin, B. M. 2011. Fast food restaurants and food stores: longitudinal associations with diet in young to middle-aged adults: the Cardia study. *Arch Intern Med,* 171, 1162–1170.

Brown, T., Moore, T. H., Hooper, L., Gao, Y., Zayegh, A., Ijaz, S., Elwenspoek, M., Foxen, S. C., Magee, L., O'Malley, C., Waters, E. & Summerbell, C. D. 2019. Interventions for preventing obesity in children. *Cochrane Database Syst Rev,* 7, Cd001871.

Caro, J. J., Briggs, A. H., Siebert, U., Kuntz, K. M. & Force, I.-S. M. G. R. P. T. 2012. Modeling good research practices--overview: a report of the Ispor-Smdm Modeling Good Research Practices Task Force-1. *Med Decis Making,* 32, 667–677.

Cobiac, L. J., Tam, K., Veerman, L. & Blakely, T. 2017. Taxes and subsidies for improving diet and population health in Australia: a cost-effectiveness modelling study. *PLoS Med,* 14, e1002232.

Cornelsen, L., Mytton, O. T., Adams, J., Gasparrini, A., Iskander, D., Knai, C., Petticrew, M., Scott, C., Smith, R., Thompson, C., White, M. & Cummins, S. 2017. Change in non-alcoholic beverage sales following a 10-pence levy on sugar-sweetened beverages within a national chain of restaurants in the UK: interrupted time series analysis of a natural experiment. *J Epidemiol Commun Health,* 71, 1107–1112.

Ejlerskov, K., Sharp, S. J., Stead, M., Adamson, A. J., White, M. & Adams, J. 2018. Socio-economic and age variations in response to supermarket-led checkout food policies: a repeated measures analysis. *Int J Behav Nutr Phys Act,* 15, 125.

Evans, C. E., Christian, M. S., Cleghorn, C. L., Greenwood, D. C. & Cade, J. E. 2012. Systematic review and meta-analysis of school-based interventions to improve daily fruit and vegetable intake in children aged 5 to 12 y. *Am J Clin Nutr,* 96, 889–901.

Evans, C. E. L., Melia, K. E., Rippin, H. L., Hancock, N. & Cade, J. 2020. A repeated cross-sectional survey assessing changes in diet and nutrient quality of English primary school children's packed lunches between 2006 and 2016. *BMJ Open,* 10, e029688.

Federici, C., Detzel, P., Petracca, F., Dainelli, L. & Fattore, G. 2019. The impact of food reformulation on nutrient intakes and health, a systematic review of modelling studies. *BMC Nutr,* 5, 2.

Feng, X., Astell-Burt, T., Badland, H., Mavoa, S. & Giles-Corti, B. 2018. Modest ratios of fast food outlets to supermarkets and green grocers are associated with higher body mass index: longitudinal analysis of a sample of 15,229 Australians aged 45 years and older in the Australian National Liveability Study. *Health Place,* 49, 101–110.

GBD Obesity Collaborators. 2017. Health effects of overweight and obesity in 195 countries over 25 years. *N Engl J Med.* 377, 13–27.

Gibson, D. M. 2011. The neighborhood food environment and adult weight status: estimates from longitudinal data. *Am J Public Health,* 101, 71–78.

Giles, E. L., Robalino, S., Mccoll, E., Sniehotta, F. F. & Adams, J. 2014. The effectiveness of financial incentives for health behaviour change: systematic review and meta-analysis. *PLoS One,* 9, e90347.

Glanz, K., Johnson, L., Yaroch, A. L., Phillips, M., Ayala, G. X. & Davis, E. L. 2016. Measures of retail food Store environments and sales: review and implications for healthy eating initiatives. *J Nutr Educ Behav,* 48 (4), 280–288 (e281)

Gunther, C., Rogers, C., Holloman, C., Hopkins, L. C., Anderson, S. E., Miller, C. K., Copeland, K. A., Dollahite, J. S., Pratt, K. J., Webster, A., Labyk, A. N. & Penicka, C. 2019. Child diet and health outcomes of the simple suppers program: a 10-week, 2-group quasi-experimental family meals trial. *BMC Public Health,* 19, 1657.

Hearst, M. O., Lytle, L. A., Pasch, K. E. & Heitzler, C. D. 2009. Inventory versus checklist approach to assess middle school a la carte food availability. *J Sch Health,* 79, 593–598; quiz 603–605.

Higgins, J., Green, S. 2020. *Cochrane Handbook for Systematic Reviews of Interventions.* Hoboken, NJ: John Wiley & Sons.

Hughes, R. & Margetts, B. 2012. The public health nutrition intervention management bi-cycle: a model for training and practice improvement. *Public Health Nutr,* 15, 1981–1988.

Katagiri, R., Sawada, N., Goto, A., Yamaji, T., Iwasaki, M., Noda, M., Iso, H., Tsugane, S. & Japan Public Health Center-Based Prospective Study, G. 2020. Association of soy and fermented soy product intake with total and cause specific mortality: prospective cohort study. *BMJ,* 368, m34.

Li, T. & Hashimoto, H. 2019. Household dietary salt consumption and mortality from cardiovascular diseases: an ecological panel analysis in Japan. *Eur J Public Health,* 29, 826–832.

Li, B., Pallan, M., Liu, W. J., Hemming, K., Frew, E., Lin, R., Liu, W., Martin, J., Zanganeh, M., Hurley, K., Cheng, K. K. & Adab, P. 2019. The Chirpy Dragon intervention in preventing obesity in Chinese primary-school--aged children: a cluster-randomised controlled trial. *PLoS Med,* 16, e1002971.

Lovegrove, J. A., Hodson, L., Sharma, S. & Lanham-New, S. A. 2015. *Nutrition Research Methodologies*. Hoboken, NJ: Wiley-Blackwell.

Lytle, L. A. & Sokol, R. L. 2017. Measures of the food environment: a systematic review of the field, 2007–2015. *Health Place,* 44, 18–34.

Miyawaki, A., Lee, J. S. & Kobayashi, Y. 2019. Impact of the school lunch program on overweight and obesity among junior high school students: a nationwide study in Japan. *J Public Health (Oxf),* 41, 362–370.

Nagata, C. 2000. Ecological study of the association between soy product intake and mortality from cancer and heart disease in Japan. *Int J Epidemiol,* 29, 832–836.

Nagata, C., Takatsuka, N., Kawakami, N. & Shimizu, H. 2002. A prospective cohort study of soy product intake and stomach cancer death. *Br J Cancer,* 87, 31–36.

Ransley, J. K., Greenwood, D. C., Cade, J. E., Blenkinsop, S., Schagen, I., Teeman, D., Scott, E., White, G. & Schagen, S. 2007. Does the school fruit and vegetable scheme improve children's diet? A non-randomised controlled trial. *J Epidemiol Commun Health,* 61, 699–703.

Regmi, K. & Gee, I. (eds.) 2016. *Public Health Intelligence: Issues of Measure and Method,* Switzerland: Springer International Publishing.

Reichardt, C. S. 2019. *Quasi-Experimentation a Guide to Design and Analysis*, New York, The Guilford Press.

Robinson-O'brien, R., Story, M. & Heim, S. 2009. Impact of garden-based youth nutrition intervention programs: a review. *J Am Diet Assoc,* 109, 273–280.

Sahota, P., Rudolf, M. C., Dixey, R., Hill, A. J., Barth, J. H. & Cade, J. 2001. Randomised controlled trial of primary school based intervention to reduce risk factors for obesity. *BMJ,* 323, 1029–1032.

Sanigorski, A. M., Bell, A. C., Kremer, P. J., Cuttler, R. & Swinburn, B. A. 2008. Reducing unhealthy weight gain in children through community capacity-building: results of a quasi-experimental intervention program, be active eat well. *Int J Obes (Lond),* 32, 1060–1067.

Scarborough, P., Adhikari, V., Harrington, R. A., Elhussein, A., Briggs, A., Rayner, M., Adams, J., Cummins, S., Penney, T. & White, M. 2020. Impact of the announcement and implementation of the UK Soft Drinks Industry Levy on sugar content, price, product size and number of available soft drinks in the UK, 2015–2019: a controlled interrupted time series analysis. *PLoS Med,* 17, e1003025.

Scientific Advisory Committee on Nutrition (SACN). 2020. Framework for the evaluation of evidence.

Springmann, M., Sacks, G., Ananthapavan, J. & Scarborough, P. 2018a. Carbon pricing of food in Australia: an analysis of the health, environmental and public finance impacts. *Aust N Z J Public Health,* 42, 523–529.

Springmann, M., Wiebe, K., Mason-D'croz, D., Sulser, T. B., Rayner, M. & Scarborough, P. 2018b. Health and nutritional aspects of sustainable diet strategies and their association with environmental impacts: a global modelling analysis with country-level detail. *Lancet Planet Health,* 2, e451–e461.

University of Otago & University of Melbourne. 2019. Anz-Hilt: Australia and New Zealand Health Intervention League Table (Version 2.0) [Online]. Available: https://www.otago.ac.nz/wellington/departments/publichealth/research/bode3/otago693006.html [Accessed].

Wrieden, W. L. & Levy, L. B. 2016. 'Change4Life smart swaps': quasi-experimental evaluation of a natural experiment. *Public Health Nutr,* 19, 2388–2392.

# 20 Systems Approaches to Improve the Food Environment for Disease Prevention

*Tarra L. Penney and Chloe Clifford Astbury*
York University

*Emma Strachan*
Leeds City Council

**CONTENTS**



## 20.1 INTRODUCTION TO SYSTEMS APPROACHES

A public health approach that seeks to 'shift the curve' of dietary risk for everyone, rather than focussing on specific high-risk groups (Rose, 2008), requires understanding how both physical and socio-structural factors shape individual-level behaviour (Bronfenbrenner, 1979; McLeroy et al., 1998). This preventive approach therefore includes a focus not only on the role that food environments play in disease prevention but on how the application of systems thinking and complexity science as a heuristic, theoretical foundation and/or set of methods could improve our understanding of how food systems shape behaviour and health (Langellier et al., 2019a).

Systems thinking can be described as a way of conceptualising the world that incorporates a set of principles designed to understand change as a process that

DOI: 10.1201/9781003043720-20

**TABLE 20.1**
**Example Characteristics of Complex Systems**

| Term | Definition |
|---|---|
| Non-linear relationships | A relationship between two elements in a system where the cause does not produce a proportional effect |
| Feedback loops | A closed chain of causal connections resulting in the output of a system or system element feeding *back into* itself |
| Delays | An interval of time between a cause and effect, which can create instability and fluctuations in system behaviour |

*Source:* Adapted from Meadows (2008), Sterman (2006), and Systems Thinking for Health Systems Strengthening (2009).

drives the behaviour of a system (i.e. a collection of elements) (Carey et al., 2015). Key among these principles are (Reynolds et al., 2016):

1. Interrelationships (connections between elements of the system);
2. Multiple perspectives (the acknowledgement that explicating a system requires understanding the system from different points of view) and
3. Boundaries (what lies within and outside of the system of interest).

Complex adaptive systems such as the food system are characterised by specific elements and relationships (Table 20.1). These characteristics can make the behaviour of these systems difficult to predict using more conventional methods and models for generating evidence (Rutter et al., 2017).

The application of these principles to understanding how healthy diets can be supported or undermined by features and functions of a wider food environment, or how social, political and economic systems interact with food systems, could provide novel forms of evidence. While systems thinking and complexity science are longstanding fields, the application of these approaches and methods to public and population health is still in an early stage of development. However, there is significant interest in the potential to inform programmes and policies with evidence capable of dealing with the inherent complexity and dynamism within and between these systems.

## 20.2 UNDERSTANDING FOOD ENVIRONMENTS AND FOOD SYSTEMS

Food environments and food systems can be characterised as complex systems, having properties such as those described in Table 20.1 (Langellier et al., 2019a). Given these properties, approaches informed by systems thinking can be useful in understanding food environments. For example, in Latin America, stakeholders modelled the food environment as a driver of urban health in cities including Lima and São Paulo, as shown in Figure 20.1 (Langellier et al., 2019b). Participants developed a model highlighting the systems properties shaping the urban food environment, including feedback loops and delays. For example, food industry spending on marketing led to an increasing preference for ultra-processed food (UPF) among consumers, which in

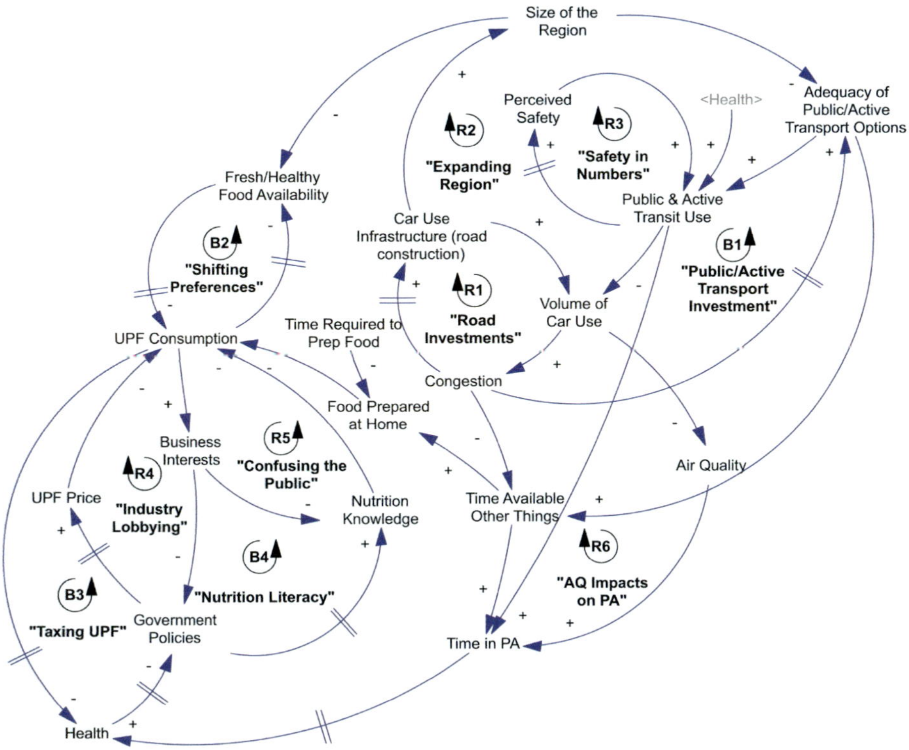


**FIGURE 20.1** An example of a systems map. (From Langellier et al. (2019b).)

turn reduced the incentives for vendors to stock fresh, healthy options. This reduced availability of healthy options further increased the consumption of UPF.

Meanwhile, increasing sales of UPF meant the food industry had more money to invest in marketing and lobbying the government. While the food industry was seen as agile, rapidly investing its profits to protect and augment its interests, the feedback loop driving government activity was characterised by a number of delays: it took time for increased UPF consumption to be reflected in the government's perception of overall population health, and it also took time for government to implement policies to reduce UPF consumption. While several Latin American governments have now implemented ambitious policies to improve population-level dietary intake, these systems insights help to explain secular increases in UPF consumption, and the sometimes-slow response of government to these changes.

A number of systems approaches involve participatory modelling, providing an opportunity for different stakeholders to come together and develop a model of the system they all belong to. This can be particularly useful in the context of the food environment, where there are many stakeholders who may have different roles and aims. These stakeholders include commercial actors in the food system, including producers, distributors and vendors; policy actors, such as planning and public health departments; as well as local residents (Mui et al., 2019). Participatory approaches can make for a more inclusive process, incorporating multiple perspectives into a systems model.

Participatory system dynamics modelling has been used to model local food environments. In Baltimore, a participatory model of the local food environment highlighted the structuring role played by crime: local 'chicken box shops' were sometimes subsidised by illicit drug dealers in return for a sheltered space in which to conduct their operations (Mui et al., 2019). These subsidies contributed to the sustained financial viability of these shops, increasing the availability of the unhealthy products typically sold there. Meanwhile, independently owned corner stores typically made minimal profits, which were further reduced by costs attributed to robbery and vandalism. In this context, selling healthier products were seen by storeowners as 'risky', as these items might go unsold and have to be discarded. Given the already narrow profit margins, many storeowners were unwilling to take this risk, decreasing the availability of healthy products at the local level (Mui et al., 2019). Without the participation of local community members and small business owners, these dynamics might have gone unnoticed.

## 20.3 INTERVENING WITHIN FOOD ENVIRONMENTS

Where the systems properties of food environments are poorly understood, policies and other interventions may lead to unintended consequences (Meadows, 2008). Understanding food environments as complex systems can be key to developing interventions that achieve the desired outcomes. Where programmes and policies aimed at changing specific outcomes are implemented within complex food systems, these key outcomes may change in unexpected ways (Jou and Techakehakij, 2012; Langellier et al., 2019a), and there may be knock-on effects on a range of other factors (MacDiarmid et al., 2011). A systems perspective can be helpful in identifying relationships that may lead to unexpected results, and participatory methods in particular highlight the range of variables that a food environment policy might impact (MacDiarmid et al., 2011).

In the first instance, a systems perspective can be useful in identifying 'leverage points' within a food environment or food system: places in the system where interventions can have the largest impact (Meadows, 2008). For example, the intervention-level framework (ILF) has been used to identify leverage points to make complex food systems more healthy, green, fair and affordable (Johnston et al., 2014; Malhi et al., 2009). The ILF delineates the various elements of a system that can be targeted, ranging from structural elements, such as the actors and physical elements in a system, to paradigms, defined as the system's deepest held beliefs, and the source of its goals, rules and structures (Johnston et al., 2014). Structural elements are easier to target through policies such as taxes and subsidies but in isolation are less likely to create system-wide change. At the other end of the spectrum, paradigms can be difficult to intervene upon, but changes at this level can create radical shifts.

With regard to the food system, changes to structural elements tend to be compatible, as many proposed changes are specific to the different subsystems impacting health, affordability, equity and sustainability (Malhi et al., 2009). However, the paradigms underlying these different aims can be in conflict. For example, while having food prices that reflect the true environmental cost of food production was deemed important in achieving a sustainable food system, the resulting increase in price would likely jeopardise the aim of affordability (Malhi et al., 2009). In order to reconcile the multiple aims we hope the food system will be able to achieve, these functions may have to be substantially revised.

Participatory approaches can also be useful in trying to intervene in the food environment. As well as facilitating a more inclusive process, participatory approaches can be key to facilitating change, as they promote stakeholder buy-in and consensus-building. This can be particularly important in intervening in food systems, where many different actors have a role (see Case Study where Food Wise Leeds engaged partners from the public sector, businesses, academics and the charitable sector). In particular, systems approaches encourage stakeholders to visualise their mental models of a system, which provides a useful opportunity for system level understandings to be compared and discrepancies discussed (Meadows, 2008; Stroh, 2015). Convening diverse stakeholders to build a shared model of a system allows not only for the identification of leverage points and effective interventions but also for generating enthusiasm and commitment from participants, which can be key to changing policy (Freebairn et al., 2017; Loyo et al., 2013).

Whole systems approaches have successfully reduced the prevalence of overweight and obesity in children in Amsterdam. The Amsterdam Healthy Weight Approach (AHWA), coming up to its tenth anniversary, has reduced prevalence of childhood overweight and obesity from 21% to 18.7%, a rare achievement in cities (Sawyer et al., 2021). The whole system approach identified key modifiable influences in the local environment and took into consideration local political, physical, social, educational and healthcare drivers. The aim of the programme was to implement multi-level action through a wide range of stakeholders so that "simultaneous capability, opportunity and motivation to perform the desired behaviour" occurred (Sawyer et al., 2021). The development team also highlights the importance of adaptation to enable response to emerging relationships. A variety of initiatives or interventions have been implemented within specified clusters including school, environment, neighbourhood and community. Examples include the JUMP-in programme for schools to improve school food and food education as well as physical activity and a community based 1-day festival on healthy meal planning. Importantly, schools that register for the JUMP-in programme must commit to the programme in its entirety rather than a few components. Another strength of the programme is that by focussing on areas of need, it has narrowed inequalities in childhood obesity, a rare achievement indeed (Sawyer et al., 2021).

Recognising the system properties of food environments can also be important when modelling how policies may operate in specific contexts. Agent-based models (ABMs) and system dynamics models (SDMs), both quantitative approaches to complex systems modelling, have frequently been used for this purpose.

ABM is a simulation method that models the behaviour of individual agents. The agents' behaviour is driven by simple decision rules, individual characteristics and interactions with other agents and their environment (Railsback and Grimm, 2019). For example, a model might take individuals or households as its agents and include a simple decision rule such as: 'when households run out of food, they buy more' (Widener et al., 2013). There might also be assumptions in the model around how different populations do their food shopping (households with less disposable income go to less expensive stores) or how the environment impacts these behaviours (people are more likely to shop close to their home or workplace). From these simple sets of rules, complex behaviours emerge. ABMs simulate the independent behaviours of individual actors in specific circumstances. As a result, they can be used to model the impacts of different policy scenarios aimed at changing the food environment. For example, ABMs can be used to model and compare the impacts of different strategies to improve the local food environment, including increasing the probability of convenience stores stocking fresh produce and implementing a mobile market distribution system (Widener et al., 2013).

SDMs model a system of 'stock' variables, such as populations, capital or resources, which accumulate and dissipate at different rates depending on the rates of inward and outward 'flows' (Meadows, 2008). SDMs have been used to model certain policies aimed at improving the wider food environment, such as sugar-sweetened beverage taxes (Liu et al., 2016). With this type of policy, several stock variables are in play: populations with different health characteristics (e.g. with and without obesity or related diseases, such as diabetes), as well as tax revenue, which then becomes capital that may be spent elsewhere by government (Liu et al., 2016). SDMs allow these multiple variables, and the relationships between them, to be incorporated into models of policy impact.

Finally, systems approaches can also be applied in evaluating interventions aimed at improving the food environment. A systems perspective on evaluation can be helpful in identifying a comprehensive range of outcome and process indicators that may be impacted by an intervention and integrating the evidence collected as part of an evaluation (Knai et al., 2018). In the evaluation of the UK's Public Health Responsibility Deal, Knai and colleagues used a qualitative system dynamics model to integrate the various components of their evaluation and provide an explanation for the policy's lack of impact on health-relevant systems, including the food system (Knai et al., 2018). The Public Health Responsibility Deal, consisting of voluntary pledges to undertake actions beneficial to public health, left the broader commercial system largely unchanged, through different mechanisms such as substantial industry leadership in the policy's implementation, the lack of involvement of public health experts and the lack of accountability, monitoring and enforcement (Knai et al., 2018). The systems approach to this evaluation allowed findings to go beyond whether or not the policy achieved its stated aim, providing further insight into the 'how' and 'why' of its limited success.

## 20.4 CASE STUDY: SUPPORTING FOOD SYSTEMS WORKING – THE LEEDS WAY

Food is a complex issue with many interlinked factors at policy, community and individual level. Since 2008, Leeds, a large city in the North of England with a population of ~800,000 and more than 2,000 food outlets, has had different food-related strategies in place. The purpose of the food strategy from 2008 to 2014 was to promote a co-ordinated and sustainable approach to increase people's ability to make healthy food choices in Leeds. During the life of the food strategy, progress was made to build relationships amongst some food systems actors such as local authority teams, but businesses were identified as a gap. Since the strategy expired, the wider landscape in which food exists has moved on. Obesity has risen further in profile as a major threat to public health, food security is a growing concern and climate change and sustainability are ever-increasing priorities.

The original food strategy was replaced with new plans including the Best Council Plan 2020–2025 which sets out the ambitions of Leeds City Council. Food continues to be a cross-cutting priority for Leeds City Council and across the spectrum this includes obesity, other diet-related ill-health, nutritional care, poverty, waste, climate change, tourism and public safety. At the same time, the plan aims for Leeds to be fair, open and welcoming with an economy that is both prosperous and sustainable so all our communities are successful. Food has a strong role to play in supporting the achievement of this ambition, balancing the needs to improve health and wellbeing while at the same time supporting businesses. Food is not only at the core of some of the city's greatest problems but is also a vital part of the solution.

Leeds City Council has adopted the Food Active, Healthy Weight Declaration (foodactive.org.uk/) which includes a specific focus on promoting a healthier food environment and is incorporated into the Best Council Plan. In addition to the Best Council Plan, Food Wise Leeds was initiated in April 2018, following a deputation to Full Council outlining the need for a strategic approach to food. Background work was led by Leeds City Council, to engage partners and develop a city vision for Food known as the "Leeds Food Charter". Food Wise Leeds aims to celebrate good food and contribute to city priorities by addressing health inequalities, reducing food poverty, supporting local food businesses, reducing the environmental impact of food production, influencing trade and consumption of food and promoting growing and cooking skills. Food Wise Leeds is following the Sustainable Food places model (https://www.sustainablefoodplaces.org/) which helps cities to raise the profile and explore solutions to food issues across six principles with the goal of promoting healthy and sustainable food to the public:

1. Taking a strategic and collaborative approach to good food governance and action
2. Building public awareness, active food citizenship and a local good food movement
3. Tackling food poverty and diet-related ill health and increasing access to affordable healthy food
4. Creating a vibrant, prosperous and diverse sustainable food economy
5. Transforming catering and procurement and revitalising local and sustainable food supply chains
6. Tackling the climate and nature emergency through sustainable food and farming and an end to food waste

Food Wise Leeds has been successful in engaging different partners from the public sector, businesses, academics and the charitable sector to work together as part of a cross-sector partnership. The partnership's work across a range of food issues, from food poverty and nutrition to supporting local businesses, earnt the partnership a Sustainable Food Cities Bronze award in 2019 and the group continue to work towards silver ambitions.

Over the last 2 years, Food Wise Leeds has developed a number of projects, including a Rainbow Rocks campaign to encourage families to eat more fruit and vegetables, and has worked to support food access models that look to longer-term sustainability and support local businesses, such as Lean Lunch, a local independent business delivering healthy meals and produce to Leeds businesses and households. Most recently, Food Wise Leeds has led the development of a Building Food Resilience toolkit for food aid providers to support residents back to food independence by having helpful conversations, considering their models of food aid provision and signposting to support services. Additional projects led by Leeds City Council involve improving the content of snacks in vending machines (https://foodactive.org.uk/guest-blog-healthier-snack-provision-in-vending-machines-findings-from-leeds-city-council-trial/).

Looking to the future, Food Wise Leeds will continue to build a good food movement in Leeds, encouraging individuals, organisations and businesses to contribute to a healthier, fairer and more sustainable food system for everyone.

## 20.5 NEXT STEPS IN SYSTEMS APPROACHES

The use of methods informed by systems thinking to address complex public health problems is increasing rapidly (Carey et al., 2015; Langellier et al., 2019a; Rusoja et al., 2018). This growing body of research involves methodological innovations as well as novel applications, such as understanding and intervening within food environments and systems. The existing evidence around systems approaches, the food environment and disease prevention policy spans a number of different methods and contexts, particularly in high-income countries, and in policy at the national and local level.

However, there are also a number of gaps in this literature. In particular, there is limited application of these methods to policy at the international level. Research at this level will be especially important for understanding and improving the food system given the complex global network of trade that makes up the food system; the borderless nature of key threats such as climate change; and the international nature of many key actors, including international agencies such as the World Trade Organization and the Food and Agriculture Organization, as well as the multi-national food and beverage companies which provide food to most of the world's populations.

In addition, research using systems approaches to understand and improve the food environment is predominantly undertaken in high-income countries. While some of the lessons learnt from this work may be useful to researchers and policymakers in low- and middle-income countries, context-specific applications and evidence are important.

## 20.6 CHALLENGES AND OPPORTUNITIES

A key challenge in the application of systems approaches lies in ensuring stakeholder buy-in. Systems approaches can be time-consuming and resource-intensive, and stakeholders working in policy and practice sometimes see them as a cost rather than an opportunity (Barbrook-Johnson et al., 2020). An important aspect of engaging stakeholders will be to develop better evaluative evidence of the benefits of systems approaches.

While challenges remain in fostering stakeholder engagement in systems approaches, these approaches also present a number of opportunities for understanding and improving the food system through policy. First, they can support the creation of evidence-informed policy by generating tailored and dynamic evidence that can be incorporated into different stages of the policy process. Second, systems approaches may facilitate coherence in implementing and making policy by taking a more holistic view of the food environment and the different elements and actors that constitute it. Finally, systems approaches may facilitate a more inclusive and democratic policy process, which may be particularly important in food environment policy which involves both powerful stakeholders, such as those representing industry, and less powerful stakeholders, such as members of marginalised communities.

## 20.7 CONCLUSIONS

The food environment may be understood as a complex system, with multiple levels of influences ranging from global trade to local retail, and multiple actors seeking to optimise for sometimes contradictory outcomes. In light of these properties, systems approaches may be usefully applied to understanding and improving the food environment. The emergent body of work in this area has the potential to facilitate policymaking that is inclusive, coherent and evidence informed.

## REFERENCES

Barbrook-Johnson, P., Proctor, A., Giorgi, S., Phillipson, J., 2020. How do policy evaluators understand complexity? *Evaluation* 26, 315–332. doi: 10.1177/1356389020930053.

Bronfenbrenner, U., 1979. *The Ecology of Human Development: Experiments by Nature and Design*. Harvard University Press, London, England.

Carey, G., Malbon, E., Carey, N., Joyce, A., Crammond, B., Carey, A., 2015. Systems science and systems thinking for public health: a systematic review of the field. *BMJ Open* 5, e009002. doi: 10.1136/bmjopen-2015-009002.

Freebairn, L., Rychetnik, L., Atkinson, J.-A., Kelly, P., McDonnell, G., Roberts, N., Whittall, C., Redman, S., 2017. Knowledge mobilisation for policy development: implementing systems approaches through participatory dynamic simulation modelling. *Health Research Policy and Systems* 15, 83. doi: 10.1186/s12961-017-0245-1.

Johnston, L.M., Matteson, C.L., Finegood, D.T., 2014. Systems science and obesity policy: a novel framework for analyzing and rethinking population-level planning. *American Journal of Public Health* 104, 1270–1278. doi: 10.2105/AJPH.2014.301884.

Jou, J., Techakehakij, W., 2012. International application of sugar-sweetened beverage (SSB) taxation in obesity reduction: factors that may influence policy effectiveness in country-specific contexts. *Health Policy* 107, 83–90. doi: 10.1016/j.healthpol.2012.05.011.

Knai, C., Petticrew, M., Douglas, N., Durand, M.A., Eastmure, E., Nolte, E., Mays, N., 2018. The public health responsibility deal: using a systems-level analysis to understand the lack of impact on alcohol, food, physical activity, and workplace health sub-systems. *International Journal of Environmental Research and Public Health* 15, 2895. doi: 10.3390/ijerph15122895.

Langellier, B.A., Bilal, U., Montes, F., Meisel, J.D., de-Oliveira Cardoso, L., Hammond, R.A., 2019a. Complex systems approaches to diet: a systematic review. *American Journal of Preventive Medicine* 57, 273–281. doi: 10.1016/j.amepre.2019.03.017.

Langellier, B.A., Kuhlberg, J.A., Ballard, E.A., Slesinski, S.C., Stankov, I., Gouveia, N., Meisel, J.D., Kroker-Lobos, M.F., Sarmiento, O.L., Caiaffa, W.T., Diez Roux, A.V., SALURBAL Group, 2019b. Using community-based system dynamics modeling to understand the complex systems that influence health in cities: the SALURBAL study. *Health Place* 60, 102215. doi: 10.1016/j.healthplace.2019.102215.

Liu, S., Osgood, N., Gao, Q., Xue, H., Wang, Y., 2016. Systems simulation model for assessing the sustainability and synergistic impacts of sugar-sweetened beverages tax and revenue recycling on childhood obesity prevention. *Journal of the Operational Research Society* 67, 708–721. doi: 10.1057/jors.2015.99.

Loyo, H.K., Batcher, C., Wile, K., Huang, P., Orenstein, D., Milstein, B., 2013. From model to action: using a system dynamics model of chronic disease risks to align community action. *Health Promotion Practice* 14, 53–61. doi: 10.1177/1524839910390305.

MacDiarmid, J.I., Loe, J., Douglas, F., Ludbrook, A., Comerford, C., McNeill, G., 2011. Developing a timeline for evaluating public health nutrition policy interventions. What are the outcomes and when should we expect to see them? *Public Health Nutrition* 14, 729–739. doi: 10.1017/S1368980010002168.

Malhi, L., Karanfil, Ö., Merth, T., Acheson, M., Palmer, A., Finegood, D.T., 2009. Places to intervene to make complex food systems more healthy, green, fair, and affordable. *Journal of Hunger & Environmental Nutrition* 4, 466–476. doi: 10.1080/19320240903346448.

McLeroy, K., Bibeau, D., Steckler, A., Glanz, K., 1998. An ecological perspective on health promotion programs. *Health Education Quarterly* 15, 351–377.

Meadows, D.H., 2008. *Thinking in Systems: A Primer.* Chelsea, VT: Chelsea Green Publishing.

Mui, Y., Ballard, E., Lopatin, E., Thornton, R.L.J., Porter, K.M.P., Gittelsohn, J., 2019. A community-based system dynamics approach suggests solutions for improving healthy food access in a low-income urban environment. *PLoS One* 14, e0216985. doi: 10.1371/journal.pone.0216985.

Railsback, S.F., Grimm, V., 2019. *Agent-Based and Individual-Based Modeling: A Practical Introduction*, Second Edition. Princeton, NJ: Princeton University Press.

Reynolds, M., Gates, E., Hummelbrunner, R., Marra, M., Williams, B., 2016. Towards systemic evaluation. *Systems Research and Behavioral Science* 33, 662–673. doi: 10.1002/sres.2423.

Rose, G., 2008. *Rose's Strategy of Preventive Medicine.* Oxford: Oxford University Press.

Rusoja, E., Haynie, D., Sievers, J., Mustafee, N., Nelson, F., Reynolds, M., Sarriot, E., Swanson, R.C., Williams, B., 2018. Thinking about complexity in health: a systematic review of the key systems thinking and complexity ideas in health. *Journal of Evaluation in Clinical Practice* 24, 600–606. doi: 10.1111/jep.12856.

Rutter, H., Savona, N., Glonti, K., Bibby, J., Cummins, S., Finegood, D.T., Greaves, F., Harper, L., Hawe, P., Moore, L., Petticrew, M., Rehfuess, E., Shiell, A., Thomas, J., White, M., 2017. The need for a complex systems model of evidence for public health. *The Lancet* 390, 2602–2604. doi: 10.1016/S0140-6736(17)31267-9.

Sawyer, A., den Hertog, K., Verhoeff, A.P., Busch, V., Stronks, K., 2021. Developing the logic framework underpinning a whole-systems approach to childhood overweight and obesity prevention: Amsterdam Healthy Weight Approach. *Obesity Science & Practice* n/a, 1–15. doi: 10.1002/osp4.505.

Sterman, J.D., 2006. Learning from evidence in a complex world. *American Journal of Public Health* 96, 505–514. doi: 10.2105/AJPH.2005.066043.

Stroh, D.P., 2015. *Systems Thinking for Social Change: A Practical Guide to Solving Complex Problems, Avoiding Unintended Consequences, and Achieving Lasting Results.* Chelsea, VT: Chelsea Green Publishing.

Systems Thinking for Health Systems Strengthening, 2009. Alliance for health policy and systems research , World Health Organization, Geneva.

Widener, M.J., Metcalf, S.S., Bar-Yam, Y., 2013. Agent-based modeling of policies to improve urban food access for low-income populations. *Applied Geography* 40, 1–10. doi: 10.1016/j.apgeog.2013.01.003.

# 21 Conclusions and Next Steps in Improving Food Environments

*Charlotte E.L. Evans*
University of Leeds

*Jayne V. Woodside*
Queen's University

*Janet E. Cade*
University of Leeds

*Maria J. Bryant*
University of York

*Carolyn I. Auma*
University of Leeds

**CONTENTS**



## 21.1 INTRODUCTION

This book fills a gaping void in relation to our understanding of the food environment. For the first time, the components of our food environment, including home, school, retailers, industry, as well as community food provision in places of worship and sports venues, are discussed, together with different methodologies

DOI: 10.1201/9781003043720-21

which integrate individual, environmental and social factors. The importance of the food environment in relation to reducing inequalities in diet and consequently health, as well as sustainability issues, are also discussed here. Although the importance of healthy food environments is now recognised at the highest levels, the influential United Nations report published in 2016 titled "Influencing food environments for healthy diets" maintains that only healthy food environments will ensure safe, nutritious and sufficient food (Food and Agriculture Organization of the United Nations (FAO), 2016); progress has been slow in the UK and elsewhere and we reflect on the reasons why this is the case.

## 21.2 SUMMARY OF WHAT WORKS IN DIFFERENT FOOD ENVIRONMENTS

There have been notable successes outlined in this book, both in terms of increasing nutrient-dense foods such as fruit and vegetables and reducing energy-dense foods and drinks high in fats and/or sugars. Such successes can inform our knowledge of *places* where food environment change can lead to meaningful shifts in consumption and the most successful methods to implement.

Children spend a large proportion of their day at school, and therefore the school food environment can have an important influence on diet quality and food preferences. Chapter 3 explores the complexity of the school food environment, with marked heterogeneity in school food systems globally. UK school meal standards have improved canteen-provided meal quality in terms of increasing fruits and vegetables and reducing energy-dense foods and drinks and students in different countries generally agree that improving school food is beneficial (Rose et al., 2021). However, in many countries, packed/bag lunches are the norm, which can be lower in quality. The school food system also has broader influence, e.g. many schools will offer breakfast, after school clubs and school gardens, while classroom-based education around food and nutrition can contribute to a whole school food policy. Like schools, adults spend a large proportion of each day at work, and modifications to workplace food environments can substantially alter eating behaviours; Chapter 4 provides good practice examples of initiatives involving vending provision and more comprehensive changes targeting access and availability of healthy food options, and the social and physical environment.

Chapter 5 explores the retail environment, which of course exerts major influence on food choice and purchase, with potential for a wide range of interventions, e.g. around price promotions, reducing availability/variety of unhealthy foods, display/positioning, all of which can produce changes in purchasing behaviour. This in turn impacts on consumption at home. Availability of fruit and vegetables within the home environment (Chapter 2), alongside repeated exposure and increased familiarity, has been shown to shape children's liking for them, with similar associations observed for energy-dense foods, although this is influenced more through interventions focussed on individuals such as caregivers rather than national or regional policies. Evidence indicates a key role for caregivers, the food they provide, their own eating behaviours and their rules around eating (e.g. eating as a family), in establishing healthy food environments for children.

The growth in out-of-home eating (in 2018, 44% of all food spending was on food away from home in the UK) means that planning at regional level could influence the number of less healthy food outlets such as fast food outlets. This is a challenging area, particularly with the growth in food delivery and 'dark kitchens' delivering food but with no shopfront and the balancing of business and health at local government level. Opportunities for intervention also exist in other out-of-home eating environments. In the UK, calorie labelling is mandatory for all restaurants, pubs and cafes with more than 250 employees from April 2022. The importance of controlling portion size is considered in Chapter 15 in all settings, but particularly out of home. Likewise, food is widely available in community spaces such as sports centres and transport hubs, with concessions or vending machines tending to offer a higher proportion of energy-dense foods. Chapter 9 highlights the intervention opportunities in these types of setting.

The potential contribution of the food industry to improve diet quality is explored in Chapters 6 and 7. Progress has been made in reformulation, e.g. reducing sugar content of sugar-sweetened beverages in response to the UK soft drinks industry levy and reducing trans-fats across many product categories. These products have wide reach and therefore, they have potential to reduce diet-related health inequalities. On the other hand, the drive for food companies to make a profit means that decisions which drive sales rather than improve diet quality have led to distrust and unease amongst non-commercial players.

## 21.3 WHICH METHODOLOGIES ARE MOST SUCCESSFUL?

The previous section demonstrates the importance of *place*, but *methodologies* to achieve environment and, ultimately, behaviour change differ in intensity and likely potential impact; as classified according to the Nuffield ladder of interventions. The main findings of this book are visualised in the synthesis map (see Figure 21.1) with stronger interventions at the top of the pyramid. Places where evidence exists on improvements in nutrient-dense foods (e.g. fruit and veg) are on the left while places where evidence exists on reducing energy-dense foods are on the right of the pyramid. Also denoted on the map is where there is evidence that progress has been made to reduce diet inequalities (orange donut rings).

There is strong evidence that increasing availability of nutrient-dense foods such as vegetables and restricting availability of energy-dense foods improves diet quality in different environments. This includes restricting availability of marketing of energy-dense foods. Financial incentives and disincentives such as reducing the price of vegetables and taxing energy-dense foods also offer real potential for purchasing and consumption change. Nudge/choice architecture interventions offer promise and the evidence is particularly strong for fruits and vegetables. However, nudging appears to be less effective for energy-dense foods with stronger interventions needed focussing on availability and price of these foods. In addition, there is a role for responsible media representation of nutrition information, as well as mandatory labelling, with accompanying education, to help drive healthier choices.

The relationships between food environments and eating behaviour are complex. Systems mapping (Chapter 20) is a novel method which can help us understand the

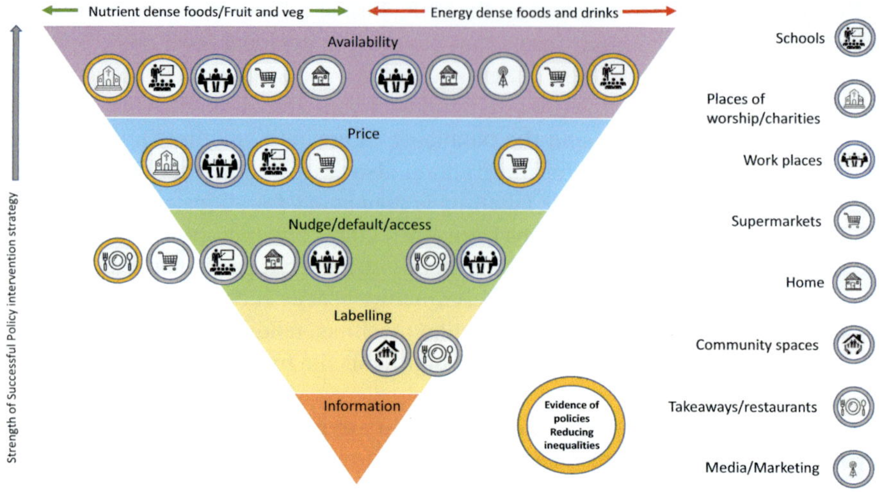


**FIGURE 21.1** Evidence Synthesis map. Circles indicate success of different types of interventions and policies to change diet behaviour. Stronger intervention approaches are at the top of the diagram and milder interventions at the bottom. The right side of the pyramid provides evidence for energy dense foods high in fats and sugars in different food environments and the left side provides evidence on nutrient dense foods such as fruits and vegetables. An orange ring indicates evidence of reduction in inequalities in diet is reported.

key factors influencing this complexity. Ultimately, a range of intervention strategies are likely to be needed to bring about real and sustained environment and behaviour change.

## 21.4 HOW TO REDUCE DIET INEQUALITIES

High-quality food environments provide easy access to nutritious, affordable and palatable food; however, inequalities in food access persist in many areas. More deprived communities in some countries, such as the UK, are more likely to experience poor quality food environments such as increased access to fast food outlets (Chapter 8) and less access to high-quality food retail outlets selling nutrient-dense foods (Chapter 5). This has led to some areas, in the UK and the US for example, being characterised as "food swamps" when there is a high density of fast food outlets or "food deserts" with a lack of access to healthy foods such as fresh fruit and vegetables (Cooksey-Stowers et al., 2017). This situation continues to worsen rather than improve, exacerbated by COVID-19 when restrictions resulted in restaurants closing and takeaways dominating the out-of-home food sector. The evidence put forward in this book suggests stronger interventions are needed to improve fast food environments (see Figure 21.1) such as improving availability and price to ensure food consumption is more equitable both inside and outside the home. Promising findings were reported from a nudging intervention to increase vegetables (Chapter 16). Less evidence is available on reducing inequalities in consumption of energy-dense foods but changing the default (item or portion size) in food outlets of all kinds in addition to restricting availability and increasing price are plausible approaches.

Success in reducing inequalities is evident in this book in a number of environments. Schools in many countries have played a key role in providing free school meals, milk and fruit to children living in low-income households (Chapter 3). Vouchers providing free fruit, vegetables and milk to families with young children have the potential to also improve home environments (Chapter 2 and 17). Places of worship, as well as religious-based charities, also play a pivotal role in many communities freely providing nutritious food to prepare at home (Chapter 11), as well as free hot meals to those in need (Chapter 10). Furthermore, reformulation by the food industry to eliminate artificial trans-fats has reduced inequalities in consumption of trans-fats (Chapter 6). Some policies suggest that inequalities in diet aren't further widened such as the soft drinks industry levy in the UK, and may possibly reduce inequalities in health when further evaluation is completed. Chapter 19 highlights the importance of rigorous evaluation.

## 21.5 IMPROVING FOOD ENVIRONMENTS IN LOW- AND MIDDLE-INCOME COUNTRIES

Inequalities between, as well as within, countries exist. In many sub-Saharan African countries, children's health is a priority and school meals are provided but standards are either absent or are misaligned with dietary recommendations (Food and Agriculture Organization of the United Nations (FAO), 2018). Nutritionally adequate school feeding policies can be framed, implemented and monitored at country level through a multi-sectoral approach, incorporating lessons, for example, from Brazil's National School Feeding Program (Programa Nacional de Alimentação Escolar). Many workers in low- and middle-income countries are informally employed, accessing food at their workplaces through informal and poorly regulated food sectors, such as street food. In such countries, priority should be given to the regulation of street food by streamlining standards, including nutritional labelling, food safety and nutrition education messaging. Evidence from the UK illustrates the positive impact of standards in school food environments. Food marketing and advertising are largely associated with large multinationals, in many high-income countries. In many European countries, these aspects of the macro-food environment are regulated by clear standards, e.g. defining when and what can be advertised to children. Conversely, in many low- and middle-income countries, some multinationals coexist with 'localised' fast food retailers. Here, gaps exist regarding who advertises and the extent of their reach, who the advertising targets and whether regulatory mechanisms exist. This evidence must be prioritised to guide the design and implementation of appropriate, country-specific fast food marketing and advertising policies. The emergence of mobile phone applications and online delivery platforms, e.g. Jumia Food, has influenced access to fast foods in urban areas in sub-Saharan African countries, e.g. Kenya, Uganda, and Nigeria. A dearth of evidence exists on the availability of healthy options, the extent of their reach and nutrition labelling on such online platforms. Lastly, while high-income countries show the efficacy of Sugar Sweetened Beverages (SSB) taxation, implementation in sub-Saharan Africa falls behind (Laar, 2021; Ndlovu and Swinburn, 2021). Here, imperative to implementation is an understanding of the country's health priorities, negotiating opportunity costs between policy and the food industry, and enhancing political will and policy and legal frameworks.

## 21.6 SUSTAINABLE FOOD ENVIRONMENTS

It would be inconceivable to consider the future of our food environment without including food sustainability issues. The UN Sustainable Development Goals, approved in 2015, aim to end malnutrition, address nutritional needs throughout the life course and provide access to safe, healthy and sustainable food (see Chapter 10). Recently, the issues of nutrition and sustainability have become a greater priority across the globe and perhaps brought more to the limelight as a result of the COVID pandemic. For the first time, whole populations were able to see first-hand how reliant we are on global food production and distribution, encouraging discussion on the impact of food systems on planetary health.

While sustainability is the specific focus of Chapter 18, it is widely embedded throughout. For example, Chapter 3 highlights the importance of schools to support equity and sustainability through the offer of high-quality, locally produced foods, culturally enhanced environments and learning about (and with) food across the whole school day (including opportunities to grow food). Chapter 5 summarises evidence of the influence of retail geography, where areas of the highest deprivation are most likely to be exposed to outlets selling poorer quality, higher processed foods compared to more affluent areas. There is a recognised need and opportunity to consider transforming food systems to better promote sustainable food. In the UK, the National Food Strategy was published in 2021 (https://www.nationalfoodstrategy.org/) which recommended 14 actions including sugar and salt taxes, school- and community-based initiatives, support for low-income families to increase nutrient-dense foods and improved government procurement; all highlighted as important in this book.

The role that industry plays, and will continue to play, in our food systems is substantial. We have learnt that over 80% of the food that is sold in supermarkets is processed; much of which being defined as 'ultra-processed'. Retailers propose that much of this is being driven by an expectation of year round availability; however, placing the responsibility on consumers is neither effective nor ethical. Chapter 6 sets out actions required to transform retail environments to improve health, reduce inequalities and ensure sustainability. It's likely that appreciable change in this area will only happen more rapidly via legislation (e.g. sugar and salt reduction policies); however, there is also a responsibility for retail, including community facilities (Chapter 9), to enhance their offer via improved procurement policies which offer locally produced, affordable food. Considerably more radical food pricing policies might emerge in the coming years (Fujimori et al., 2019), not as a direct response to the need for better dietary health but from the growing clamour for tougher international action to tackle GHG emissions from food production (e.g. meat and dairy produce).

While there is a positive movement towards consumer demand for more plant-based foods, our food offer needs to shift towards one in which seasonal, local foods are dominant and the 'default' offer. Not only will this have potential to benefit health, it can optimise air quality, reduce water use, mitigate biodiversity loss and improve land use. Shared targets like this increase our likelihood of the greatest impact provided they are driven by clear policies.

Research transforming food systems and sustainable development goals are gaining momentum, but there is still much to do. Major policy change relies on a robust evidence base and a good amount of advocacy which engages stakeholders. This in turn has the potential to benefit environmental as well as population health, ensuring there are equal opportunities for everyone to access healthy, affordable and palatable food which also benefits the planet.

## 21.7 BARRIERS TO PROGRESS

Despite general agreement that the food environment is important in terms of diet and health, progress has been slow which may be due to many reasons. Our exposure to the food environment, as described in this book, touches on every part of life; and yet, we do not have any well-defined, valid approaches to measure this complex construct. Too often, nutrition is ignored in the assessment of food provision, with many high-level evaluations simply relying on agricultural production volumes of foods. If we want to improve the health of the population through food behaviour change, we need to take account of the food environment as a whole system.

The food environment is constantly evolving and changing as dietary habits shift and industry innovates but what prevents us from improving our food environments? As well as a lack of measurement tools, there is a lack of a standards framework against which we can compare our situation to evaluate whether our food environment is healthy or not. In the UK, an expert panel designed a policy index which includes information on fast food and access to fruits and vegetables (The Food Foundation, 2016), but the tool has not yet been validated which limits its use. We do have metrics to assess the nutritional quality of foods (as opposed to food systems) such as nutrient profiling models (Chapter 14), which have been used to restrict foods advertised on television, though these vary by country/industry. Food advertising is now frequently seen through unverified sources such as blogs and social media (Chapter 12). Food labelling (Chapter 13) may be ignored by the consumer or misunderstood; just providing information is not enough to create change.

If we cannot access healthy food, we cannot eat it. The industry and retailers have a major role in ensuring everyone in society can afford to eat healthily and can easily find familiar, healthy products (Chapter 5). Product reformulation can lead to an improved food environment and demonising all processed foods is not helpful; however, the food industry needs to implement improvements in the nutrient profile of their products to provide a more equitable reach of healthy products (Chapters 6 and 7). Challenges remain around packaging and food waste for perishable products.

Whose responsibility is it to improve food environments? In the home (Chapter 2), support is needed, particularly to help provide positive experiences to young children to increase diet quality, but home environments are hard to reach. Chapter 3 discusses the innovative Japanese concept in schools of Kyu-shoku which embeds healthy eating with education highlighting that cultural factors are important and a cultural shift is needed. Changes, such as reducing portion sizes, need to be introduced gradually to allow populations to adapt to new cultural norms. Leaders in sports or social media need to play a role as trusted role models, but messages must be consistent to be taken seriously (Chapter 12). The government has overall responsibility for population health; however, commercial interests can conflict with public health. Nudging (Chapter 16) is unlikely to be as effective as taxation (Chapter 17) to promote behaviour change and a combination of approaches is usually necessary.

## 21.8 FINAL WORDS AND NEXT STEPS

There is a growing realisation that building healthy food environments to improve food availability, affordability, access and choice is important in countries of all income levels, although issues have been raised about how ill-equipped current food systems are to deal with the wide range of food-related challenges we now face including agriculture, food poverty, sustainability and health (De Schutter, 2020). More research is needed, particularly in food environments where strong interventions have not been tested and evaluated such as in community spaces. Building on the work presented here, we need to generate rigorous and valid measurement tools to provide comprehensive evaluations of food environments. This will enable us to track progress and provide greater understanding of how the environment influences food choices linked to population health. Action is needed to reduce availability of energy-dense foods and increase availability of fruits and vegetables, particularly where large inequalities in diet and health exist. A reluctance to improve unhealthy food environments will inevitably increase the financial burden on health care systems in order to manage the resulting diet-related chronic diseases (Lobstein, 2015). The next decade provides exciting opportunities to increase the quality of a wide range of food environments to improve our health with both sustainability and equity as key features.

## ACKNOWLEDGEMENTS

We are grateful to Carmen Piernas-Sanchez and Stephen Leather for their expert help and feedback on the evidence synthesis map.

## REFERENCES

Cooksey-Stowers, K., Schwartz, M. B. & Brownell, K. D. 2017. Food swamps predict obesity rates better than food deserts in the United States. *International Journal of Environmental Research and Public Health,* 14, 1366.

De Schutter, O., Jacobs, N. & Clement, C. 2020. A 'Common Food Policy' for Europe: How governance reforms can spark a shift to healthy diets and sustainable food systems. *Food Policy,* 96.

Food and Agriculture Organization of the United Nations (FAO). 2016. Influencing food environments for healthy diets. https://www.fao.org/3/i6484e/i6484e.pdf

FAO. 2018. Regional overview of national school food and nutrition programmes in Africa. http://www.fao.org/3/I8063EN/i8063en.PDF.

Fujimori, S., Hasegawa, T., Krey, V., Riahi, K., Bertram, C., Bodirsky, B. L., Bosetti, V., Callen, J., Després, J., Doelman, J., Drouet, L., Emmerling, J., Frank, S., Fricko, O., Havlik, P., Humpenöder, F., Koopman, J. F. L., Van Meijl, H., Ochi, Y., Popp, A., Schmitz, A., Takahashi, K. & Van Vuuren, D. 2019. A multi-model assessment of food security implications of climate change mitigation. *Nature Sustainability,* 2, 386–396.

Laar, A. 2021. The role of food environment policies in making unhealthy foods unattractive and healthy foods available in Africa. *EClinicalMedicine,* 36, 100908.

Lobstein, T. 2015. Prevalence and costs of obesity. *Medicine,* 43, 77–79.

Ndlovu, N. & Swinburn, B. 2021. Readiness for sugar sweetened beverage taxation in sub-Saharan Africa. *Global Health Action,* 14, 1917801.

Rose, K., O'Malley, C., Eskandari, F., Lake, A. A., Brown, L. & Ells, L. J. 2021. The impact of, and views on, school food intervention and policy in young people aged 11–18 years in Europe: A mixed methods systematic review. *Obesity Review,* 22, e13186.

The Food Foundation. 2016. Food Environment Policy Index (Food-EPI) for England. https://foodfoundation.org.uk/publication/food-environment-policy-index

# Index

Note: **Bold** page numbers refer to tables, *Italic* page numbers refer to figures and page number followed by "n" refer to end notes.

For Product Safety Concerns and Information please contact our
EU representative GPSR@taylorandfrancis.com Taylor & Francis
Verlag GmbH, Kaufingerstraße 24, 80331 München, Germany